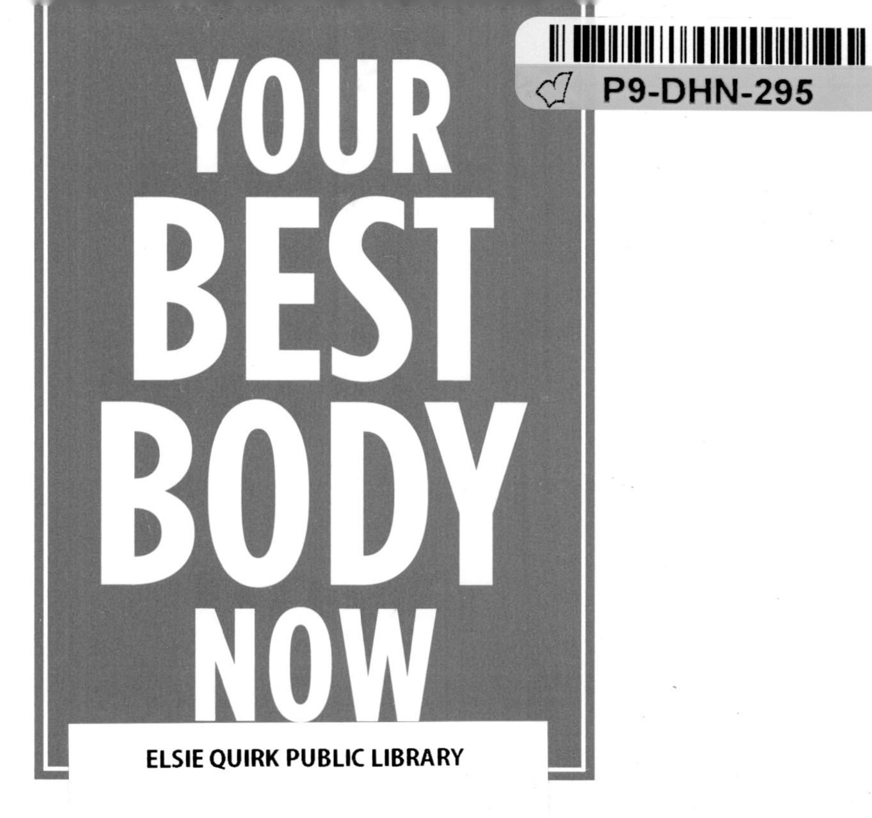
YOUR
BEST
BODY
NOW

Also by Tosca Reno

The Eat-Clean Diet

The Eat-Clean Diet Cookbook

Tosca Reno's Eat-Clean Cookbook

The Eat-Clean Diet Companion

The Eat-Clean Diet for Men

The Eat-Clean Diet for Family and Kids

The Eat-Clean Diet Workout

The Eat-Clean Diet Workout Journal

The Butt Book

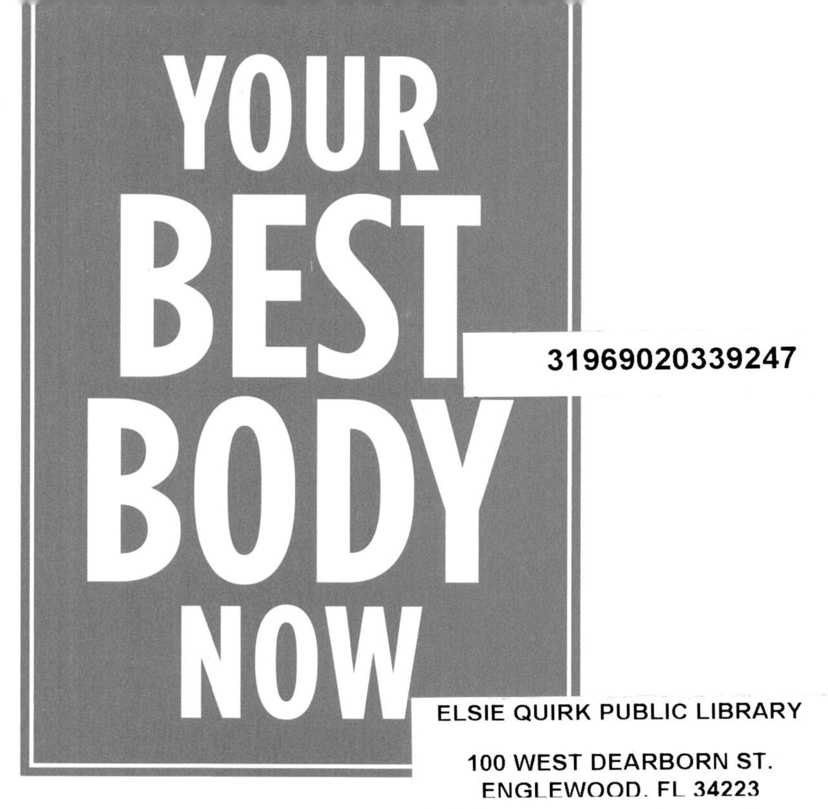

Look and Feel Fabulous at Any Age the Eat-Clean Way

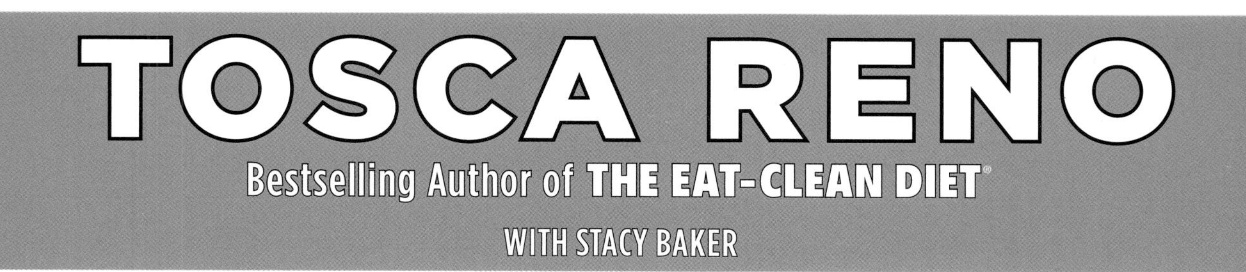

Jacket and interior photos of Tosca Reno by Paul Buceta
Recipe and select food photography by Donna Griffith

HARLEQUIN™

Your Best Body Now
ISBN-13: 978-0-373-89224-2

The health advice presented in this book is intended only as an informative resource guide to help you make informed decisions; it is not meant to replace the advice of a physician or to serve as a guide to self-treatment. Always seek competent medical help for any health condition or if there is any question about the appropriateness of a procedure or health recommendation.

Library of Congress Cataloging-in-Publication Data
Reno, Tosca, 1959—
Your best body now : look and feel fabulous at any age the eat clean way / Tosca Reno ; with Stacy Baker.
p. cm.
Includes index.
ISBN 978-0-373-89224-2 (pbk.)
1. Middle-aged women—Health and hygiene. 2. Health. 3. Physical fitness.
I. Baker, Stacy. II. Title.
RA778.R36 2010
613'.04244—dc22
2010005769

Tosca Reno jacket makeup by Sabrina Rinaldi
Tosca Reno jacket styling by Rachel Matthews
Before-and-after photos of Christine Cmolik, by Jennifer Fohrenkamm
Before-and-after photos of Julio Van Acker by Roger Cox
Recipe development by Kelsey-Lynn Corradetti

Oxygen January 2010 cover photo (page 22) by Paul Buceta, reprinted with permission from Robert Kennedy Publishing

Celebrity photos:
Page 24: INF/The Canadian Press (Scott Kirkland)
Page 34: The Canadian Press (Jim Cooper)
Pages 42 & 84: Rex Features/The Canadian Press (Picture Perfect)
Pages 144 & 285: Rex Features/The Canadian Press (BDG)
Pages 176 & 207: Rex Features/The Canadian Press (David Fisher)
Page 242: INF/The Canadian Press (Devan)

www.eHarlequin.com

Printed in U.S.A.

CONTENTS

Your Best Body Now Tool Kit

PART 3

FOREWORD

IT'S NEVER TOO LATE TO BECOME A BETTER YOU

I FIRST CROSSED PATHS WITH TOSCA about a year and a half ago when I discovered her *Eat-Clean* book on Amazon.com. When the book arrived, I dove right in, curious to see if Tosca would have the answer to my never-ending quest to lose weight (10 extra pounds that I swear have been with me since high school). I read the book cover to cover, and when I was done, I was overwhelmed with emotion. Here seemed to lie the answer that I'd been looking for: how to feed my body and not starve (I'll never throw out my low-cut jeans in favor of "mom jeans").

A few days later, I called Tosca to tell her how much I loved the book, and we quickly bonded over our shared passion for clean eating and fitness. We agreed that being "middle-aged" carries a lot of negative stereotypes—too many baby boomers throw in the towel, mistakenly assuming that the best years of their lives are over. But the fact is that these years can be the very best ones of your life. Tosca is proof positive of this fact—she transformed her body and her life when she turned forty.

During one of our many subsequent chats, I told Tosca she should write a book for us women over forty that addressed the fitness, nutrition and well-being challenges that we face as we get older. Now that I was in my early fifties, many of the rules and strategies that had worked for me in my thirties and forties no longer applied. I wanted a new program that would work for me now.

In *Your Best Body Now*, Tosca offers concrete, easy-to-follow guidelines that actually make a difference. This book is not about hype. It's about substance. And most important, it acknowledges that we're always changing. It offers clear action plans for every decade of life.

Tosca and I agree that it's important to focus on the present and not on the past. It's never too late to become a better you. Enjoy the journey, and always remember to be who you are.

— Bobbi Brown
CEO and founder
of Bobbi Brown Cosmetics

The Road to a Fabulous New You—At Any Age

PART

1

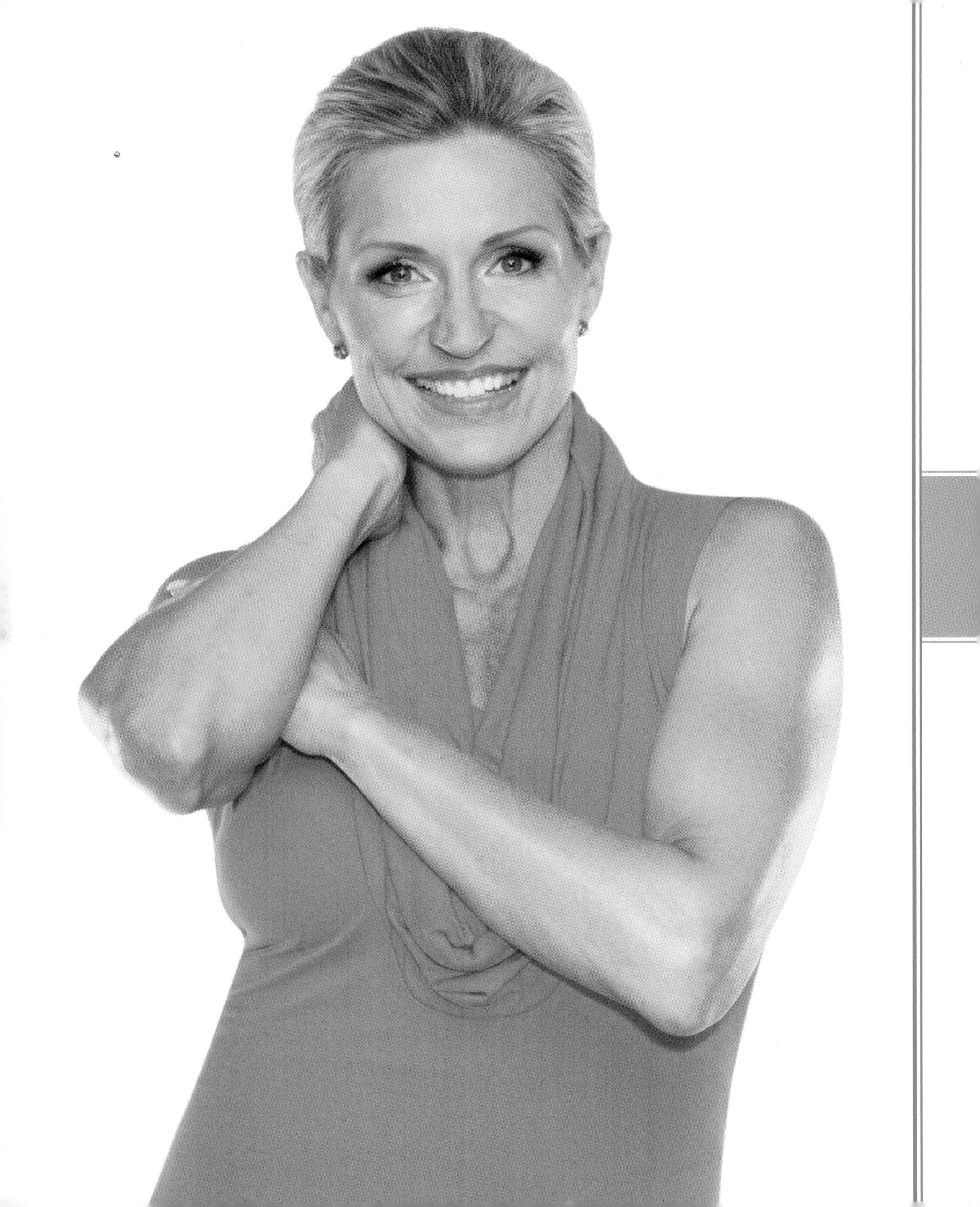

My Journey: How I Created My Best Body Now

1

LOOKING AT ME, YOU MIGHT THINK, "IT'S EASY FOR TOSCA TO talk about eating well or exercising more. Look at how fit she is." The truth is, I look and feel healthy because *every day* I make the conscious choice to look and feel this way. I live better than ever before at fifty because I made the mental shift ten years ago to finally treat myself with confidence, respect and the same amount of love, forgiveness and dedication I've given to my family.

I wasn't born a swimsuit model. I didn't take a magic pill or win the "great body" lottery. I struggled with my weight, energy levels and self-esteem like many of you. It wasn't until I hit my personal rock bottom that I embraced a new way of living. Step by step I changed my habits, from what I ate to how often I exercised to my inner dialogue about being good enough, thin enough and young enough.

> I wasn't born a swimsuit model. I didn't take a magic pill or win the "great body" lottery.

Many of you have asked how I've done it—transformed myself head to toe, both internally and externally, at forty. I've packaged my insights and strategies into *Your Best Body Now* so that you learn not only that there's another way to live but also that it is possible for you to experience it—beginning *now*.

Your Best Body Now was created to share with you in detail how I made my total-body transformation and what I do on a daily basis to stick with my goals to live better and healthier. The results of my very simple, commonsense program have given me not just a healthier relationship with food but also a more beautiful body, stronger self-esteem, newfound energy and a sexiness that comes from truly knowing who you are. (The fact that I look ten years younger is also a bonus!)

The specifics of this program, the Best Body Now transformation, include a decade-by-decade look at how our bodies evolve in our thirties, forties, fifties and beyond, plus tailored guidelines to age-proof your body through nutrition, exercise, health, beauty and motivation. I'll offer real-life tips, tricks and tools—personally test-driven by me

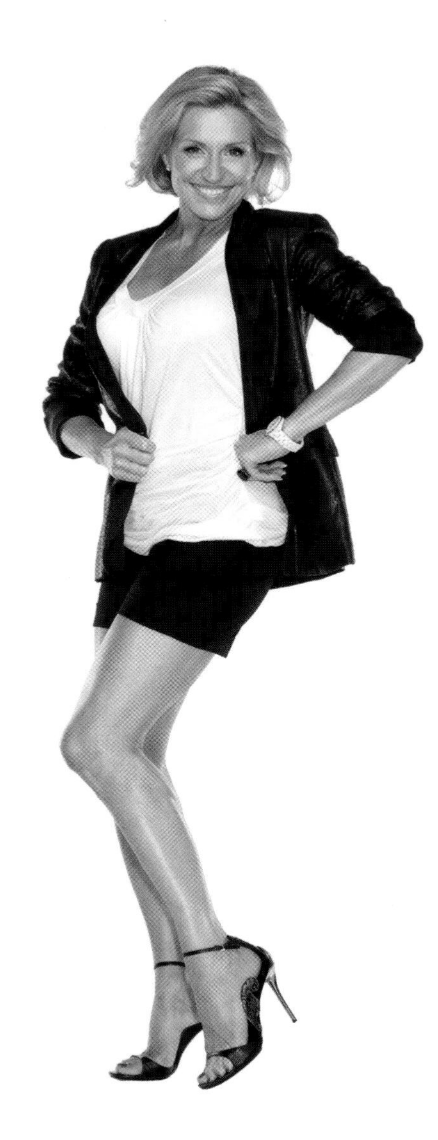

over the past decade—for overcoming challenges, banishing unhealthy habits and arming yourself with the know-how and inspiration you need to reach your goals.

My dream is that my program (and my personal success with it!) serves as a reality check for those of you who believe that your best years are behind you. Whether you need to lose 5 pounds or 200, whether you're a gym rat or a novice, work these principles into your life where you need them most and you will see results. I'm living proof that it is possible to live more beautifully and confidently than ever, no matter what you, your current situation or your life looks like in this exact moment. I did it, naturally—you can, too!

Whether you need to lose 5 pounds or 200, whether you're a gym rat or a novice, work these principles into your life and you will see results.

I invite you to partner with me in the Best Body Now transformation and start having the time of your life right now. The possibilities are endless and entirely within your control. Come on, join me—we'll do it together!

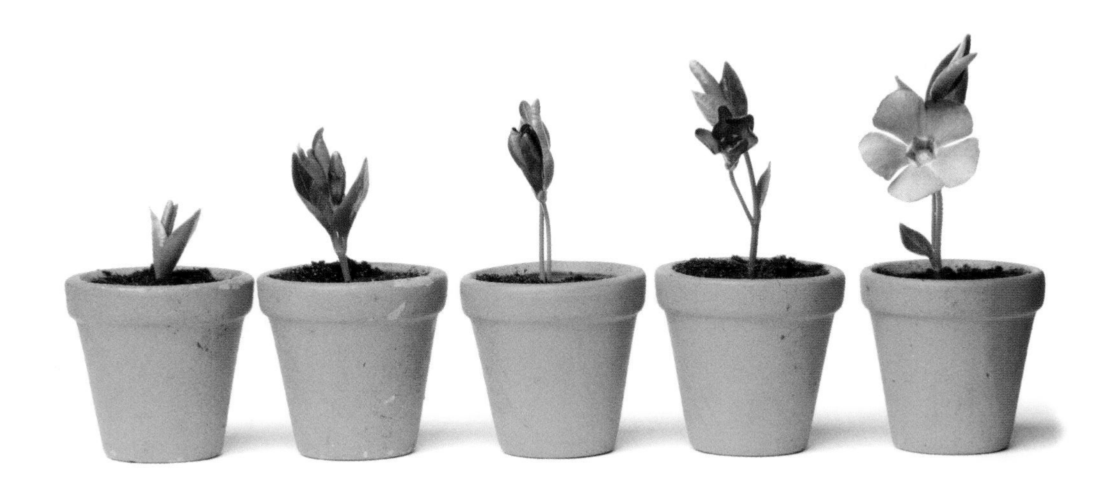

The Seedlings of a Personal Revolution

IT MIGHT BE EASY FOR YOU TO THINK that I've always been a great athlete or had a particular passion for sports—natural abilities that have made my road to a fabulous fifty more attainable. That's far from the truth. My childhood was probably a lot like most kids' back then—I was active, carefree and happy. My days were spent swimming, tooling around on a bicycle, playing soccer with friends or simply adventuring at my family's cottage.

I did fairly well in school, which ultimately led me to university. In terms of beauty, I'd never thought of myself as anything but average. Arriving at university on that first brilliant day of classes in September 1977, a group of senior boys held up numbered flash cards as freshman girls walked down the streets toward campus. They sat on rooftops and balconies flashing numbers, rating our looks from 1 to 10. I got a 10 but was too clueless to realize what that meant. When my sister filled me in, it was a complete surprise for this tall, skinny girl, standing 5' 8" and weighing 127 pounds, wearing my favorite jeans and a Disney sweatshirt, without a care in the world.

University got the better of me and my "perfect 10" figure. Student life was exciting, as was the freedom of living on campus. With all that fun and hedonism, my weight became an issue all too soon. By my second year, my weight climbed to its heaviest, a shocking discovery I learned while attending a Weight Watchers class out of frustration at not being able to fit in my clothes. I still remember the sick, sinking feeling in my stomach during the mandatory weigh-in while I stood on the scale, staring dumbfounded at the number: 204 pounds! On many people that might look bad, but somehow on me, it didn't look as bad as it should have. I was tall, and those 77 extra pounds coated me all over, like a thick blanket. Thankfully, overalls—the perfect weight hider—were all the rage and soon became my everyday go-to "uniform."

Now officially *fat*, what was I going to do?

Weight Watchers wasn't a long-term option, mostly because it was too embarrassing being the youngest one there. Instead, the most obvious solutions seemed to be starvation and relocation. The plan? To drop weight quickly and move to a place where no one remembered the formerly fat me. So, I stopped eating and changed cities, from Queen's University in my hometown of Kingston, Ontario, to continue my studies in Edmonton, Alberta, where my boyfriend at the time lived.

Starving myself worked well, thanks to wonderful self-discipline. When I make up my mind to do something, I do it with a vengeance. In no time, 60 pounds were gone! I walked everywhere on campus, learned to ski, played soccer and even coached a women's soccer team. My weight plummeted back to an exhilarating 127 pounds. I had won, or so it seemed.

Although my body didn't look unhealthy, this desperate way of dieting created a condition called hypoglycemia, which results from low blood sugar caused by a poor diet or not eating enough. The illness hit hard, often causing me to pass out, sometimes in inappropriate places such as the produce aisle. Rather than talk to my doctor, I handled the situation alone. When dizziness struck, I simply ate or drank something sugary to stop me from passing out. It was an easy fix, and one that allowed me to keep cutting calories.

Life moved forward and I checked the boxes: graduation, first job, marriage, kids. At twenty-two, after completing university, I did a short stint as a pharmaceutical sales representative. But my professional life ended quickly. At a Rod Stewart concert my boyfriend proposed to me and a year later we married. The next year, our first daughter, Rachel, was born on November 27, 1984. She came early, after I'd gained just 22 pounds. Pregnancy terrified me—I feared regaining the 77 pounds I'd just struggled to lose. As it turned out, morning sickness took its toll—I'd lost 10 pounds the first trimester, so I concentrated on staying healthy, taking vitamins and following the advice of my doctor.

When Rachel was still a baby, my husband got a promising job opportunity and our little family moved to a different town. Even though it was only four hours away, it felt like the other side of the earth to an inexperienced mother with an infant and no clue how to handle this new life chapter. Despite the stress and challenges, my weight stayed in check, and I launched myself into decorating a new home and taking care of my precious baby girl.

Family photographs from this time show a happy young mom sailing, biking, hiking, gardening and swimming with her daughter. This role as a mother and wife kept me busy and joyful. Even so, in the back of my mind, a niggling thought would creep in every once in a while: "I went to college. Am I wasting my God-given abilities? Should I be doing more?" But I threw myself into motherhood and homemaking with a vengeance because in order to be fulfilled at anything, I'd have to become very good at it.

Before long, it was time to relocate again. My life began to take on a pattern of moves and pregnancies. Kiersten arrived February 9, 1988, and Kelsey-Lynn April 26, 1991. With each event came another

> The weight fluctuations hid the real problem: *I* disappeared little by little with each change.

new city and a job promotion for my husband, along with a drastic transformation in my weight, which not so surprisingly coincided with my emotional stress. Sometimes I would become too skinny, weighing only 115 pounds. Other times I'd be heavy again, weighing 165 pounds. The weight fluctuations hid the real problem: *I* disappeared little by little with each change, buried behind my husband's success and the challenge of adjusting a family to each new city.

My children became my greatest source of joy and pride, both in their accomplishments and in my commitment to raising them well. The exhilaration I felt from being a young mother to these three beautiful girls carried me to the happiest moments of my early thirties. I wanted to make their lives joyful and rich with positive memories. Being this "supermom" meant not only acting the role but looking it as well.

My relationship with my husband, however, wasn't as successful. When I looked my best—carrying little excess weight, if any—I still felt like I was never good enough. He used his thumb and forefinger to encircle my wrist and measure how "big" I was. Often he would embarrass me by putting on my jeans and making fun of the fact that he could fit in them. Rather than recognizing that he acted like this because of his own insecurities, the message in my mind was clear: "Something is wrong with me."

> He used his thumb and forefinger to encircle my wrist and measure how "big" I was. I felt like I was never good enough.

It wasn't just my size—no matter how clean I kept the house or how many perfect meals I prepared, I wasn't good enough. Our home was beautiful, we had three healthy children, he made a good living, and life should have been happy, but it definitely wasn't. There was a deep, dark bottomless pit in him that couldn't be filled, and as a result, I took the blame for whatever didn't satisfy him. The more dissatisfied he was with our life, the more I disappeared emotionally. I vividly remember choosing to turn myself off, shut down from my husband, and be entirely present for my girls. This decision—combined with food "therapy"—seemed the perfect coping strategy for an empty relationship. Thinking back over the years, I have no real sense of when I was fat or skinny. So immersed in being the caregiver and so oblivious to my own needs, I truly have no idea which were my "heavy years." In fact, at the time, I took my cues from photographs.

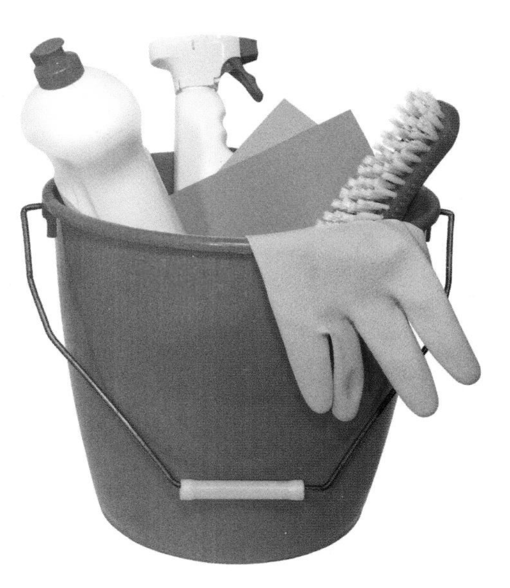

> My children became my greatest source of joy and pride.

If I saw a picture and thought I looked overweight, I'd start cutting out food. My sense of self depended on what others said about me: when my husband said I was too fat, I tried to lose weight; if my in-laws told me I was too skinny during pregnancy, I was careful to eat more. A true sense of self—of *me*—never emerged.

> My sense of self depended on what others said about me. A true sense of self—of *me*—never emerged.

My "Now What" Moment

MY JOURNEY BEGAN AT AN AGE WHEN many women find themselves looking back at who they used to be and wishing they still had the looks, the energy, the health and the opportunities they had in their twenties or thirties.

I was that woman, too.

My childbearing years were behind me. I was thirty-five—my third and last daughter was three years old—and feeling uncertain of the direction my life would take. Gone were the days of diapers and bottles, leaving me with more free time than I'd had in years. For what, I didn't know.

> Instead of joy, I felt only a vacuum, an empty space where happiness should have lived.

My wake-up call came on what would otherwise have been a normal day. My husband shared what should've been a reason to celebrate: he had just been promoted to an impressive new position, complete with a smashing new title, a hefty boost in salary and the spiffy executive office—a dream come true and the payoff for his hard work and dedication to the job.

Naturally, he was beaming. I, however, was not.

> I was thirty-five but felt sixty, and looked like a tired, baby-weight-carrying mother who hadn't remembered to nurture *herself*.

He looked at me for a response, the shared excitement and pride a wife would *want* to feel, but I was numb. Instead of joy, I felt only a vacuum, an empty space where happiness should have lived. This void settled within me. Maybe it had always been there, just pushed aside by never-ending to-do lists and the nonstop "go" mentality of running a household. Either way, this feeling wasn't going away. By the next morning, after my newly promoted husband left the house, sporting his three-piece suit, a shiny leather briefcase and a spring in his step, I shut the door behind him and, in my frumpy sweat pants and T-shirt, crumpled down onto the entryway floor and let out the cry that had been buried deep inside for years.

Maybe it was the resounding clap of the door or just the shock of realizing my situation, but something awakened in me. A leaden silence settled on my shoulders that morning. I'd already given birth to our children—that chapter of life had ended, as did the newness and the firsts that come with it. No more babies. No more first steps. No more plans. On my horizon...*nothing*. My husband's life moved forward with great success, as did my children's, while mine seemed to be standing still. I was thirty-five but felt sixty, and looked like a tired, baby-weight-carrying mother who hadn't remembered to nurture *herself* with the passion, guts and tenacity she'd always used to care for her family. By putting myself second (or third or fourth), I was no longer my best self. In fact, I didn't know who I was at all.

And there it was—my "now what" moment. What would I do, I wondered, now that my children were getting older and the years when I was supposed to thrive were slipping away?

> By putting myself second (or third or fourth), I was no longer my best self. I didn't know who I was at all.

A plan B? An opportunity to recapture, reinvigorate and reinspire myself? I didn't have one. In fact, I didn't even know that a new way of living was an option. My husband's continued success only sharpened the lack of mine. I'd completely disappeared—the era of having babies had ended, and nothing remained to identify with. I had lived through raising my children, checking off my daily tasks, managing a busy family schedule and doing miscellaneous *stuff*. Underneath it all, there was nothing left of me. I had become a human *doing*, not a human being.

> Weight has always been a battle. Food was my weapon of choice.

My life was defined by being a mom, a perfect housewife who could cook, bake and clean like no one else. Long gone was the young, vibrant, intelligent twentysomething college student I'd once been. Somewhere, somehow in the course of living, I'd lost the essence of me. This recognition became the beacon that helped me find my way back again.

Despite this epiphany, I didn't have the courage to change just yet. Instead, I remained on autopilot, leaving my world unchanged. The years crept forward to yet another job-related move, our fifth. But despite my fear, a surge of inner rebellion began brewing—the role of "good mother" and "happy homemaker" wasn't enough anymore. There had to be more. At birthday celebrations, I wished for an answer—a way out. When I blew out the candles on a cake, I would always secretly wish for "promise, possibilities and rescue." Nothing happened...but underneath it all, my spirit stirred. I was slowly building up the confidence and motivation to change.

My only dependable companion was food. It's the obvious, convenient addiction, always available in abundance. There's the loving ritual of meals—you plan them, shop for them and prepare them for your family. It's no wonder food is the ubiquitous drug of every lonely, unhappy housewife. There couldn't be anything easier for me, the mother and caregiver in my family, than to fill my emptiness with the contents of the refrigerator, and so it began. Eating led to more misery and extra pounds. Weight has always been a battle. Food was my weapon of choice.

These feelings of resentment jump-started a cycle of dissatisfaction, worry and tears that was difficult to stop. Ice cream, peanut butter and cheese became my so-called anti-depressants. Food numbed me, like a drug that prevented me from showing up to take care of myself. The trouble with it was that the high didn't last long. Tough situations test the real you. Life's a breeze when nothing goes wrong; it's during the struggles that you need to be present to truly discover the stuff of which you are made. Unfortunately, when you ease pain by eating, rather than addressing the underlying issues, the real you never heals.

> My only dependable companion was food. It's the obvious, convenient addiction, always available in abundance. It's the ubiquitous drug of every lonely, unhappy housewife.

My thinking was shortsighted. What purpose does eating to fill the emotional void accomplish? Sure, there's the quick rush of satisfaction, but ultimately as your waistline expands, so does the self-loathing.

As time went on, I became more resentful of my husband's success and myself. Here I was, a woman with a university degree, doing the most important job of all, raising our family, and yet where was my raise? My reward? My promotion? Would I ever get recognition for outstanding performance, high achievement and selfless dedication, honors that my husband received for giving 110 percent to the company? This may sound selfish, but many mothers have felt unappreciated and undervalued, regardless of how confident and fulfilled they are in their roles or how deeply they love their kids. I punished myself for feeling this way but couldn't shake it, no matter how hard I tried.

The truth is my life didn't change until the moment I decided to take charge—there wasn't a single earth-shattering event or catastrophic power from the outside that forced my hand. In fact, it was the absence of growth that finally motivated me. My life lurched to a standstill, so the options were to either face the truth or continue denying the reality I'd buried for years. "It's time for Tosca to show up in her own life," I told

> Ice cream, peanut butter and cheese became my so-called antidepressants.

> My life didn't change until the moment I decided to take charge.

myself. Of course, that meant addressing the failure of a seventeen-year marriage. Yes, we raised three beautiful children, certainly a triumph, but there was no happiness between husband and wife. No sharing of life and love. My body was empty, yet full at the same time—devoid of emotion, but satiated by poisonous foods I'd consumed to fill that hole. The time had come to do something about it.

My Journey to Forty: Creating the Best Body of My Life

DURING THE SUMMER OF 2001, I ENDED the marriage. We'd tried counseling and even separated for a while, but nothing rekindled the love that grounds a healthy marriage. Neither of us was happy, nor were our children. I had to leave to take my life back. It felt like learning how to breathe again. I focused on being optimistic, grateful and successful, rather than bitter and vindictive, because doing so would deliver the best results for everyone in the long run. After all, we both deserved to be happy and loved. I truly believed that.

When the dust settled and the papers were signed, I learned to take my first few steps as a fortysomething mother of three without a steady income, as well as the stumbles that come with it. It was terrifying and exhilarating all at once. The learning curve was steep. I was still going to be the mother I'd always been, but many things had to change, including the fact that I'd have to have a turn at living, too. Innately I understood it was also time to take better care of myself. Although I was good at taking care of my children, I was terrible at taking care of myself. I was always last on the to-do list. My biggest challenge

> Although I was good at taking care of my children, I was terrible at taking care of myself. I was always last on the to-do list.

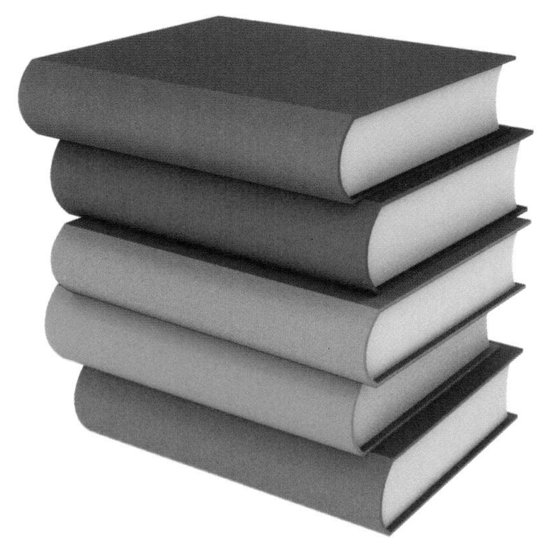

was this shift in mind-set: How was I supposed to accomplish putting myself first? Could I really learn how to take care of *me*?

To prep for life as a single mom, I took a leap of faith and began a year-long teacher training program. The degree was more than a piece of paper. It was an entry back into the job market, a way to financially support my children and a small step in taking back my self-confidence. As a mature thirty-nine-year-old student, I took a crash course in time management—it was quite the juggling act raising three daughters, driving them to dance lessons and competitions, and managing my studies at the same time. I'd leave the house with the girls in the morning, go to school all day, then come home to be a mother again. After the children were tucked into bed, I'd start my homework. Pulling all-nighters when you're forty is much different than when you're twenty! There were many sleep-challenged nights and long, tiring days, but when May rolled around, I graduated with a teaching degree in hand and finally felt the stirrings of pride again.

Late nights and studying can be the formula for weight gain, and at that point I had no time or money for the gym. Like most college students, I gained the "freshman 15." Nutrition got put on the mental back burner. Although I started the school year weighing 157 pounds (and not looking too bad, either), it wasn't long before my weight shot back up. My graduation photo shows me as broad-shouldered, heavy and "big-boned"—adjectives people use to describe you when they don't want to say you're fat, and the way my ex-husband had always described me. Though the words hurt, it wasn't enough motivation to eat better...at least not yet. I was still celebrating my achievement of a teaching degree—a goal I'd reached by myself, for myself.

Unfortunately, amidst my celebration, my hypoglycemia came back in full force. On more than one occasion, a severe episode of low blood sugar would cause me to pass out, then sleep for at least an hour. It could happen anywhere from my children's dance studio to the grocery store to a family vacation in Niagara Falls. My children remember finding me passed out from hypoglycemia, asking me if I'd eaten and giving me sugar. It was exhausting and embarrassing—my own children knew I was neglecting my body. My constant battle with food continued to

> I was looking at a family photograph from a summer vacation at the beach. I saw an overweight mom bookended by three lean, tanned and healthy-looking girls. What would happen to them if something were to happen to me?"

damage my health. I hated how I felt—sweaty, clammy and out of control.

I began to worry about my health and getting back into shape. My father had been ill most of his life with epilepsy and heart disease. The extra weight I'd carried, lost and regained over and over again had put a strain on my health as well. I already had trouble climbing the stairs in our old Victorian home—those steps were steep and narrow—and hypoglycemia continued taking its toll. This reality check, combined with my family medical history, prompted me to seriously consider joining a gym.

There were three other enormously important factors: my daughters, Rachel, Kiersten and Kelsey-Lynn. When people ask me how I first got myself off the couch and into running, swimming and weight lifting I always answer the same way: "I was looking at a family photograph from a summer vacation at the beach. I saw an overweight mom bookended by three lean, tanned and healthy-looking girls. What would happen to them if something were to happen to me?" That photo scared me into action. I realized that if I took good care of myself, I'd have a better chance of living a long, healthy life with them. I'd experience the wonderful opportunity of watching them grow up to be the purposeful young women they were meant to be. Terrified of squandering that opportunity, I finally bought a gym membership and jump-started what would become my Best Body Now transformation. From that moment, I never looked back.

> I finally bought a gym membership and jump-started what would become my Best Body Now transformation. From that moment, I never looked back.

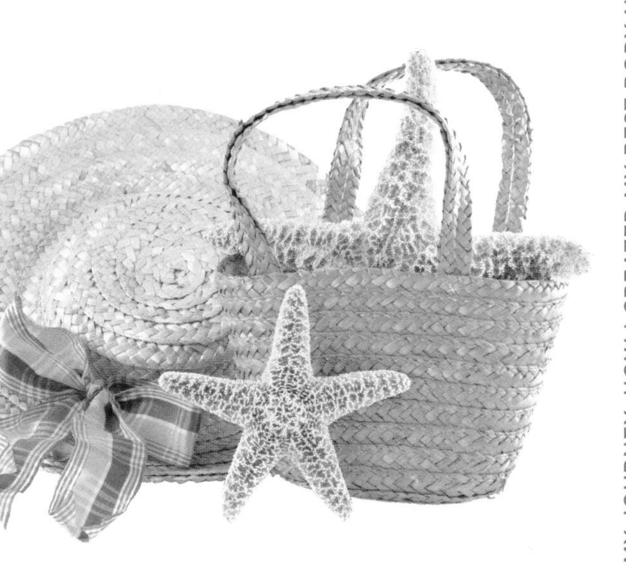

Finding My Way Around the Gym

My Best Body Now transformation started at the gym. But there was one huge problem: the gym had pretty much always been a foreign place to me. It always felt like one more obligation on the to-do list and unnecessary time away from my children. Most women can identify well with this "bottom of the heap" mentality—it's part of our natural need to care for others before ourselves. By the time I was forty, however, my kids were old enough to take care of themselves, and I was out of excuses. Putting my body through a tough workout seemed like the obvious first step to take. How hard could it be?

Step 1: lace up the gym shoes. Step 2: shore up the self-esteem. That was the plan. For me, "going to the gym" meant lacing up a pair of running shoes and doing cardio on a treadmill. Honestly, it scared the crap out of me. I dreaded the idea of running, sweating and looking ridiculous because I was laughably out of shape. It worried me that the regular gym rats would laugh at my pathetic efforts. But you have to start somewhere, and running seemed far less intimidating than anything over in that other part of the gym where the weights were.

My earliest efforts involved spending no more than thirty minutes at the gym. That was relatively easy, and it got me out the door before too many people noticed me. My uniform? Loose-fitting T-shirts and baggy sweatpants—no one was getting a peek at parts of me I didn't want them to see!

This was where my transformation started, on a treadmill with the earphones jammed into my ears and my hands gripping the handles of the Star Trac. The volume was turned up loud enough to drown out my moans and groans. Apparently it was quite motivating. (Note to self: don't turn up the speed on the treadmill until you have the lungs to match—yes, I was one of those clueless types who fell off the back while running.) Too proud to ask for help, I figured it out on my own. One perk of being an unemployed mom was that I could work out during the quiet hours, so I could embarrass myself all I wanted!

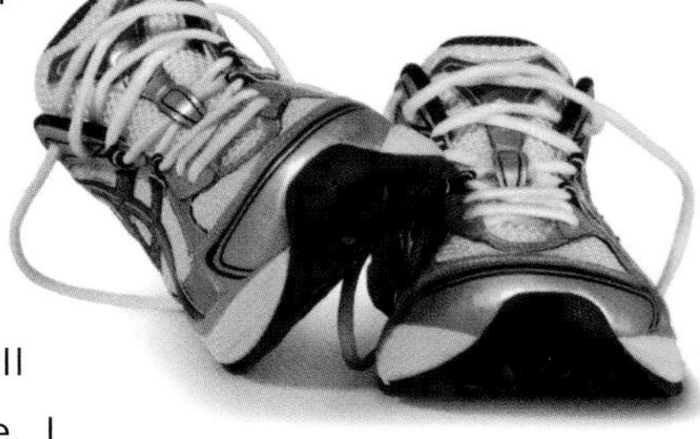

As I stuck with it, my thirty-minute rule fell by the wayside. I began logging forty-five- and sixty-minute runs—I'd had no idea I would love it so much! And not just the treadmill—the elliptical machine and the Stairmaster also became my cardio favorites. When I got started, nothing could stop me. "Whoo! Look at me! I'm running! I feel amazing!" I would chant

Step 1: lace up the gym shoes. Step 2: shore up the self-esteem.

to myself as I sweated. The whining had stopped. Instead of punishment, the gym became a beautiful sanctuary where remarkable changes turned a broken-down housewife with no clear direction into a confident woman who took pride in herself. My self-esteem bounced back. I even shed the baggy T-shirts and sweatpants and began to wear jog bras and dance pants for my sweat sessions. This was exciting stuff!

Somewhere around this time came my yearly physical. I love my family physician. She was the voice of reason during many tough times. While she prodded, poked and tested me, she asked how things were going with my divorce and whether I needed a prescription for antidepressants, assuring me that this is common for women going through such a traumatic and difficult situation. I told her that I was taking care of myself physically and emotionally by working out and didn't need drugs. I was right.

Regular training and better nutrition also improved my health stats. My blood pressure dropped back to a healthy range of 110/60 and my LDL and HDL showed marked improvement. My LDL was initially bordering on the unhealthy at 167 mg/dL and my HDL stood at 41 mg/dL. Now I was getting readings of less than 100 mg/dL for my LDL levels and way up above 60 mg/dL for my HDL levels. Where I'd struggled with bowel movements most of my life, going as infrequently as once every three days or so, this was no longer an issue. And, of course, the scale showed a steady drop in weight.

I left the doctor's office feeling stronger and prouder than ever before. My life was beginning to turn around.

> Instead of punishment, the gym became a beautiful sanctuary where remarkable changes turned a broken-down housewife with no clear direction into a confident woman who took pride in herself.

Fate has a way of interjecting itself into life. Although I'd always wanted to teach, whenever jobs came my way, as luck would have it, so did better opportunities. While completing teaching placement, I met a young girl named Chelsea in one of my first-grade classes; her father, Robert Kennedy, was the one and only bona fide icon in bodybuilding. Of course, I had no idea who he was; we just chatted on the playground occasionally when he took his daughter to school.

Instead of diving right into my teaching career, I put my previous interior design training to the test and undertook the renovation and design of Robert's new home. I had studied interior design while living in the United States during my thirties. I loved to create beautiful spaces and had had plenty of practice doing this with the numerous moves we endured as a result of my then husband's career. I loved it—and it turned out I was good at it! What a surprise! I figured the work would be a great way to add some cash to my depleted bank account, plus give me the summer off with my girls, and I could jump back into teaching in the fall. But as it happens, life got in the way of my plans.

Learning to Eat More, Not Less

When I first began working out, cardio made bold, drastic changes to my body, but somehow it wasn't enough—I basically became a skinny version of my formerly fat self, an envelope with saggy bits inside. Marathoners aside, you can't run yourself into being toned and tight. I wanted to see shape. I started reading health and fitness magazines and realized that training with weights was the secret behind all the gorgeous women in the pages. I wanted to take it to the next level, to gain a more beautiful shape, so I got a personal trainer who showed me how to use the equipment and the weights, which kick-started my confidence over in the "other part" of the gym.

Unfortunately, because I hadn't started Eating Clean, progress was slower than desired, and my hypoglycemia wasn't entirely under control. I wanted more. I wanted to be healthy, feminine and curvy. I also shared with Robert my commitment to changing my body. I'd been working out at the gym for a year or two and had seen amazing progress, but I wasn't achieving the results I desired.

I wanted more. I wanted to be healthy, feminine and curvy.

Robert asked, "Want to have a little adventure? How about doing a bodybuilding contest?" I laughed. He didn't.

He offered me the opportunity to train with him. I quickly learned that when you're lifting weights, you're *reshaping* your body. Soon I was training with him all the time, rather than the personal trainer at my original gym. What I didn't know is that while working with me, he'd been quietly assessing my determination, commitment and strength level. Did I have what it takes to prepare for an amateur bodybuilding competition? While training together, Robert would test me to see if I could do a certain exercise: "Tosca, do 12 reps with 40 pounds." I would always do more reps at a higher weight than he asked, not for any reason other than I liked the personal challenge.

One day I'd just finished some arm training and was leaning back on a piece of equipment. Out of the blue, Robert asked, "Want to have a little adventure? How about doing a bodybuilding contest?" I laughed. He didn't. "I think you're ready. We can make

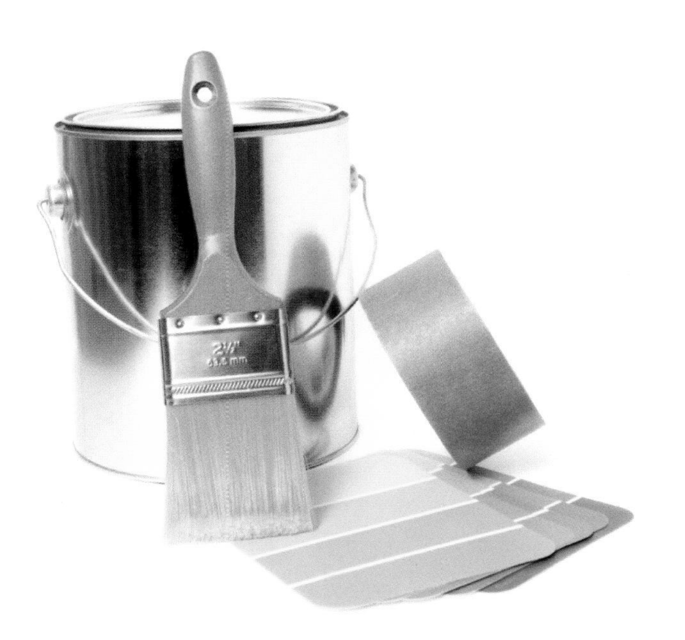

this happen." Of course, I said yes to Robert's bodybuilding challenge. Call me naive or overly ambitious, but either way, this man was giving me an opportunity, and all I had to do was eat well and train—where was the downside?

When we began, Robert taught me the oddest thing I'd ever heard in my messed-up food world of deprivation and overeating. "To lose weight, you must eat *more*," he told me. Surely he was kidding, I thought. No one advises a woman who's dieting to up her calories. But I wasn't in a position to question his expertise. When Robert first started training me as a bodybuilder, he had one condition: "Do everything I ask you to do and don't question me." In that sentence, he took on the job of both teaching me how to change my eating habits—the very same approach I'll teach you in this book—and coaching me through a bodybuilding competition.

So there I was, in the exact place I'd asked to be. I'd hoped and prayed for *more*, and my wish was coming true. I first learned what that word meant while preparing for the competition, which proved to be a masterful stroke of genius on Robert's part. "More" came in the form of a new way of eating. The program, based on a diet of unprocessed foods eaten in several small meals throughout the day, came to be called Eating Clean, which I explain in my previous book *The Eat-Clean Diet*.

Honestly, I was scared. I didn't want to look like those freaky, veiny, over-muscled men in the muscle mags. This was a real paradigm shift, to realize that bodybuilding doesn't have to be about über-muscular, vein-popping, manly women. Weight lifting is really body *shaping* and *sculpting*, finding your gorgeous feminine physique, and it's a process that can benefit anyone at any age or strength level. In fact, when I think of beautifully lean, sculpted muscle outside of competition, I think Kelly Ripa or Jennifer Aniston, who are skinny, toned and lean.

So at forty-two, I began a several-month journey of preparing for my first physique contest, transforming my body entirely from frumpy to shapely. This took more discipline and dedication than nearly anything I'd ever done. And I noticed that Eating Clean—eschewing sugars, fats, cheese, ice cream, soda, bread and so on in favor of lean protein and complex carbohydrates—made me look and feel younger.

My doctor noted my transformation in my blood work during my yearly physical—my blood chemistry was amazing. I was lean. My hair was thick and shiny. My skin was taut and glowing, and it showed few fine lines.

> I noticed that Eating Clean—eschewing sugars, fats, cheese, ice cream, soda, bread and so on in favor of lean protein and complex carbohydrates—made me look and feel younger.

My fingernails grew beautifully. My immune system was rock solid—I was never sick, and the hypoglycemia had disappeared! People who had not seen me in a few months or years wondered what I'd done to make such a remarkable change. The answer, of course, was my new method of eating, partnered with weight training—the basis of the Best Body Now program.

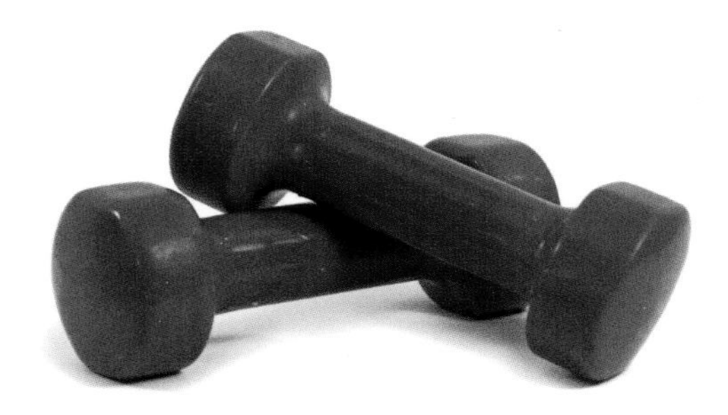

Discovering My Best Body Now

As I prepared for the contest, I realized this was my opportunity to refocus on me. Exercise and good nutrition allowed me to undo the damage of self-neglect step by step through reps, sets, intervals and daily discipline. I wrote the words "If you can imagine it, you can do it" nearly everywhere I could as a constant reminder.

My former inner dialogue was replaced by motivational, loving mantras that pushed me forward rather than holding me back. It was a brave new world. I learned that my brain and mind are stronger than my body. I can push myself further than what is expected or demanded of me. In fact, even when starting at the gym, I always considered each day a new contest: "What new exercises will I do today? What test can I push against? How far can I go?"

> Exercise is never punishment; it's always the reward I'm giving to myself. It's how I take care of *me* every single day.

Even now, when I'm in the gym, I think of it as taking care of myself, and it's about time! Exercise is never punishment; it's always the reward I'm giving to myself. It's how I take care of *me* every single day. Through training I was finally able to think about Tosca, to find myself, the part of me that was lost for years because I chose to sacrifice me for others. The results speak for themselves!

Now I had curves where there were none before.

Not only that, but I was rebuilding my very damaged self-esteem. Instead of constantly doubting myself, I felt a renewed sense of strength. Getting out of an unhealthy relationship, combined with new eating and training habits, helped repair the heaviest damage.

Soon the person I was always meant to be, the person who had gone into hiding for so many years, began to emerge. My body was improving in the same way my self-esteem was. Now I had curves where there were none before, particularly in the glutes. This was truly magic! The truth is that you don't need a pill or any "magic" food to get rid of fat and create lean muscle; you just need to train correctly. I slowly placed more emphasis on strength training than cardio, which gives your heart and lungs a good workout but does little to change your physique: you'll still be a smaller, flabby version of yourself. With weight training, my body was tighter and leaner (even if the scale did not reflect that with numbers) as well as stronger, curvier and healthier.

While we trained for the competition, Robert offered me the opportunity to stretch my writing skills. He was redesigning *Oxygen* and wanted to have a fortysomething voice speaking about the very changes I was going through. What started as a few assignments quickly grew into a regular column called "Raise the Bar," which turned out to be as inspirational for others as it was for me. Suddenly I was getting regular feedback from women about how my own success motivated them to reach deeper within themselves to make changes. Women (and men for that matter) in their thirties, forties and fifties were finding hope and confidence in my journey. We were flooded with feedback—we'd tapped into something very real. I was finding my voice.

With weight training, my body was tighter and leaner as well as stronger, curvier and healthier.

Soon I came to realize what I'd always felt in my bones—I was a teacher. I can inspire others to make changes in their lives. What I do now as a columnist and fitness expert is more than just having a lean, toned physique—what motivates me every day is knowing that I can inspire others to make positive changes in their lives. I know that I have a purpose that feels good and right for me. It just so happens that I found my stride when many people are reaching an age when they hang up their gym shoes, rather than try them on for the first time. The decision

> As my forties raced by, I learned so much about myself. I finally met the real me and with that discovered my life's true purpose.

to make positive changes was relatively easy once I took the first challenging step. And as my forties raced by, I learned so much about myself. I finally met the real me and with that discovered my life's true purpose.

Through my writing and appearances at health expos and conferences I kept hearing women say how difficult they found their forties to be. They moaned about going through menopause and dealing with terrible symptoms such as hair loss, aging skin, hot flashes, weight gain, cravings, lack of libido, meno-pot (that tummy pouch that happens postmenopause) and illnesses of all sorts. I kept getting letters from women, desperate for advice on how to handle all the new challenges they faced with age. As I fielded the questions, I realized something much more important. Here I was in my forties, right along with so many of these women, yet I was *not* experiencing any of these symptoms. I felt so good it was almost criminal. I'd stumbled onto something with my new way of eating and weight training—by following the program, I sailed through menopause. I didn't face the same aches and pains of aging thanks to my new healthy habits.

So I ask you: if you knew that you could transform your body by eating delicious, nutrient-dense foods throughout the day and never going hungry, wouldn't you? The answer is *yes*! The good news is that you don't need to be convinced—I'm living proof that it works!

It's funny, because I don't think this journey could have happened any other way. All those years of personal neglect, unhealthiness and rock-bottom self-esteem led me to a place of self-appreciation, personal challenge and gratitude. I'm in a place that I never could have gotten to had I not struggled to truly find my purpose. I've realized I'm not alone—and neither are you! Many women, from actresses to politicians to medical experts, only begin to make their mark in the world after thirty-five. Think Julia Child, Sharon Stone, Iman, Goldie Hawn, Halle Berry and countless other gorgeous fortysomethings who are winning Oscars, landing magazine covers, reinventing and rebranding themselves as sexy, decades after their so-called youth.

> Shouldn't it stand to reason that you would be *more* likely to be able to excel at it with *more* life experience, with the perspective that comes with life after thirty-five?

What makes these women any different than you? Whatever your talent, shouldn't it stand to reason that you would be *more* likely to be able to excel at it with *more* life experience, with the perspective that comes with life after thirty-five? I discovered this was true for me and countless women like me. And regardless of your talents, is there any reason why this shouldn't be the case for you, too? Pause for a moment. Are you thinking about all the reasons why you cannot do what I have done? The money, your current commitments, your perceived limitations? This book is about helping you get past this initial self-doubt and providing you with the knowledge and the strategies you need to forge ahead nonetheless.

The Road to Fifty: Discovering a Still-Better Body and Fuller Life

A DECADE AFTER MY PERSONAL REVOLU-tion, I've truly discovered that fifty *is* the new thirty. I've finally learned to live a purposeful life, and I feel more alive than ever. Each day is full of possibilities, rather than minefields. Knowing that the opportunities are limitless feels enormously empowering. It's the inspiration that still fuels me to share my message with women who feel life ends at a certain age. Thank goodness that's not true, otherwise I'd never have really lived!

What's even more beautiful about my road to fifty is that I'm not worrying about what happened in the past or what's in store for me tomorrow—instead I'm focused on life in this moment. One thing is clear, however: my fifties have been filled with purpose and meaning in a way that continues to bring me new challenges and powerful, life-altering experiences. This was not true in prior decades of my life.

> I've truly discovered that fifty is the new thirty.

In my twenties, I lived to please others, even my parents, instead of actually listening to my heart. It was a decade of beginnings: I went to university, fell in love for the first time, became a mother and topped out at my heaviest weight—204 pounds. Although

TOSCA TIDBIT

A masterpiece, a true work of art, has the quality of being created slowly, lovingly and with passion, then bursting into life. You're the masterpiece you're creating right now!

I'm not worrying what happened in the past or what's in store for me tomorrow—instead I'm focused on life in this moment.

young in years, I felt and looked much older than I actually was. My thirties were really all about being a mother to my three daughters. Learning to take good care of my daughters was an incredible experience. No, it wasn't easy. Sure, it wasn't laughter and fun all the time, but I gave it everything I had, always putting myself last.

By the time I hit my forties, I had launched my personal reinvention. Reinvention is really about rescuing yourself—changing myself from the woman I was to the woman I am today gave me a new lease on life. At the end of my seventeen-year marriage, which coincided with the end of my thirties, I realized I was in dire need of an overhaul physically, emotionally and personally. That reinvention would be the hallmark of my forties.

I would also encourage women (and men) to put themselves first. Just as on an airplane, you need to put the oxygen mask on yourself before assisting others. That's a simple rule of lifesaving—you can't take care of others unless you take care of yourself. Regular exercise combined with a diet of whole, unprocessed foods has become so habitual, just like brushing my teeth, that I hardly recognize them as habits anymore. Rather, they are what must be done every day for me to be at my best. I can't live without them. I'm miserable, grouchy and constipated if I ignore any aspect of these healthy habits.

Just months away from fifty, I was selected to be on the January 2010 *Oxygen* cover in a bikini, five years after my first time on the magazine's cover, proving that the Best Body Now program isn't just a diet or a workout but a powerful antiaging program. Exercise really is the fountain of youth. I haven't found one better; have you?

I wandered through life before. Now I charge through it. Perseverance comes from knowing you have something important to do and doing it. Motivation comes from fear—what would happen if I did not take care of myself? Inspiration comes from results—I was not born with this body, I created it. Once I discovered this truth I could not stop myself from embarking on the voyage of my life.

At 50, I still rely on the formula that transformed my body in its forties: 80% nutrition + 10% training + 10% genetics = Beautiful and Healthy Body

The quality of my life has changed incredibly. Where I had no voice before, I now have one, and others want to hear it. Where my life had no purpose, there is now meaning. I have boundless energy. My health and physique are closer to those of a twenty-five-year-old than a fifty-year-old.

Now, at fifty, I'm filled with energy and vitality each and every day. I know what I want, and I get it. My head is full of ideas, and I'm filled with passion and energy—I literally can't wait for the next day. Fifty is all about infinite possibilities and boundless opportunities. Fifty is hot!

Fifty is all about infinite possibilities and boundless opportunities. Fifty is hot!

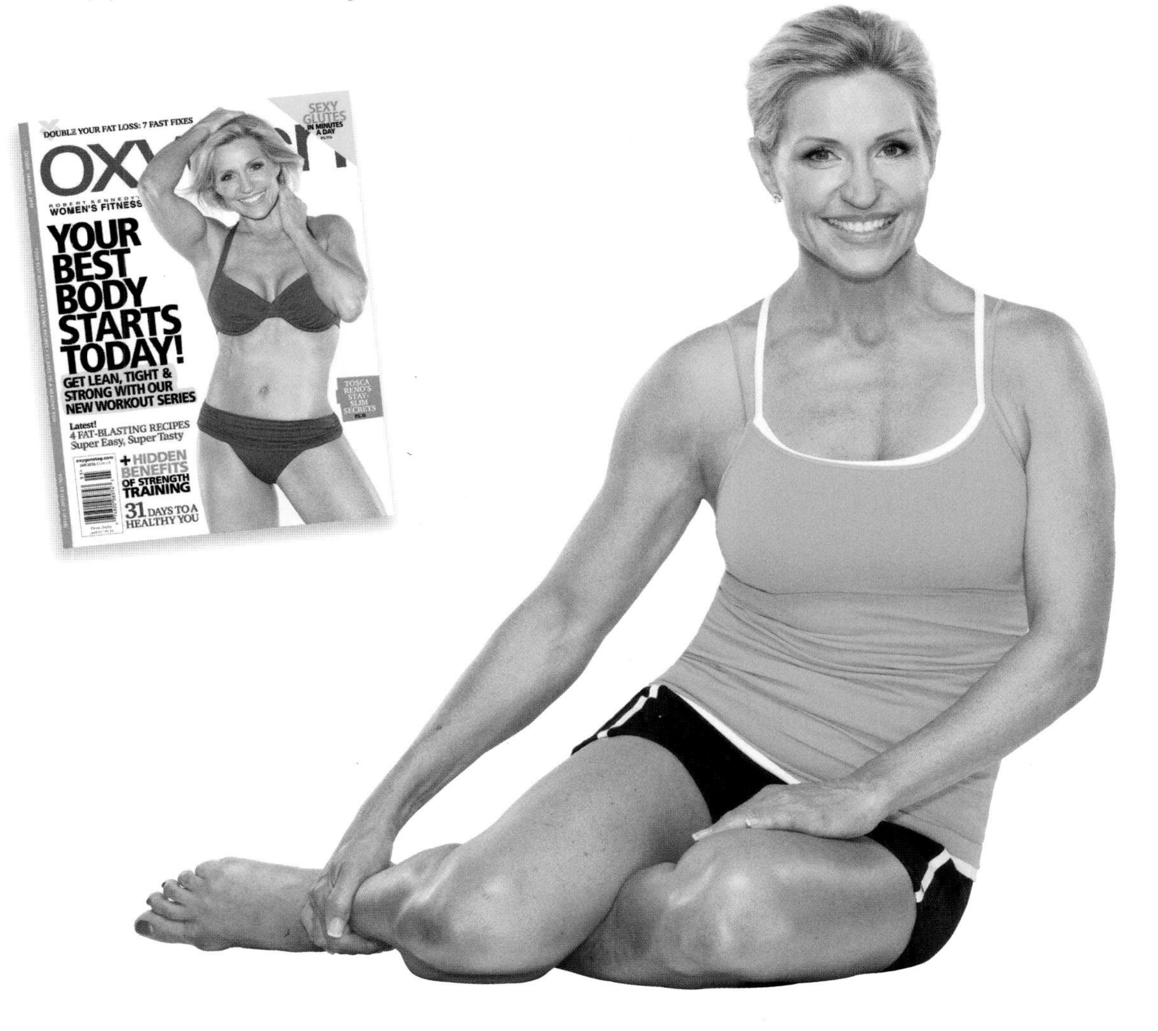

Discover Your Best Body Now

THE BEAUTY OF THE BEST BODY NOW program is that it covers all areas of your life—I discovered that Eating Clean and weight training could reshape my body, but in order to keep myself looking and feeling my best year after year, I had to tackle my health habits and beauty routine and make sure I was motivating myself every step of the way. This book will walk you through all five parts of the Best Body Now program: diet, fitness, health, beauty and inspiration. These are the tactics that I use every day to look and feel my best—and trust me, they work!

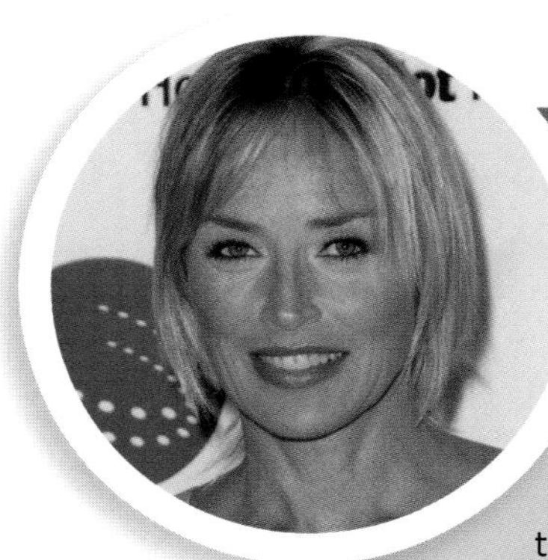

The "H" Factor: A-List Proof That Life Gets Better at 40

The Best Body Now mind-set is finally blossoming in the celebrity scene, as many of the hottest big-screen stars and music mavens have proven that it's possible to thrive after their "now what" moment—and long after their industry has counted them out as being too old to be sexy leading ladies or serious rock stars.

One of my favorites? Sharon Stone. Is it just me or does she get noticeably sexier every single day? What I love most about Sharon is that she completely transformed her reputation from being known by casting agents as a reliable but unremarkable supporting actress to one of the sexiest screen sirens ever. The turning point? She passed thirty, overhauled her diet and began working out for the first time in her life. The results speak for themselves: she earned top marquee billing and inclusion in countless "Most Beautiful" and "Sexiest People" lists that continue into age fifty and over. Love it!

If you're not a believer, if you think life is over because you are thirty-five, forty, fifty, sixty, whatever the magic number, think again. Now's the time to explore aspects of yourself that may have been shelved for job and family obligations, and seize the abundance of opportunities that exist in every moment. Why wait? Have you followed your heart? Have you danced with reckless abandon? Have you given yourself the time you deserve to eat, exercise and live better? If you begin today with even the smallest step, imagine what you will have achieved by year-end.

Come on, I'm with you every step of the way! Let's get started!

> If you think life is over because you are thirty-five, forty, fifty, sixty, whatever the magic number, think again.

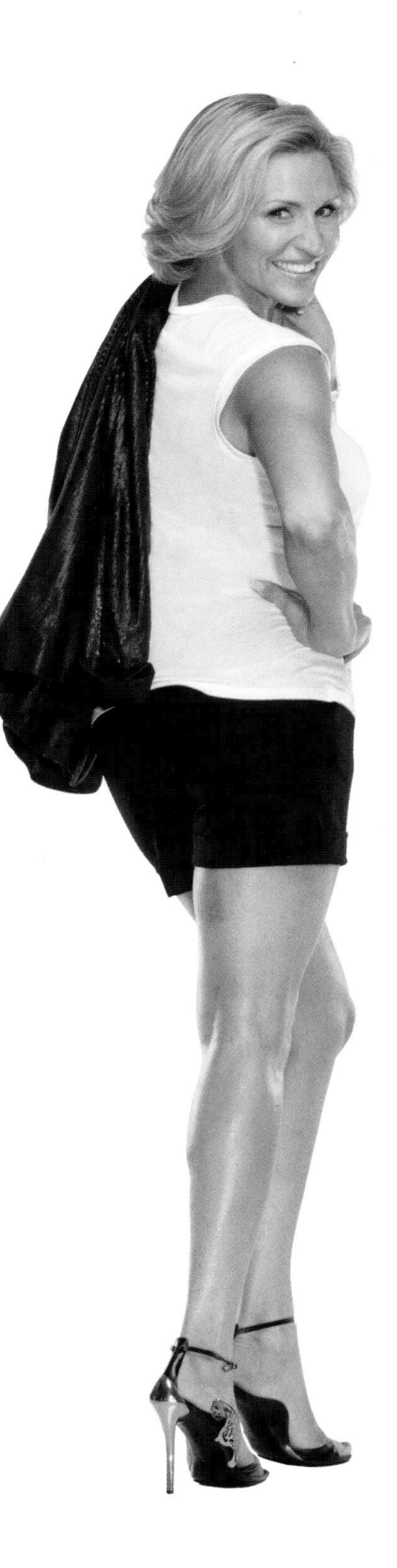

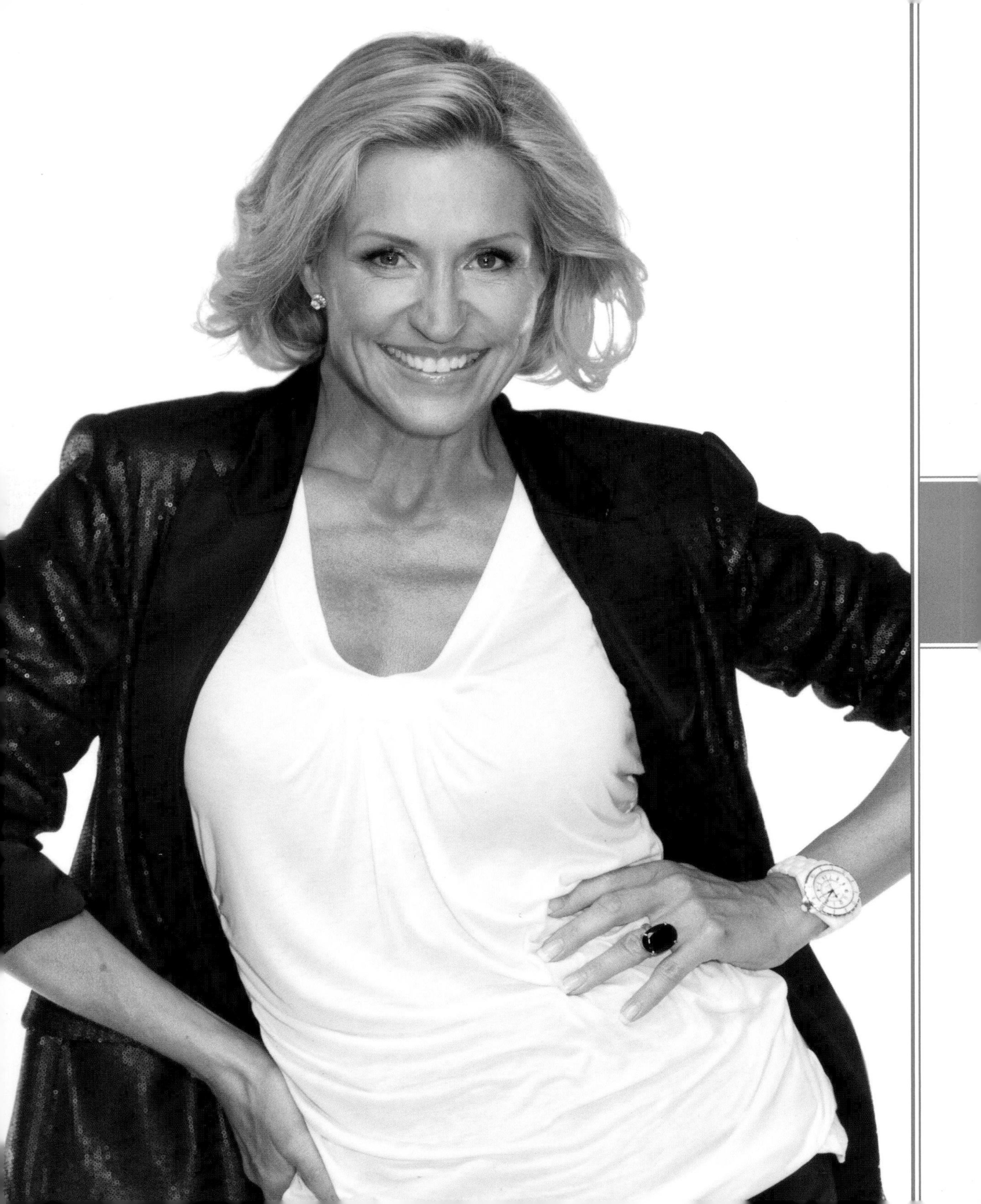

Champion a "New You": *Allow* Yourself to Live Better

2

MY MESSAGE DOESN'T COME FROM THE IMPECCABLE WAY I lived my life—my journey has been filled with potholes, U-turns and some messy, impossible-to-navigate streets. Rather, the strength of my words comes from how I allowed myself to change my mind-set, corrected my many mistakes and used a bad situation to inspire a massive life makeover. If an ordinary woman can walk fearlessly through the maze and find her way out of it with a degree of dignity, a heart full of hope and a newfound sense of self, you can, too. I'm that ordinary person. I'm not a celebrity, a superhero, nor a woman with a pedigreed last name or a pocket full of cash with which I can hire doctors to transform my body.

I'm simply someone on the heels of fifty who wants to turn the tables on the middle-age mind-set for women who think living better than ever is impossible.

We all face our forties and fifties with hesitation. After all, our children are gaining independence and even raising families of their own, so what happens to us? Who do we become? In an interview with Oprah, California First Lady Maria Shriver shared her own fears and insecurities about life after her husband, Arnold Schwarzenegger, was nominated as governor and she lost her job as an NBC news anchor as a result. "I got lost in my own life," she confessed. When she lost her job with the network, she felt she had lost her identity.

I related to her statement so well, because I, too, felt unentitled to live my own life. But here was this fifty-two-year-old woman sharing her own doubts and fears about who she was. "Women today need to make a name for themselves," she said.

I agree. No matter how big or small the name, it just has to ring true for the real you. The biggest first step you need to take, the one that will allow you to embrace everything you're about to read and fully embody the Best Body Now principles, is this very simple mind-set shift: give yourself *permission* to change.

> Give yourself permission to change.

This split-second decision will ground everything you're about to do and help you continue to make the best choices for you every single moment of the day.

Empower Yourself

I KNOW MANY OF YOU ARE LIKE ME: YOUR lives are complicated, and maybe you have a long way to go. You're balancing an entire life, from kids to career to marriage to home, and flipping your mind-set switch might not necessarily get everyone in your clan on board. That's okay. This is about *you.*

Any type of change can be scary, but I guarantee, a new energetic, happy you will be a positive force in everyone's life.

If you are like me when I first started my Best Body Now journey, you probably have a whole list of roadblocks—mental and physical—that make this first step the hardest one to take. How do I push myself through these types of speed bumps? I act big but start small. I break down each seemingly unsurpassable challenge into little, manageable pieces that I can wrap my mind—and my solutions!—around. It's

> I'm my number one cheerleader.

so much easier to tackle a huge issue when you divide and conquer.

For example, in the beginning of my journey, I couldn't think, "I have to lose 70 pounds." It was too overwhelming. Instead, I woke each morning with an action plan for that day. Not only are you downsizing the stress factor, but you're also giving yourself the chance to celebrate mini victories along the way. You'll see my test-driven strategies throughout each chapter, and I invite you to explore them all, as well as add your own to the mix!

The other strategy I use is to empower myself with nurturing, I-can-do-this statements that support my progress rather than thwart it. I'm my number one cheerleader. This trick still helps me push to greater heights no matter what I'm trying to achieve. For example, when running long distances, I tell myself, "Just ten more minutes. No problem!" The thoughts running through our heads are 75 percent of what it takes to make absolutely anything happen. That's why you can't afford to let your inner critic have a say in your transformation. Instead, *be* the pep rally that gets you up and moving each day, and reward yourself each night by recounting *every single* positive choice you made. Did you trade a trip to the vending machine for an apple with peanut butter? Ask a friend to switch your spa day to a bike adventure? Post an uplifting "I can do it!" note on your bathroom mirror? Small or big, remind yourself before you sleep that you are your own hero.

> The thoughts running through our heads are 75 percent of what it takes to make absolutely anything happen.

These same principles work when dealing with people or events that may give you opportunities to test your new mind-set. (I think of them as my mental toughness personal trainers!) You'll be surprised to discover that once the people around you see that your new lifestyle and mental toughness are here to stay, they'll climb on board. To get you prepped, I've listed some of the bigger challenges you may face with those in your support network, and how to sidestep them with confidence and strength.

TOSCA TIDBIT

Great masterpieces don't have to be works of art in the traditional sense. Think Elizabeth I's England, Abigail Adams' co-presidency with John Adams, Jane Goodall's departure from her mentor Louis Leakey, Katherine Graham's late-in-life emergence from an abused housewife to a successful newspaper publisher. We can all be masterpieces if we first change how we think about ourselves.

Your Kids: Do They Want You "Fabulous"?

THE ANSWER: OF COURSE! THE KEY WITH kids is the "slow and steady" game, along with complete transparency. I don't hit them over the head with my plans to Eat Clean and live a healthier life; I lead quietly, by example. This means I buy no junk food for the house, for example, and when dining out, I ask the waiter for smart substitutions like steamed or broiled fish instead of fried. Our kitchen is stocked with Clean foods that are plant-based, nutrient-dense and unprocessed. If my kids want junk, they choose to buy it. I won't. I commit to exercise daily and invite my family to participate when possible. I treat myself with respect through my language and my actions. In other words, I walk the talk. Others have the choice to journey with me, or not. But either way, I'm full steam ahead.

Your goal is to champion your own changes. Live and breathe your new you each and every day. Sure, it's natural for kids to initially resist what's new or different, but you must embody your principles and mind-set and consistently show commitment to your new lifestyle. Answer their questions, be honest, experiment with family changes together and breathe a healthy curiosity into their world. It may take time, but eventually they will see that you've made a very powerful, completely unshakable decision to live better.

If your kids don't support you at first, consider this another opportunity to show how passionate you are about this good-health cause and how basically nothing can stop you from doing what's best for your mind and body.

My girls didn't initially support the changes I was making—they were used to their mother one way, and were scared about what would happen if I changed—but I refused to stop. What message would I be sending if I buckled under pressure because my kids didn't like my Best Body Now lifestyle? Instead, I showed them that their mom isn't a coward and can stand tall and powerful in the face of tough challenges. Eventually, they saw that they weren't losing their mom; I was actually upgrading to Mom 2.0, a stronger, more powerful version of the person I once was, with more energy and happiness to share.

I was actually upgrading to Mom 2.0, a stronger, more powerful version of the person I once was, with more energy and happiness to share.

Your Husband: Can He Support a New You?

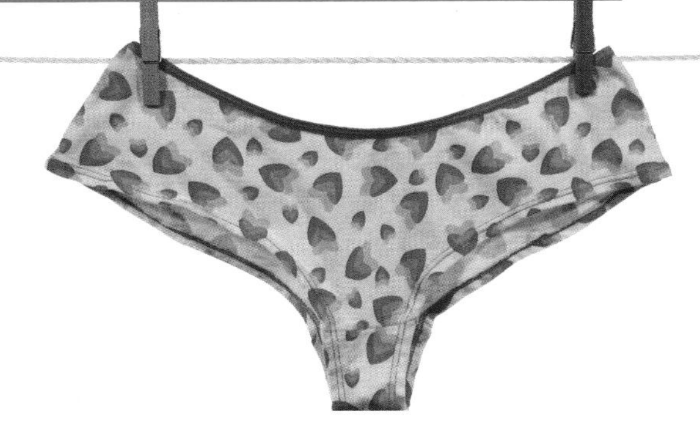

THE ANSWER: ABSOLUTELY! FROM THE thousands of reader stories I've read, partners are ecstatic to see their wives taking better care of themselves. The benefits are innumerable, but the most popular seems to be a renewed interest in sex! And why not—he's got a leaner, more toned wife who is happier, healthier and hotter than ever. What's not to love?

> If he feels like he's part of the transformation, he'll be more likely to jump on board.

Sure, some husbands become cranky initially, but usually it's because they feel threatened by the idea that their partners may soon become more attractive and that hubby may have to make some changes, too! Fragile egos don't like to be pressured. And, yes, it's true that it takes a strong, self-assured man to want his wife to look newly sleek and sexy.

How do you make sure your partner feels more secure? Start slowly and involve him in the process. If he feels like he's part of the transformation, he'll be more likely to jump on board. Not only that, you need a strong, supportive partner when going through such an exciting and massive makeover, so his involvement is critical.

Ask for his support and be specific about what you need—can he take the kids to school in the mornings while you hit the gym, help plan healthy meals you'll both enjoy, join in energizing family activities like hiking rather than renting movies, even motivate you on days you're feeling sluggish? Be clear that you'll be a better person, and partner, if you're healthy and that his encouragement and help is key to your success. At the same time, he should know that this is *for you* and *about you*, so while you would love his buy-in, you're committed to health and wellness.

> Ask for his support and be specific about what you need.

Your Friends: Will They Honor Your Driven New Lifestyle?

THE ANSWER: GIVE THEM THE CHANCE! Some friends are totally supportive, while others want you to be successful but not outshine them. That's normal. Your goal is to stick to the principles that resonate with you and the dreams that burn inside. I'm lucky to have a great group of supportive pals who have not only encouraged me to be brave and soar but also stayed with me through the journey. Make sure to surround yourself with positive, like-minded people.

The best way to bring friends on board is to share this process with them so they can understand and support your efforts—you want friends who are going to realize that your gym time, for example, is sacred, so they'll plan something that doesn't conflict with your schedule rather than making you feel guilty. Or better yet, they'll join! Another idea is to relay what you've learned so they can also become their strongest, most powerful selves. The more you give, the more you get in return! In my circle, we support each other in taking chances, doing things differently, stretching outside the comfort zone and truly seizing life. By doing it together, we guarantee our individual and collective success!

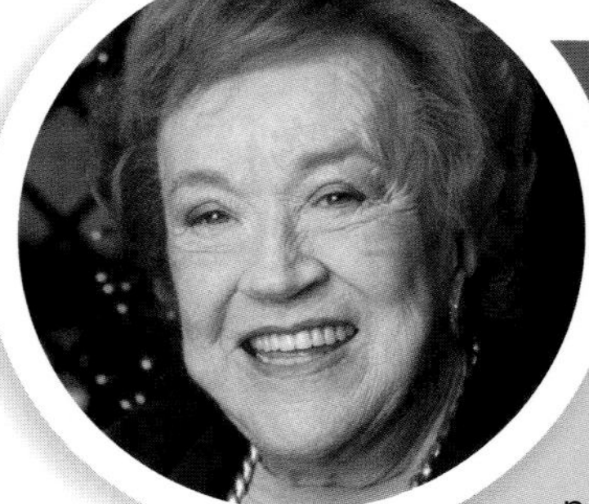

The "H" Factor: A-List Proof That Life Gets Better at 40

I adore trailblazers! The one-of-a-kind Julia Child, the powerhouse chef who brought fancy French recipes to kitchens all across North America, epitomizes the pioneering "fabulous new you" attitude. She didn't even film the pilot of her timeless cooking show until the age of forty-nine. The Julia Child we all know, and her legacy-setting contributions, were all made after the age of fifty. She proved to the world that dreaming big can start—and *spring to life*—at any age.

Your Career: How Do You Balance Work Demands With Your New Life?

THE ANSWER: PLANNING! IT'S EASY TO think that planning meals and training sessions, implementing new health and beauty strategies or even simply thinking differently about yourself and your life can be difficult, if not impossible. When people tell me this, my response is always that you haven't been taught how—you can do this in a way that (1) won't eat up your leisure time and (2) can be worked into your job demands.

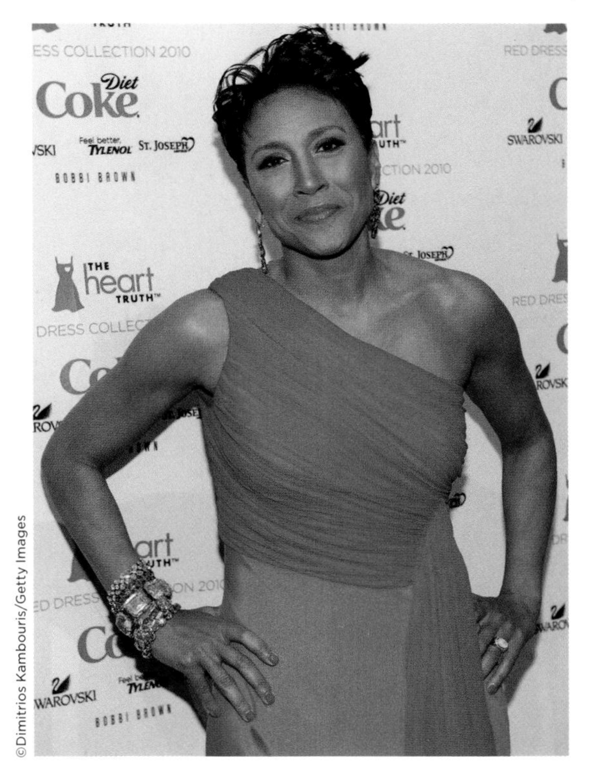

©Dimitrios Kambouris/Getty Images

Robin Roberts

TOSCA TIDBIT

Robin Roberts, the fiftysomething co-anchor of ABC's *Good Morning America* powered her way to success by following the rules and breaking them. She says, "I was a woman, I was black and I didn't care if people said I didn't belong in sports broadcasting. I pushed my way in." She became the first black female sportscaster on ESPN. Today Roberts hosts a morning show to millions, opening her heart and soul to the audience. Robin follows a guiding principle of lifting herself out of her problems by focusing on what you can do, not what is impossible. Roberts is an example to all women to push forward regardless of the obstacles, including breast cancer. As a survivor, Robin is an inspiration to all of us.

This is your five-part mission:

1 INVERT YOUR PRIORITY LIST. Remember, you are your first priority, rather than the last. You're best able to tackle an endless to-do list and the stress that comes with it when you're happy, healthy, energized. That's the goal.

2 BLOCK OFF BOTH WORK AND PLAY IN YOUR SCHEDULE, SO THAT YOU CARVE OUT TIME FOR YOURSELF AND GET THE PROPER WORK-LIFE BALANCE. Seeing this on your daily agenda will help you spot imbalances and allow you to see that play is just as important as work. Am I selfish with my time? Absolutely! Do I neglect anyone? Absolutely not, especially myself!

3 WORK AND PLAY HARD. My schedule is rigorous by design. When I'm working, I'm extremely efficient and effective so that when downtime hits, I'm able to enjoy it without worrying about what's left on my plate. I see an extra ten minutes here or there at work as opportunities to get more done. For instance, I can reach out to more readers, answer more e-mails, test-drive another recipe. When the clock is ticking, I'm humming—every minute counts! Same goes with my leisure time. It's sacred. Vacation is vacation, play is play. When you've committed yourself to time outside of work, it's yours. Read, dance, write, exercise, turn off the phone and the computer. It's just as important for you to relax and refuel as it is for you to be at max efficiency when on the job.

4 DON'T BE AFRAID TO ASK FOR HELP. Even superheroes have sidekicks. I have an entire arsenal of support...friends, family, colleagues, you name it. To stay organized and in control, I lean on the people in my circle who can do it better, faster, more efficiently.

5 PLAN AHEAD. To incorporate strong new food, exercise, health, beauty and motivational principles into your life, take time to arm yourself with the gear (a kitchen filled with unprocessed, fresh foods and a workout-ready tote), the tools (empowering inner dialogue and beauty tricks) and the mind-set ("I will do this!"). Then consider how to use your downtime to guarantee success on the job. Make meals in advance. Get up an hour early to work out. Toss out your old cosmetic bag and start fresh. This is your blank canvas. You're starting over and painting a whole new you.

It's just as important for you to relax and refuel as it is for you to be at max efficiency when on the job.

MY BEST BODY NOW

Triumph of the Not-So-Average Jane
Allison Earnst's Journey

THEN
5'6", AGE 32
189 POUNDS

NOW
AGE 34
132 POUNDS

I was a former fast-food junkie—I breezed through burger joints alone at night and tried to escape my feelings of anxiety. However, it only made things worse by adding negative self-esteem and chaos to the list. My life was out of control—I felt overwhelmed, overweight and exhausted.

I had three children under three—my youngest was just six months old—and I weighed nearly 200 pounds. I fell into a vicious cycle of gaining weight and caring less about myself. The more I weighed, the more I wanted to hide the person I was becoming. I would skip breakfast and my first meal was often a drive-through lunch, followed by a big dinner and dessert.

Then one day, I snapped. I realized I had to make a change for myself and my kids. That's when I began Eating Clean and incorporating the Best Body Now program, cutting down on fast food and incorporating whole grains, lean proteins, fruits and vegetables, and I lost a whopping 30 pounds in six months—I'm living proof that even small tweaks can lead to big success at first! At the same time, I started cardio and light strength training, gradually increasing time and weights. As I began feeling better and looking better, I realized that making myself a priority was not selfish at all. It was a vital part of who I was and of being a better wife, mother and woman. If I was not being the best I could be, I was not being true to myself or my family.

Two years after topping out at 189 pounds, I just finished my first NPC Bikini Competition with girls ten years younger! Don't be afraid to dream big. Set high goals, big challenges and go for it! My goals in the beginning seemed laughable, but I set them, believed them and accomplished them.

While it was challenging, the key was making Eating Clean and working out a priority, plus staying flexible. I would often get up early to work out before my husband left the house or even go during peak hours just to clock gym time. You're never going to reach a day and feel like you have arrived. It's a lifelong journey, and you just do the best that you can each day. You will have slip-ups, and that's okay—just jump right back in and keep on pushing!

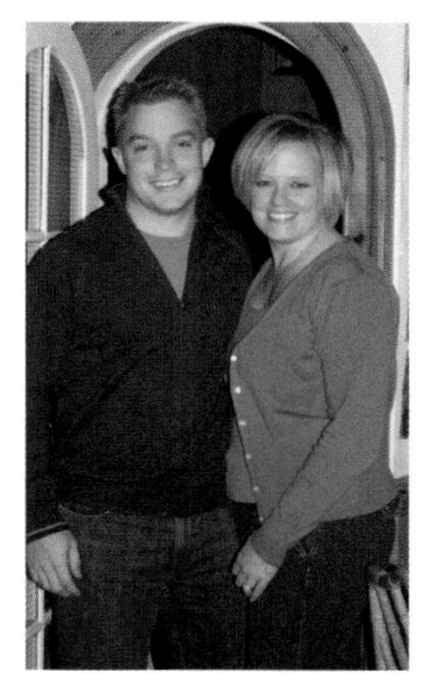

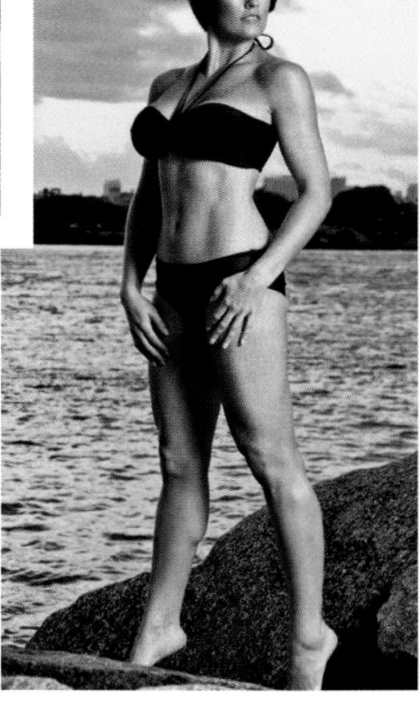

Since my transformation, I'm happier, more energetic and more fulfilled in all areas of my life. Instead of turning to food for comfort in times of stress or anxiety, I view exercise as therapy. I take great motivating music and it's my own personal time to take a break, zone out, think and sweat it out. I work out because I want to, and when I miss a day or two, I miss the positive feelings it brings out in me.

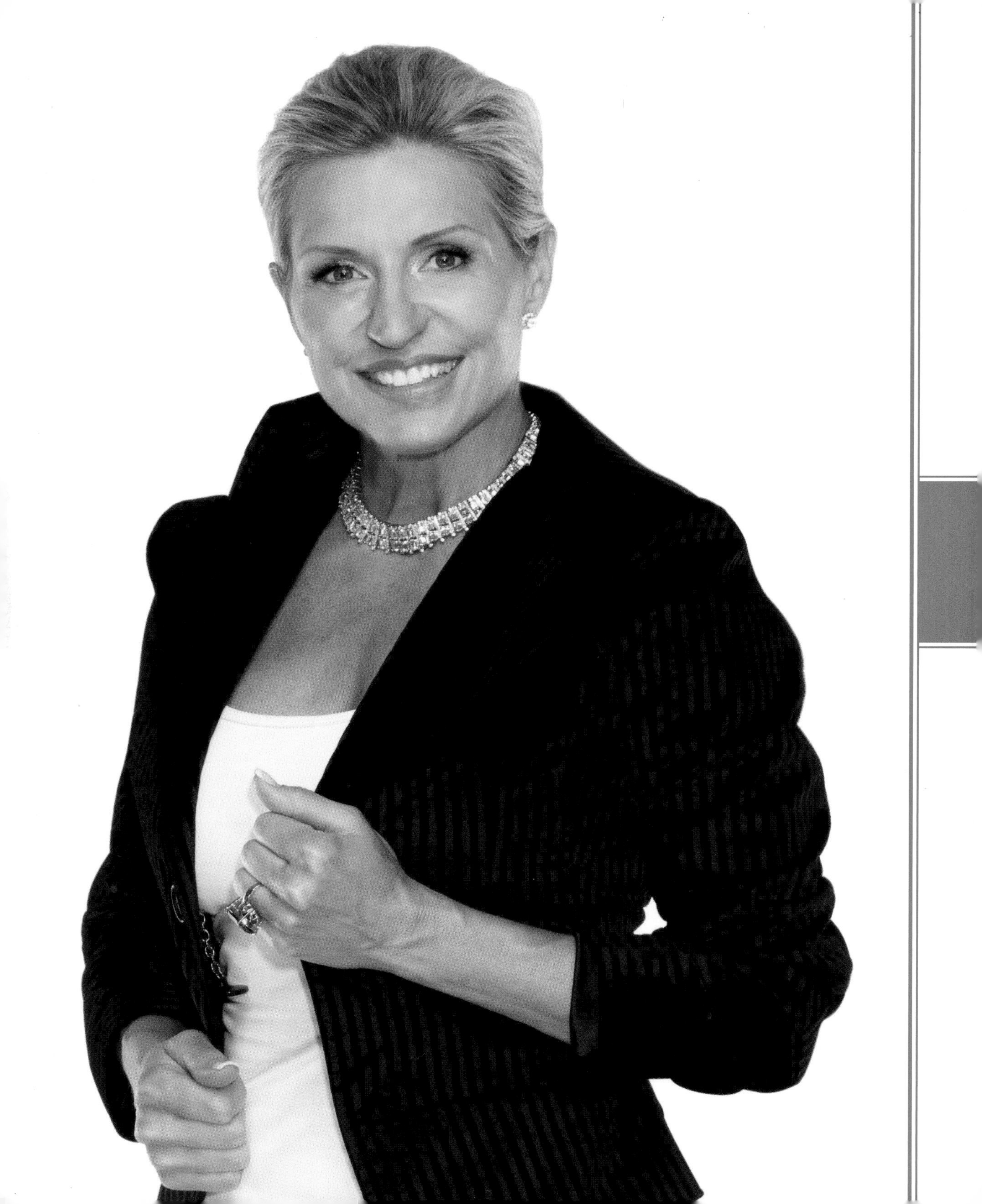

3 Jump-Start Your Best Body Now!

WHEN I BEGAN, I KEPT A LITTLE PIECE OF WISDOM AT THE TOP of my mind: take care of yourself in order to be the best person you can be, so you become the example for others to do the same—even if they don't join your transformation, they'll realize you're unstoppable. True emotional and mental health comes from believing this right to the core. An unhealthy person who neglects herself isn't equipped enough to help her kids, her spouse or her aging parents. Successful women understand this implicitly.

Get Ready to Say "Go!"

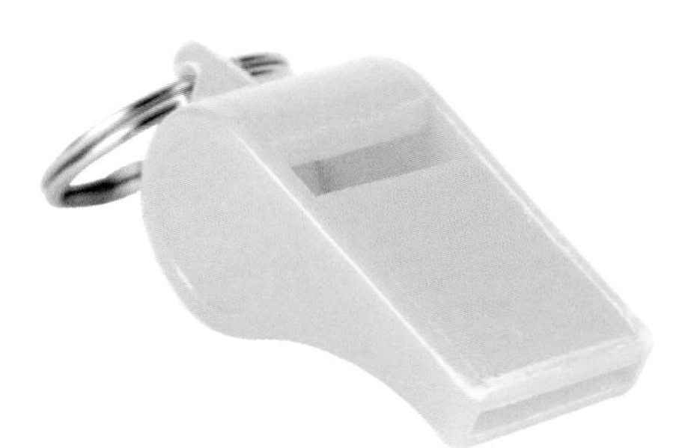

THE BONUS IS THAT THIS BELIEF SYSTEM builds you up and provides a foundation that extends into all areas of your life, rather than breaking you down. Each small success inspires you to discover more about yourself and how powerful you can be if you're willing to let go of misconceptions about your personal strength. You begin to crave challenges and push the bar of expectation even higher than you've ever imagined. It's the most deliciously frightening, wonderfully life-altering journey you'll ever begin. And despite the effort and challenge, I can't for a moment fathom how I ever could have lived another way.

So start here, start *now*. Get your brain on board and give yourself permission to unleash the gorgeous you within.

The last reminder, one I want you to keep close to your heart, is that your journey isn't one of indulgence or irresponsibility; it's a *necessity*. It's not like you're saying, "I need another new pair of stilettos." Rather, you're telling the world, "I want a strong, sexy body, an inspired mind and the energy to shape life."

> Your journey isn't one of indulgence or irresponsibility; it's a *necessity*.

Now that you're empowered, prepped for challenges and armed for an awe-inspiring new beginning, let's rock this Best Body Now journey! Remember this moment, because once you commit, you'll never want to look back. Let the jump-starting begin!

TOSCA TIDBIT

Did you know that the mulberry tree was a favored symbol during the Renaissance because it flowers late, once every few decades, bursting into bloom? Sounds just like the perfect metaphor for the sexy Best Body Now sisterhood!

Jump-Start Your Best Body Now

HOW DID I JUMP-START A FABULOUS new me? I just did it. I began *acting* as though my mind and body were already where I wanted them to be. I pushed intimidation and self-consciousness aside, and ate and exercised like I was already in top condition, even though I was 70 pounds overweight. Those small changes, combined with my rock-solid "change will happen" attitude, became the small steps that allowed me to achieve what some thought was impossible. I made my dreams a reality by embodying them.

I made my dreams a reality by embodying them.

This is where the Best Body Now journey begins. Be the healthy, vibrant, sexy person you envision.

In Parts 2 and 3 of this book, I'll go into specific detail about jump-starting the journey in all areas of the Best Body Now program—food, fitness, health, beauty and inspiration. Until then, arm yourself with these thirteen momentum-building steps for beginning your own Best Body Now transformation (most of them take just minutes):

1	Share your new commitment with your husband or partner first, and get support—ask for his involvement. Be specific, be patient, be brave!
2	Talk to your children about changes they're likely to see in you and how this will impact their own lives—invite their participation. Make your new life fun!
3	Reach out to your closest friend to discuss your new journey—maybe she would like to go on the ride, too. Ask to reshape your time together in ways that strengthen the friendship and your health. Get her support in sharing news with your circle of friends.
4	Find a community of like-minded people who have similar goals so you can motivate and challenge each other in positive ways. Can't find one? Start your own with women you know!

5 Start with a clean slate. Clear out your kitchen, medicine cabinet and cosmetic bags of unhealthy or expired products so you're not tempted to revert to old, bad habits and can start fresh.

6 Plan your first-week menu, then stock your kitchen with healthy, unprocessed options so you avoid temptation. No junk food.

7 Join a gym or create workout space in your home. This ensures you'll work out from the get-go. (Excuse-proof your workout now: squats and lunges don't require weights or much space to start.)

8 Schedule time today on your calendar for work and play during the next week. (If you're motivated, schedule your month!)

9 Look at this transformation as a *lifestyle*, not a series of events, and you'll soon create positive habits. One bad decision won't throw you off track—you're seeking lifelong change.

10 Consider "cheat" days as "treat" days. This allows you to enjoy your indulgence without feeling guilty, and to get back on the Best Body Now fast track immediately. I don't advocate that people live like monks, but keep treat days to one every week or two for the best results, especially when you're just starting.

11 Look for outside sources of inspiration—books written by a hero of yours, speaking engagements by people you admire, art galleries, inspirational documentaries. Find what inspires you and immerse yourself in it. Read a quote or two before bed and one when you wake in the morning for motivation.

12 Give yourself a big goal to work toward. I use contests to keep my mind focused on a daily basis. Other options? A charity walk or run, a marathon or triathlon, an event in your life like your anniversary. Whatever puts a date on your calendar (six months from now) and an end game (30 pounds dropped), write it down, visualize it, say it aloud every day. You can do this.

13 Be in the moment and don't look back!

One Small Change Leads to One Big Accomplishment

If you're here and already saying to yourself, "Yes, but..." and you find the whole concept too overwhelming, do this one simple thing: find your one worst habit—drinking too much, smoking, late-night snacking, eating junk food, avoiding exercise, neglecting your beauty routine—and eliminate just that single behavior. It's only one. One man I advised had had a twelve-soda-a-day habit for ten years. We eliminated just that one crutch by switching him to water and he lost 55 pounds fast, plus kick-started a complete life overhaul. This isn't a miracle—it's the result of a commitment to a baby step ("I'll drink water today instead of soda"), repeated each day. I started with small changes, too, and here are just some of the enormous life-altering payoffs that started right away:

- I dropped 37 pounds quickly—and 70 in nine months.
- Lean muscle mass replaced fat, flabby tissue.
- My body fat is down to 9 percent when competing and 12 percent when not.
- My body took on a beautiful, feminine shape.
- My skin became rejuvenated and shed signs of fatigue and aging.
- My mental clarity improved significantly.
- My nails grew beautifully, becoming stronger, healthier and chip-free.
- My energy levels skyrocketed. Today, my schedule is twice as packed as it was in my thirties, but I get out of bed with a spring in my step and power through each day without quick-fix empty calories, caffeine or catnaps.
- My hair became fuller and thicker, as it was in my twenties.
- Trigger foods no longer tempted me.
- My blood work tested in the optimal, super-healthy range (and my hypoglycemia disappeared).
- Depression lifted. Today I'm happier than ever.

- My libido kicked in and I began feeling sexier and more vibrant than I had in years.
- I sailed through menopause. (I stopped having periods at forty-eight but feel as good now—if not better—than ever before!)

> It doesn't matter where you start—just start.

One small change this very moment is one step closer to achieving more than you've ever thought possible. It doesn't matter where you start—just start. I'm with you all the way.

Get ready. This is going to be a glorious ride!

The "H" Factor: A-List Proof That Life Gets Better at 40

Like millions of other women, I consider Oprah Winfrey one of my idols. Even though this reigning grand dame of media began her life as a beauty queen, by her thirties she evolved into a nationally syndicated talk show hostess who handily eclipsed the genre's patriarch, Phil Donahue. That wasn't enough; she also landed an Academy Award nomination for her role in *The Color Purple*. And not only has she transformed her life, but she's also helped countless others change theirs. At forty-nine, Oprah became the first African American billionaire to appear on the Forbes 400. Her take on it: "I feel like turning fifty is everything you were meant to be in your life." My take? The best is yet to come for the unstoppable Oprah!

MY BEST BODY NOW

Triumph of the Not-So-Average Jane
Debbie Squizzero's Journey

My transformation was as much internal as it was external. At my highest weight of 161, I had poor eating habits, dry hair and skin, and rock-bottom self-confidence.

THEN
5'6", AGE 35
161 POUNDS

NOW
AGE 38
130 POUNDS

My meals were prepackaged and box-based: Pop Tarts, cereals, frozen entrees, cookies, pastas and hamburgers. Veggies were basically a no-show in my diet, save the occasional zucchini or corn. All of this was chased down by a pretty fierce soda habit.

Then I began Eating Clean. Before, I would eat when I was hungry and would make poor choices because I was not choosing the right foods, ones with fiber and protein, to keep me full. Now, I space my meals out every few hours in order to keep my metabolism rolling at a good pace and burning calories, and to keep my blood sugar stabilized so that my hunger is in check and I'm not hungry at all!

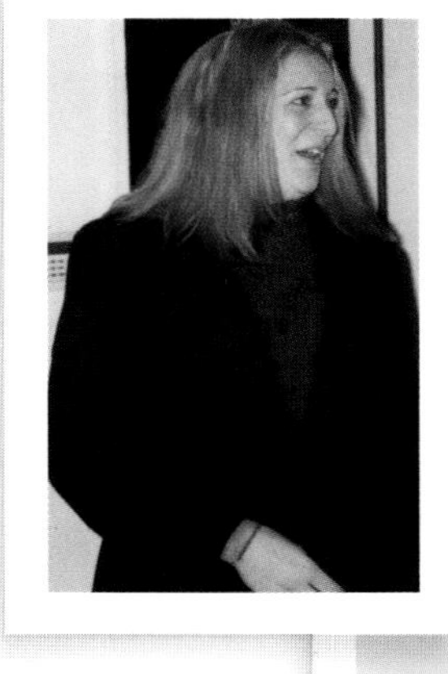

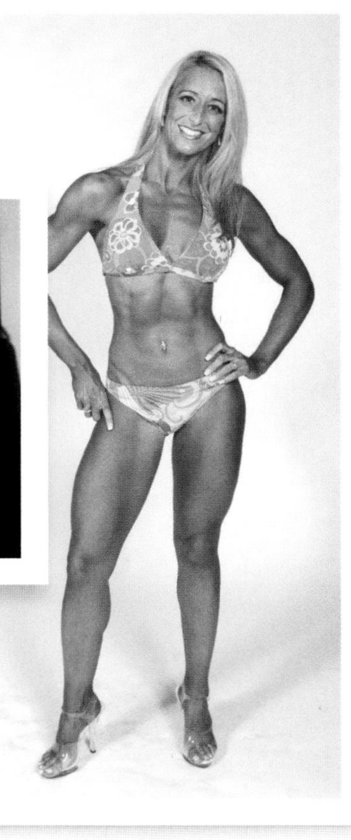

Next I incorporated weight training, and not only did the pounds come off, but my gorgeous new shape began to emerge as muscle replaced fat. My confidence soared. I felt better about myself, and I liked me—I couldn't believe I could actually look like this. I felt stronger on the inside mentally and felt I could help others who wanted to know how I got to this place of helping myself.

My trick was planning ahead! I listed everything I needed to cook for the week based on Tosca's Eating Clean recipes. I tried vegetables I never would have looked at twice but was eager to try because I was experiencing firsthand what they were doing for my body.

I became more confident in other areas of my life like my job. I spoke up more often for what I believed in and what I disagreed with, instead of holding it all in and just going with the flow.

Today, I'm a certified personal trainer who teaches others the same principles, and have also joined the bodybuilding competition circuit. I have a sense of confidence and empowerment that I never imagined was within the realm of my inner being. Just the way I look and feel every day keeps me motivated with energy and confidence. I love to help people when they ask how I obtained my goals and how they can obtain their goals with food or exercise. Being a role model or inspiration to others is such a good feeling.

Get Your Best Body Now—For Life

PART

2

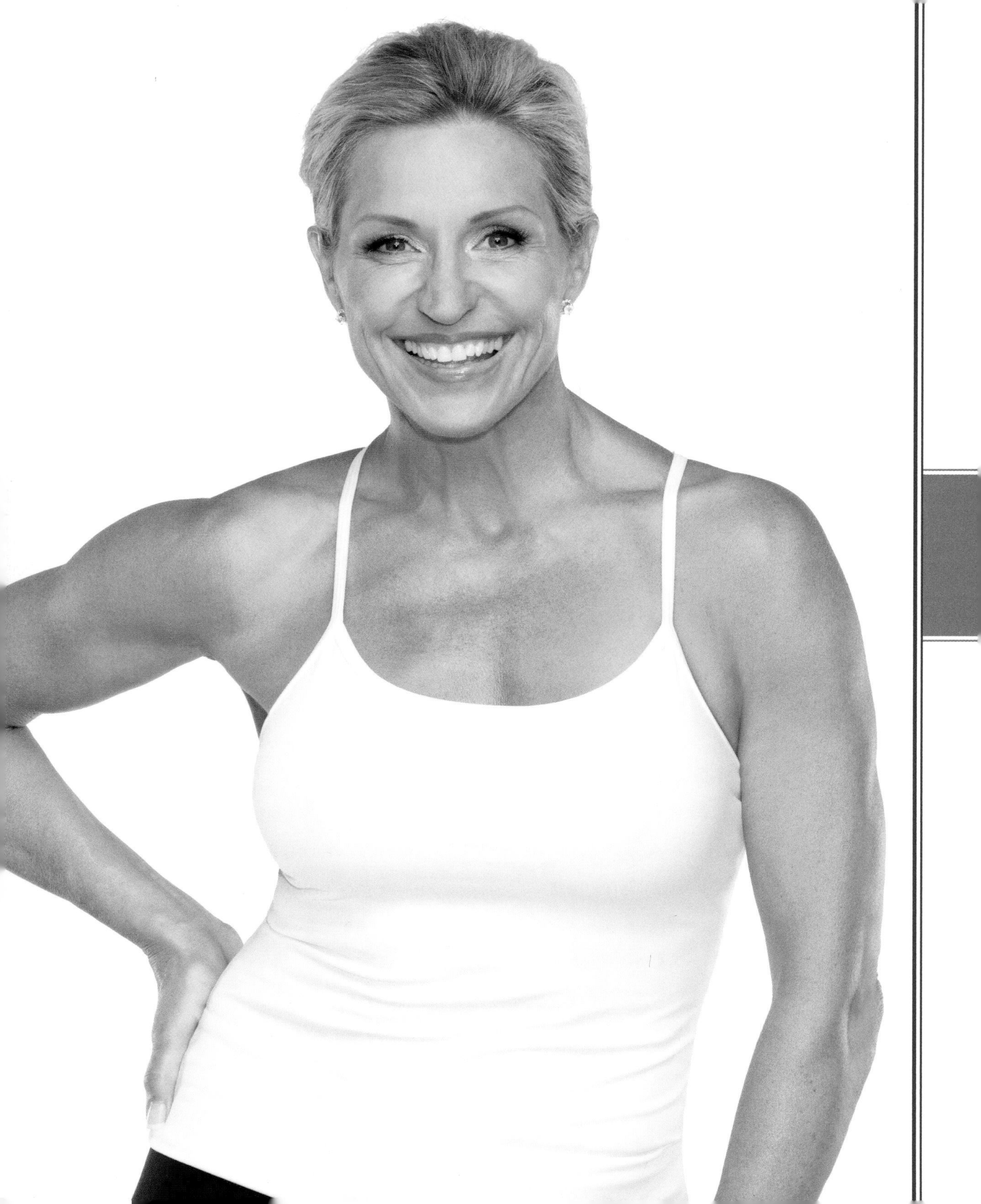

4 Best Body Now Diet

MOST EXPERTS AGREE THAT 80 PERCENT OF HOW YOUR BODY looks is based on nutrition. You can work out all you want, but if you have poor eating habits, you won't see results. That was my story—I was able to lose a small amount of weight by doing cardio, but it wasn't until I changed the way I was eating that I began to see a *real* change in the way my body looked. I sought out advice from those who had the leanest bodies around—professional weight lifters and fitness models—and adopted their lean-body strategies. Their secret and mine? A whole new approach based on eating more and making better food choices.

The plan involves eating unprocessed foods, which I call Eating Clean. It's not a diet, it's not a starvation plan, it's not a gimmick or fad. Eating Clean is a healthy approach to food, one sure to create enormous improvements in your energy levels, weight, health and more. Even better, everyone at any age can do it. The process is so simple you can begin this very moment—right now!

It wasn't until I started Eating Clean that I truly saw my body change and become leaner, stronger and sexier. As it turns out, the benefits weren't just cosmetic. What I discovered is that many of the health issues I was battling were eliminated or reduced by my new plan, and the so-called inevitable conditions or problems I had anticipated as the result of aging never happened.

It's not a diet, it's not a starvation plan, it's not a gimmick or fad.

Diet Tweaks That Get Results

THE FUNDAMENTAL TENETS OF THIS program—eating Mother Nature's healthiest offerings several times a day—are so powerful and successful because they demand that we continue to fuel our bodies throughout the day, *every* day, with all the disease-fighting, age-proofing, energy-boosting, muscle-building, body-beautifying nutrients and vitamins our bodies need to live better, longer. Eating this way is not about sacrifice, either—you won't feel deprived at all, since another tenet of this program prescribes eating smaller meals more frequently. It's about rewarding yourself with foods that satisfy you now but help you stay healthy, lean and strong for years to come.

The fundamental principles of the Best Body Now diet are simple: eat several smaller meals a day sufficient in protein, as well as fresh fruits, vegetables and whole grains. Simply put, it's eating smart. It's eating foods as close to nature as you can possibly get them. Eating this way is not about consuming less or depriving yourself. It's not even about counting calories. You never have to count calories again. It's about eating natural foods frequently and in abundance to fire up your metabolism all day long so it can do the job it was always meant to do—burn fat!

Even better? Because you're eating several times daily, my plan helps you get all the nutrients and vitamins you need to prevent, fight or reverse minor health challenges, disease and the signs of aging through a powerhouse prescription of fresh fruits and vegetables, whole grains and lean proteins—nutrients needed to build the best version of you possible.

BEST BODY NOW Diet Basics

CONSIDER FOOD AS NUTRITIONAL "MEDICINE." Everything we eat has the potential to work for our health or against it. When we "eat healthy," we're doing more than giving our bodies fuel for a day. By eating foods rich in vitamins and minerals, we're actually strengthening our cells, organs and systems so they function at their peak and arm our immune systems to fight illness, disease and age-related changes. When we eat unhealthy foods or skip meals, we're depriving our bodies of the nutrients they require to function properly and prevent health problems. Making smart food choices today will set you up for a youthful, healthy, ageless mind and body.

> Making smart food choices today will set you up for a youthful, healthy, ageless mind and body.

EAT SIX MEALS PER DAY (ONE MEAL EVERY TWO TO THREE HOURS). I know it sounds unbelievable and is the opposite of what most popular diets tell you, but eating better foods *more frequently* actually increases your metabolism and keeps energy levels high all day. Regular snacking on power foods curbs overeating by preventing you from ever becoming overly hungry and gives you more opportunities to eat nutrient-dense foods throughout the day. Eating regular small meals once every three hours also helps stabilize blood sugar levels. You'll also find the cravings will stop because you're constantly fueling your body with satisfying foods. When you eat just three meals a day, your metabolism and blood

TOSCA TIDBIT

Skipping meals and drastically undereating can put your body in starvation mode. Eat six meals each and every day to speed up your metabolism and increase fat burning.

> Breakfast eaters have better concentration, higher daily nutrient intake, greater energy levels and lower overall weight.

sugar levels dip and you're more likely to eat unhealthy foods, as well as overeat, when you're feeling very hungry and deprived.

NEVER SKIP MEALS, ESPECIALLY BREAKFAST—MAKE IT A PRIORITY. Some people believe skipping breakfast is an easy way to eat fewer total calories in a day, but doing so actually sets you up for having less energy and ultimately eating more. Many studies, including a recent one from Tufts University, have shown that consuming a nutritious breakfast increases glucose levels in the body and boosts energy levels for the entire day. You could think of breakfast as your primer meal that sets the tone for the rest of your day. Other benefits? Breakfast eaters have been shown to possess better concentration, higher daily nutrient intake, greater energy levels and lower overall weight when compared to those who skip the first meal of the day.

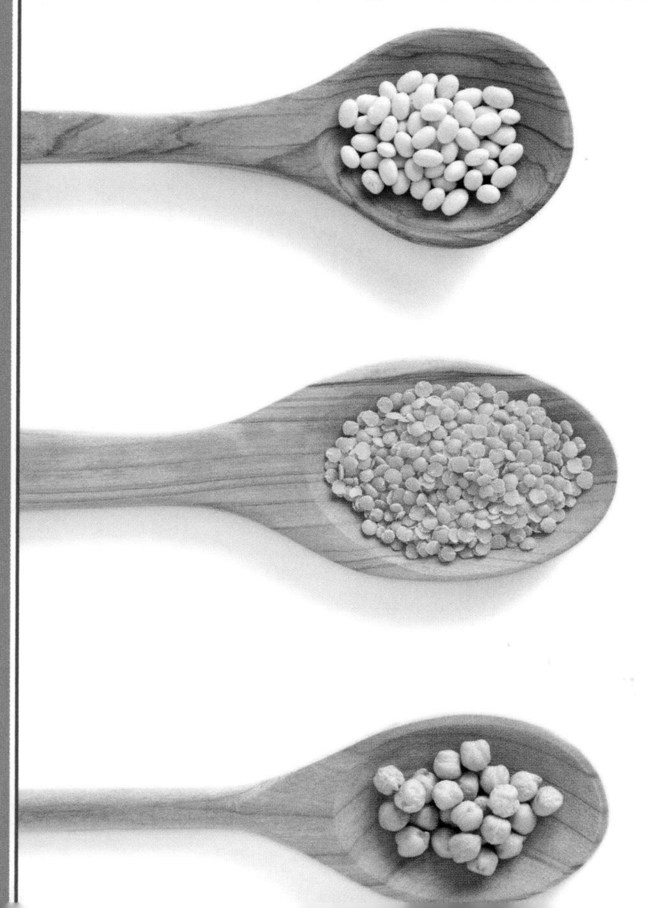

MIX PROTEINS AND COMPLEX CARBS AT EVERY MEAL. It's important not only to eat several small meals regularly throughout the day but also to make sure they consist of a healthy combination of complex carbohydrates and lean proteins from sources including poultry, eggs, dairy, soy products, beef, game, nuts, seeds and fish. The reason is these two macronutrients, when eaten together, promote a feeling of satisfaction or fullness. This helps you feel full longer while fueling your body's fat-burning process at the same time.

Carbohydrates are divided into complex and simple types—both turn to glucose (sugar) when digested and are absorbed into your bloodstream to give your body energy. Complex carbs—found in whole grains, beans and legumes, and vegetables (see the Best Body Now Foods Checklist on page 58)—are digested more slowly than simple carbohydrates because they're made of three or more linked sugars. Simple carbohydrates—including refined starches, glucose,

HEALTHFUL VS. UNHEALTHFUL FATS

FATS ARE ONE OF THREE SUBSTANCES YOUR BODY USES FOR ENERGY—CARBOHYDRATES and protein are the other two. Fats contain 9 calories per gram, while protein and carbs are about 4 grams each. Despite the higher calories, some fats are incredibly good for your body, and necessary to keep it running in top shape. These are called "functional fats."

For the Best Body Now diet, it's important to distinguish between the two types of fats: saturated and unsaturated.

Saturated fats

These are the unhealthful fats that raise your LDL, or "bad," cholesterol and contribute to heart disease. These fats include:

1. Animal products such as fatty meats, whole milk, full-fat ice cream
2. Tropical oils (excluding coconut oil, a healthful fat that I strongly advocate—it is no longer implicated in heart disease)
3. Trans fats, which are found in trace amounts in meat and dairy, but are primarily created through the hydrogenation of vegetable oils to extend their shelf life

Trans fats are particularly detrimental because in addition to raising your LDL, they may also lower your HDL, or "good" cholesterol, which puts you at risk for heart disease. You'll find them in foods such as margarine, dressings and packaged snacks such as cookies, crackers and cakes.

Unsaturated fats

Choosing these fats over unhealthful saturated fats may help reduce your LDL, according to the National Institutes of Health. The list includes coconut, palm kernel and red palm kernel oil, seed oils, olive oil, flaxseed oil and organic butter.

fructose and other sugars found in refined and processed foods such as cookies, sodas and candy—are made of one or two linked sugar molecules, contain few nutrients and are digested quickly, which is why they're typically referred to as empty calories.

Complex carbs and lean proteins, when eaten together, help you feel full longer, while fueling your body's fat-burning process.

This means that eating complex carbohydrates causes glucose to enter your blood stream much more slowly—your blood sugar levels don't see the big spikes and dips caused by refined processed foods that give you fast energy but leave you feeling sluggish and often craving more within a few hours.

When you pair complex carbs with proteins, such as chicken, fish or almonds, the protein helps slow the release of glucose into the blood sugar even further, so glucose is used as energy rather than stored as fat. At the same time, protein helps rebuild muscle and stimulates a fat-burning hormone called glucagon.

Saturated fats, trans fats and sugar lurk in surprising places.

CONSUME UNHEALTHFUL SATURATED FATS, TRANS FATS, SUGAR AND ALCOHOL SPARINGLY. These are collectively best considered as public enemy number one and have been linked to everything from obesity to heart disease to cancer. Unfortunately, saturated fats, trans fats and sugar lurk in surprising places. For example, table salt has trace amounts of sugar in it, which is why I've switched to sea salt. Traditional jarred peanut butter also contains high amounts of sugar. Even one cigarette can contain 4 grams of sugar. When I began reading labels, I was surprised at the number of foods that I thought were good for my family—even "diet," "low-calorie" or "healthful" boxed meals and

It's never too late to reverse bad habits and start fueling your body with powerful nutrients.

frozen foods—but contained large amounts of unhealthy fats, sugar and sodium. Many age-related diseases appearing in our forties and fifties are caused by eating excessive amounts of these unhealthful foods earlier in our lives. The good news is that it's never too late to reverse bad habits and start fueling your body with powerful nutrients. Make it a habit to scrutinize labels when grocery shopping so you don't unwittingly eat these killers.

DON'T EAT CALORIE-DENSE FOODS THAT OFFER NO NUTRITIONAL VALUE. Processed and fast foods, such as chips, cookies, french fries and more, are a nutritional wasteland. Most packaged foods and frozen entrées fall into this category, as does just about anything you're getting by way of a drive-through window. The calories in these foods are called "empty" because they give you a quick burst of energy, but without any vitamins, nutrients or natural ingredients, so they offer no real health benefits. After consuming them, you experience a momentary high, due to a short-lived spike in blood sugar, and you're left feeling hungry soon after. Eating anti-foods such as these generates cravings for even more empty calories because they never satisfy you, unlike eating clean, natural, nutritious foods.

> Processed and fast foods are a nutritional wasteland.

EAT *FRESH* FRUITS AND VEGETABLES. Fresh produce, an important ingredient of the Best Body Now eating plan, is chock-full of immunity-boosting fiber, nutrients, vitamins and antioxidants. Antioxidants are substances that prevent the formation of free radicals, molecules that can cause cancer, heart disease and age-related illnesses. Eating plenty of fruits and vegetables helps fuel a Best Body Now lifestyle, one that also involves plenty of physical exercise. Adding a minimum of several servings a day of these foods ensures you meet nutritional needs and ward off disease. Think of eating these foods as your proactive step toward excellent health. Don't be fooled by imposters such as store-bought juice drinks. These generally aren't a good substitute because they often contain little real fruit juice and staggering amounts of sugar.

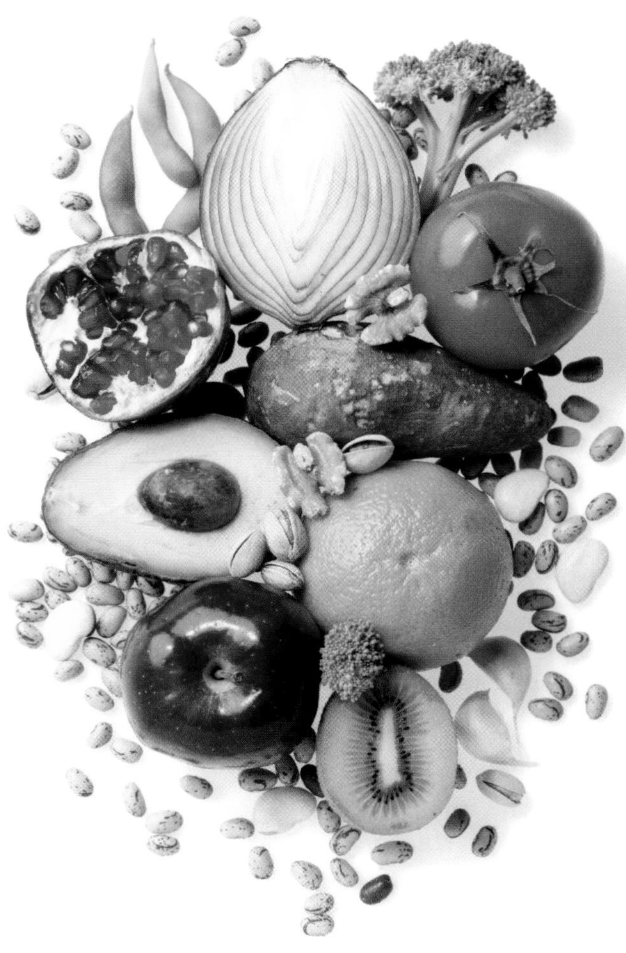

THINK ABOUT PORTION SIZES. Although the Best Body Now plan doesn't focus on counting calories, it's important to keep in mind how much fuel your body truly needs. Most of the portion sizes in restaurants are nearly twice the size of a true serving—I always ask to have half my entrée served and the other placed in a doggie bag, or else I order salads and appetizers that are more appropriate serving sizes. At home, it's easy to "clean your plate" to avoid leftovers or eat a few more bites simply because extra food is available, which is in effect overeating. In reality, each protein serving should fit in the palm of your hand and is roughly the size of a deck of cards. A serving of complex carbohydrates from grains should fit in the cup of your hand and is about the size of a tennis ball, while a serving of complex carbohydrates from veggies fits in the palm of two open hands and a serving of complex carbs from fruit should fit in one open hand.

DRINK A MINIMUM OF 8 GLASSES OF WATER A DAY (OR 2 TO 3 LITERS). Drinking plenty of clean, fresh water every day is one of the easiest, fastest and smartest ways to revitalize your body. Staying hydrated is essential to keeping your body functioning at its best. In fact, much of our body, including our brain, muscles, cells and blood, contains water and needs it to stay working efficiently and effectively. When you're low on liquids, your body lets you know through various symptoms including irritability, fatigue, headache and constipation, to name a few. When you're well hydrated, however, your energy levels soar, your skin and hair become supple and nourished, and your immune system stays strong because you're giving cells the nutrients they need to stay healthy and function properly, as well as ridding your body of toxins.

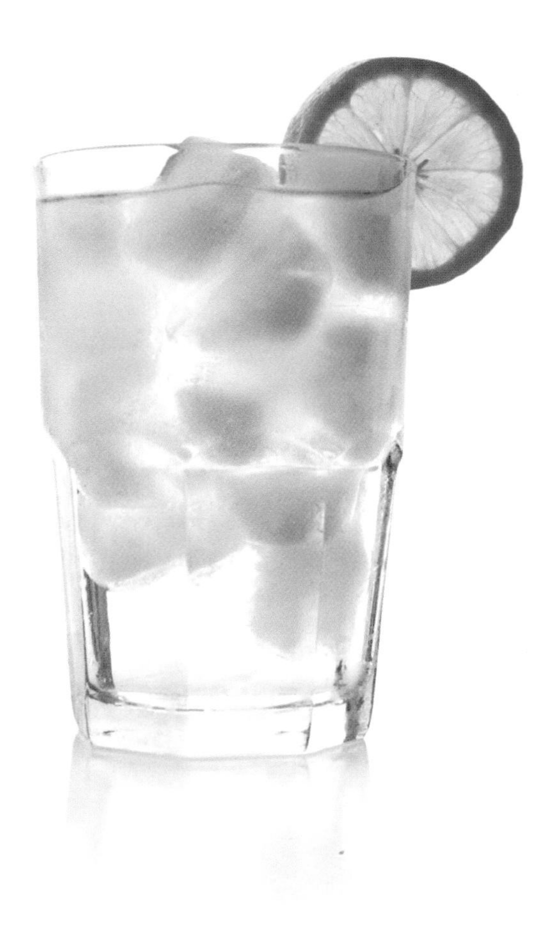

A TYPICAL DAY OF BEST BODY NOW EATING

Refer to Chapter 9 for specific recipes or inspiration for new Best Body Now dishes.

BREAKFAST	2/3 cup cooked oatmeal topped with 2 tablespoons flaxseed and 1/4 cup mixed berries, 4 hard-boiled or scrambled egg whites plus 1 yolk, with 16 ounces or 500 ml of water.
MIDMORNING MEAL	Fruit smoothie made with 1/2 cup plain low-fat yogurt, 1/2 cup fresh or frozen berries, 1/2 cup skim, rice or almond milk, 2 tablespoons flaxseed.
LUNCH	Egg salad sandwich on whole-grain bread or a wrap (my favorite brand is Ezekiel) and 16 ounces or 500 ml of water. In lieu of mayonnaise, use low-fat yogurt, yogurt cheese (see recipe on page 259) or hummus. Use 4 egg whites and 1 yolk for the egg salad. It's absolutely delicious.
MIDAFTERNOON MEAL	A handful of homemade trail mix, an apple and 16 ounces or 500 ml water.
PRE-DINNER	If you eat again later with your family: Broth-based or vegetable-puree-based soup and 16 ounces or 500 ml of water.
DINNER	Roasted skinless chicken breast with steamed asparagus and broccoli, three small red potatoes and 16 ounces or 500 ml of water.

START YOUR BEST BODY NOW

IT'S CHALLENGING TO COMPLETELY overhaul your nutrition habits all at once. Drastic reductions in food intake, as suggested in many popular fad diets, can cause the body to store fat and ultimately slow the metabolism. My secret? Make small but significant changes that are more practically and mentally manageable and over time put you on the path to eating a healthier diet of unprocessed foods at regular intervals throughout the day. That is one of the most powerful principles of the Best Body Now Diet—eating more of the healthiest foods and eating more frequently at regularly spaced intervals throughout the day.

1 **ELIMINATE SWEETS FROM YOUR DIET.** Candies, cakes and cookies are the obvious enemy of good diets. But sugar has a way of sneaking into seemingly healthy snacks, and is often the reason you can't lose those last pesky 5 pounds. Look at the nutrition labels of these secret saboteurs: processed peanut butter, sweetened yogurts, granola, canned fruits in syrup, fruit juices, protein bars and canned soups and sauces. Many salad dressings and condiments contain sugar, corn syrup or other sweeteners that stop your progress in its tracks—and you have not even enjoyed the sweet taste!

2 **REPLACE IRREGULAR SNACKING WITH SMALL HEALTHY MEALS.** Chips, crackers and other crunchy treats are often used as a way to relieve stress or anxiety. If you enjoy a crunchy texture, try smarter options such as unsalted nuts or popcorn. Fruits and veggies, including apples and carrots, can also do the trick. As part of the Best Body Now eating plan, it is always best to pair such foods with protein. So make sure to eat nuts with an apple or hard-boiled egg whites with a piece of Ryvita or a brown rice cake.

3 **SWITCH OUT WHITE CARBS FOR BROWN.** Healthy carbohydrates are whole grains including brown rice, whole-wheat pastas and 100 percent whole-wheat breads. White grains, such as white flour, pasta and rice, are refined and stripped of vitamins, fiber and iron, while whole grains are filled with disease-fighting nutrients. They also take longer to digest compared to refined grains that cause a drastic rise and fall in blood sugar levels. A food eaten in its complete state, fiber and all, delivers an entire package of healthful nutrients and benefits, something a Twinkie cannot do!

4 MIX YOUR PROTEIN SOURCES. This is the perfect way to avoid mealtime boredom and enjoy a more well-rounded diet. In addition to lean meats, chicken and fish, try vegetable-based proteins including soy foods (soy milk, edamame or tofu), quinoa, various seaweeds and spirulina. Low-fat dairy (such as yogurt and skim milk) and egg whites are smart options, too. Make sure to choose unsweetened soy products to avoid the hidden sugar in the vanilla-flavored versions often served at coffeehouses.

5 RETHINK YOUR CONDIMENTS. What is it about creamy, delicious additions such as mayonnaise, dressings or butter that make everything from sandwiches to dips to tuna salads seemingly taste scrumptious? Yet these creamy condiments are often loaded with unhealthy fats and unnecessary ingredients. Don't worry! Life won't go bare and bland without them. Throw out your mayo and fill your shelves with items such as low-fat hummus, goat cheese, avocado, fresh tomato, salsa and lemon juice. They're perfect for spreading on pitas and wraps, or moistening a yummy salad. Try making egg salad with hummus instead of mayonnaise—your taste buds won't be disappointed. I often use a wonderful food called yogurt cheese to make a creamy alternative for otherwise unhealthy condiments. (See page 259 for the recipe.) It is so versatile it can be used as either sweet or savory and it is simple to make. This protein-dense spread can be used as an alternative to those other creamy condiments you thought you couldn't live without.

6 ADD PUNCH TO YOUR WATER. Adding citrus slices, such as oranges, limes and lemons, to your water bottle infuses flavor and antioxidants. This makes 64 ounces or 1,920 ml—the daily recommended amount without exercise—go down easily.

7 USE FLAVOR BOOSTERS TO IMPROVE TASTE. Clean foods don't have to be boring. Processed foods often seem more flavorful because of all the unhealthy ingredients they add. Once you remove them from your diet, your taste buds will recalibrate and you'll find yourself reinvigorated by the intense flavors of food without the added artificial ingredients. Here are my favorite nonfat condiments that heighten taste: fresh and dried herbs, horseradish, garlic, mustards, ginger, no-sugar-added cranberry sauce, vinegars, Worcestershire sauce, citrus fruit, freshly made salsas, pureed fruit- and vegetable-based sauces, unsweetened apple butter or sauce, Bragg's All Purpose Seasoning and low-sodium soy sauce.

BEST BODY NOW FOODS CHECKLIST

Consider this list as a guideline for Best Body Now basics, but you can also refer to the shopping list in Chapter 9 for more ideas and inspiration as you stock your kitchen.

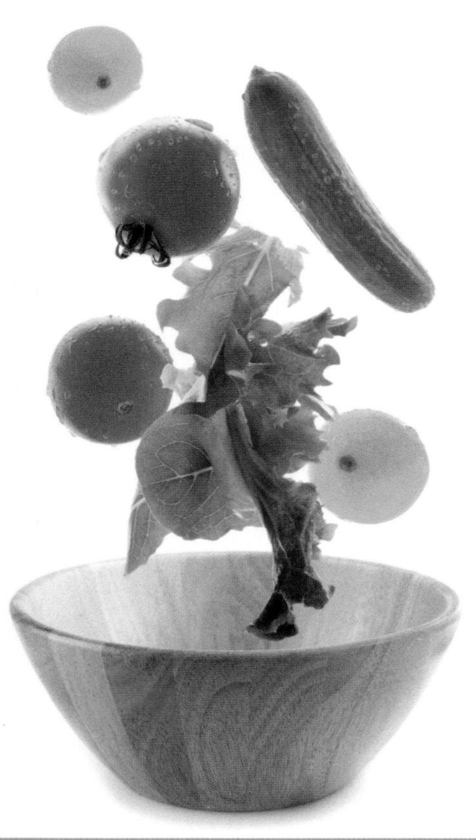

SEASONINGS AND SPICES

- ☐ Dried herbs, such as rosemary, basil, oregano, sage, mint, thyme, bay leaves, marjoram
- ☐ Spices, such as ginger, curry powder, cinnamon, paprika, cayenne or red pepper, dried chiles, turmeric, garlic powder, onion powder, nutmeg, mace
- ☐ Seeds, such as fennel, celery, cumin, anise, coriander
- ☐ Sea salt
- ☐ Black or white pepper
- ☐ Vinegars: balsamic, apple cider, sherry, wine, rice
- ☐ Low-sodium broths: chicken, vegetable, fish
- ☐ Low-sodium bouillon cubes: chicken or vegetable
- ☐ Citrus juices: lemon, grapefruit, lime
- ☐ Sweeteners: real maple syrup, honey, molasses
- ☐ Pastes: wasabi, tomato, chipotle, anchovy, chili

HEALTHY GRAINS

- ☐ Brown rice
- ☐ Wheat germ, wheat berries
- ☐ Buckwheat
- ☐ Whole oats
- ☐ Wheat bran, oat bran
- ☐ Bulgur
- ☐ Millet
- ☐ Cream of wheat
- ☐ Quinoa
- ☐ Arborio rice
- ☐ Puffed rice
- ☐ Whole-wheat bread or tortillas
- ☐ Other whole-grain wraps or bread
- ☐ Rice noodles, soba noodles

NUTS AND SEEDS

- ☐ Unsalted almonds, walnuts, pistachios, hazelnuts, cashews
- ☐ Pine nuts
- ☐ Soy nuts
- ☐ Unsalted pumpkin, sesame, sunflower seeds
- ☐ All-natural nut and seed butters, such as almond, sunflower, peanut

CEREAL

- ☐ Shredded wheat
- ☐ Kashi
- ☐ Muesli
- ☐ Weetabix
- ☐ All-Bran
- ☐ Ancient Grains
- ☐ Homemade trail mix or granola

DRIED FRUIT

- ☐ Dates
- ☐ Figs
- ☐ Cranberries
- ☐ Blueberries
- ☐ Goji berries
- ☐ Apples
- ☐ Raisins
- ☐ Prunes
- ☐ Cherries
- ☐ Apricots
- ☐ Mulberries
- ☐ Crystallized ginger

CONDIMENTS AND SAUCES

- ☐ Mustard
- ☐ Salsa
- ☐ Worcestershire
- ☐ Soy
- ☐ Hot sauce
- ☐ Fish sauce
- ☐ Oyster sauce
- ☐ Hoisin sauce

OIL

- ☐ Extra-virgin olive oil
- ☐ Coconut oil (preferably extra-virgin)
- ☐ Safflower oil (preferably cold pressed)
- ☐ Flaxseed oil
- ☐ Cold-pressed seed oils (sesame, flax, pumpkin, tomato, etc.)
- ☐ Rice bran oil

VEGETABLES

- ☐ Ginger root
- ☐ Sweet potatoes
- ☐ White, yellow, red or purple potatoes
- ☐ Onions, scallions
- ☐ Garlic, garlic scapes
- ☐ Shallots
- ☐ Squash
- ☐ Pumpkin
- ☐ Turnip
- ☐ All leafy greens
- ☐ Beans
- ☐ Beets
- ☐ Carrots
- ☐ Turnip, rutabaga
- ☐ Parsnips
- ☐ Lettuces of all kinds

DRY GOODS

- ☐ Baking soda
- ☐ Whole-wheat flour
- ☐ Vanilla
- ☐ Baking powder

TOSCA'S KITCHEN MAKEOVER

It's time to put your kitchen to the test. Have you tossed your cookies, candies, cakes and crackers? If so, it's time to stock up on the essentials for smart nutrition. My favorite Best Body Now strategy is to stock my cupboards with healthy staples including brown rice, oatmeal, eggs, quinoa, garlic, chicken and vegetable stocks, beans, vegetables and chicken breasts, always keeping a good supply on hand. Then I make a midweek trip to the grocery store to replenish perishable goods. I've listed the items you'd likely find in the Tosca household if you just popped by. Make a copy so you, too, can navigate the grocery store with sound knowledge of Best Body Now foods.

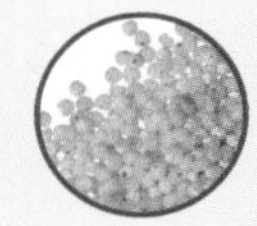

WHOLE GRAINS: brown rice, wheat germ, cream of wheat, quinoa, millet, rye, bulgur, buckwheat, oat bran, Red River cereal, spelt, kamut

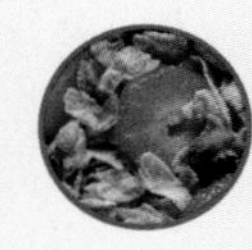

CEREALS: All-Bran, Shredded Wheat, Muesli, Ezekiel, Weetabix, Kashi

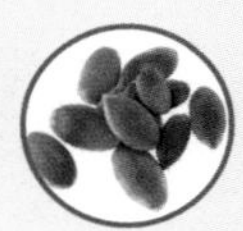

NUTS AND SEEDS: natural nut butters, cashews, sunflower, sesame, pumpkin seeds, flaxseeds, almonds, pecans, walnuts

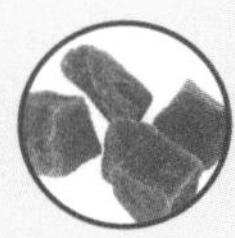

DRIED FRUIT: dates, figs, cherries, raisins, apricots, cranberries, apples, goji berries, blueberries, prunes, dried tomatoes

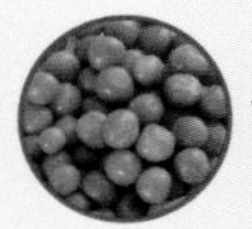

FROZEN OPTIONS: whole-grain breads and wraps, fish, edamame, chicken breasts, turkey breasts, ground chicken, ground turkey, berries, vegetables

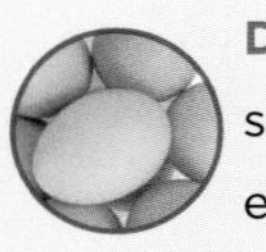

DAIRY: Low-fat soy milk, skim milk, eggs, goat cheese, plain yogurt

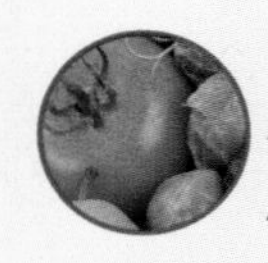

FRESH FRUITS AND VEGETABLES: Any and all—the more the better

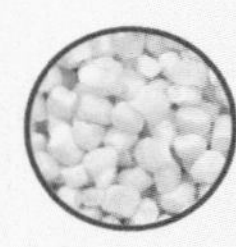

CANNED FOODS: tomatoes, tomato paste, low-sodium peas and corn, water-packed low-sodium tuna and salmon, beans

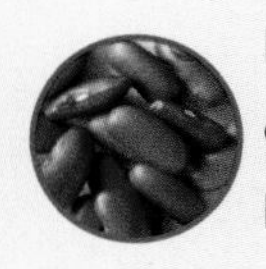

BEANS: lentils, chickpeas, kidney beans, white beans (all beans are excellent)

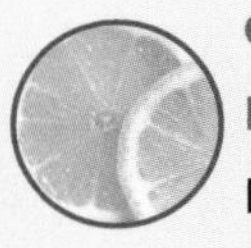

CONDIMENTS AND FLAVOR BOOSTERS: lemon and lime juice, vinegars, mustard, salsa, low-sodium vegetable or chicken broth and bouillon cubes

BEST BODY NOW RESULTS

WHAT ARE SOME OF THE BEAUTIFUL body differences you'll see from eating smart?

Many people respond immediately, noticing a revved-up metabolism, radiant skin, lustrous hair and boundless energy, all while dropping unwanted extra pounds—for good. A normal rate of weight loss is about 3 to 5 pounds per week. This is both healthy and inspiring, especially for those of you who have struggled to lose even 1 pound on a starvation or fad diet. Another welcome surprise from Eating Clean is more regular bowel movements—something many North Americans do not experience regularly today.

What are some of the beautiful body differences you'll see from eating smart?

A revved-up metabolism, radiant skin, lustrous hair and boundless energy, all while dropping unwanted extra pounds—for good.

STAY ON TRACK

IT TAKES TWENTY-ONE DAYS TO CREATE LONG-LASTING HABITS. THAT doesn't seem like long, especially considering you're making changes that will impact the rest of your life. Even so, I like to incorporate strategies that make staying on track a seamless part of my lifestyle. Try these and soon good nutrition will be as natural and simple as brushing your teeth or making the bed.

1 LIVE BY THE MENU PLAN. Removing processed foods from your diet—and eating several times a day—can take discipline at first, especially while you're learning to make it work for you. Start by planning a week's menu in advance using recipes in Chapter 9. If you know that you're buying everything you need to meet your nutrition goals for the week, you won't be tempted to stray from the shopping list.

2 BUY WHAT'S GOOD FOR YOU. I love cheese and will eat a lot of it before I can stop myself, so I know not to tempt myself. I don't purchase it at all. I've also learned to enjoy healthier substitutes, including low-fat goat or soy cheeses. You can do the same—if cookies are your biggest weakness and the quickest way to fall off the diet wagon, don't buy them. You can't eat what's not in your cupboards. Find smarter alternatives, such as treats sweetened with dried fruit or unsweetened applesauce, for special occasions or to satisfy a relentless craving.

3 SHOP THE PERIMETER OF THE STORE. The good stuff—fruits, veggies, lean proteins and dairy—always line the outer edges of the store. When you veer into the center aisles, you enter the temptation zone, where the unhealthy snack and packaged foods live.

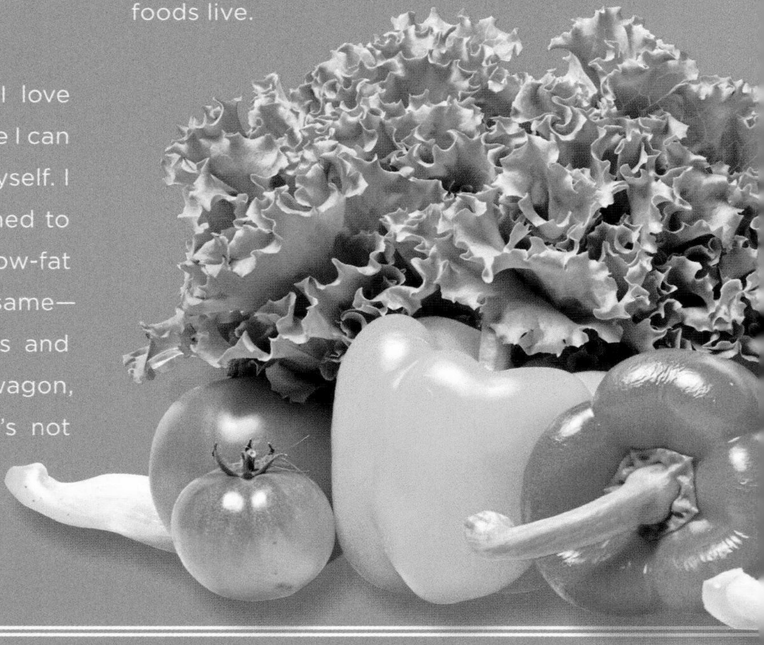

4 USE THE RAINBOW RULE WHEN BUYING PRODUCE. Your produce drawers should be filled with every color of fruits and vegetables under the sun. The greater the variety, the more vitamins and other nutrients you add to your diet. Incorporating different tastes will keep your meals interesting and flavorful so you stick with the program. Who knows? You might even learn to enjoy something new and exotic, such as mangosteens or durians.

5 FILL YOUR FRIDGE WITH HEALTHY OPTIONS. The easiest way to break your diet is to have nothing on hand when hunger strikes. A kitchen stocked with quick and easy options, however, can make sure you stay the course. My favorite "fast foods"? A whole-grain wrap with 1 tablespoon of nut butter, vegetables with hummus or salsa, fresh berries and low-fat plain yogurt. If those take too long, grab an apple along with a handful of unsalted nuts.

6 PREPARE LEFTOVERS WHENEVER YOU CAN. I love leftovers and so does my family. I grill as many as six chicken breasts at a time or a whole turkey breast, then divide it into meals. Whole grains, such as rice or oatmeal, can last as long as a week in the refrigerator. For example, I cook a lot of brown rice at the beginning of the week, and I have enough to last for a few days. Try it—you'll see how easy it'll make your life. Another strategy is creating "planned left-overs," which means to prepare extra servings of your meals so you have additional options on hand to eat over the next few days.

7 EAT MORE SOUP. Healthful soups can be a great comfort food. They're the perfect way to add extra vegetables to your diet, and it's easy to make a big pot and freeze portions for the coming weeks. When the weather gets colder I make a big pot of soup from scratch on Sunday so my family has soup on hand every day of the week. Does this sound like the perfect fast food? I think so!

TAILORED NUTRITION GUIDELINES FOR EVERY AGE

WHILE THE PRINCIPLES OF THIS EATING PLAN WON'T CHANGE MUCH, the following sections discuss how your nutritional needs differ in your thirties, forties, fifties and beyond and how to incorporate sound food habits into your daily life in order to achieve your Best Body Now at any—and every—age.

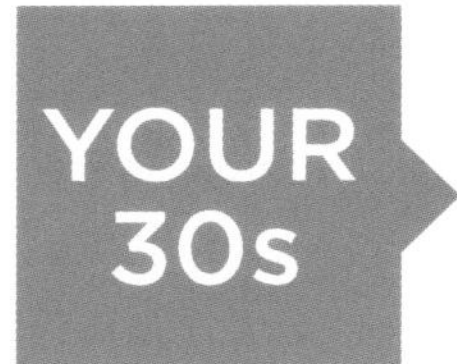

Start Disease-Fighting, Life-Enhancing, Healthy Habits

In my thirties, I didn't think a lot about what I ate or consider what effect certain foods would have on my body. I knew that I didn't want to be overweight and that overeating wasn't healthy, but that was the extent of my nutritional knowledge—that, and eat your vegetables. Our family meals contained plenty of natural ingredients, but there were times I served chicken nuggets not knowing what was in them, conventional peanut butter not thinking about its obscene sugar content, and baked goods with rancid butter, sugar and refined flour. And yes, we even ate hot dogs, something we only do now if they're made from natural ingredients.

My overall lack of nutritional knowledge was compounded by terrible habits, including:
Hefty portion sizes at home and when dining out
Eating junk
Eating sweets, cheese, peanut butter and other foods for emotional comfort
Constant snacking—huge hunks of cheese, spoonfuls of peanut butter straight from the jar
Late-night eating, including sitting in front of the TV mindlessly eating quarts of ice cream while everyone else was in bed
Disregard for unhealthy ingredients, such as sugar and sodium, which do nothing positive for my body
Cleaning my plate, especially when dining out, regardless of whether I was full or not
A lack of regard for whether or not I was eating enough fiber daily

The result? Weight gain. To compensate for the pounds I gained, I simply reduced calories or avoided entire food groups, which turned out to be a terrible strategy. Yo-yo dieting wreaked havoc on my skin, body and metabolism. I looked older, lacked energy, and ultimately developed hypoglycemia, which left me feeling weak, tired and clammy. It was after I learned what was happening to my body, both naturally and as a result of my behavior, that I was able to apply smart solutions that set me on the right track for life.

YOUR 30s — What's Happening in Your 30s That Impacts Your Nutrition Needs

- Significant life changes can heighten anxiety levels. Some of the most stressful of these include marriage, divorce, pregnancy, motherhood, raising young children, job relocations, career advancement and more, which can trigger an overpowering desire to eat food for comfort or stress release. I leaned heavily on indulging in comfort foods in my twenties and thirties, which led to my skewed relationship with food.

- A hectic, fast-paced lifestyle can make you turn to fast-food diets and unhealthy snacking simply because they seem like the quickest and easiest way to keep hunger at bay. Healthy foods, however, can be just as portable, and they help fuel your body with the energy it needs to manage your busy life.

- High-stress work schedules leave you little time to plan what to eat for lunch, so you become dependent on take-out, the communal candy jar or the office vending machine—whatever you can shove into your mouth while still working at your desk or running between meetings.

- When your life becomes incredibly busy, family, friends and obligations take priority, and exercise is usually the first item to fall off the to-do list. Working out, however, is the perfect way to give you natural energy to fight cravings and to rev up your metabolism to burn fat. And don't forget that a sweat-inducing workout can also be your saving grace emotionally and mentally. The gym was my salvation when I was going through the worst time in my life. It can do the same for you.

- More items on the to-do list also mean fewer hours available for sleep each night. Numerous studies show that sleep deprivation elevates your cravings for simple sugars, such as those found in candy, cookies and other vending machine options, as the body struggles to achieve an energy boost. Research out of the University of Chicago offers one explanation for this: lack of sleep actually increases the levels of hormones that make you feel hungry and decreases those that make you feel satiated, which can cause you to snack or overeat.

PLAN FOR BEST BODY NOW SUCCESS

ONE OF THE EASIEST WAYS TO MAKE healthy nutritional habits stick is to plan ahead. Here's how I do it:

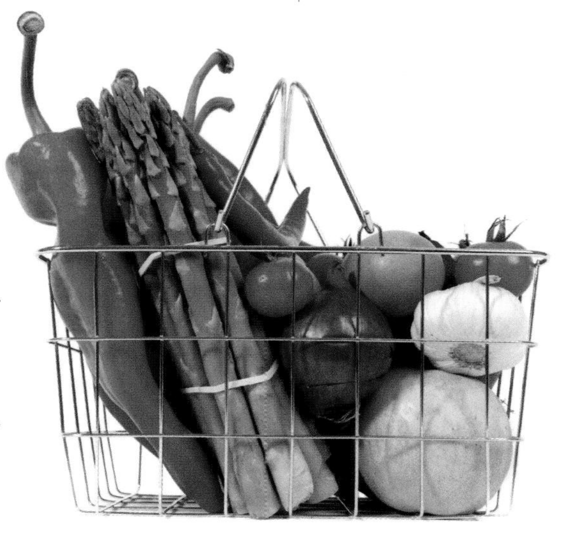

PLAN YOUR GROCERY LIST. Before going to the store, I make sure my kitchen is stocked with the items in the Best Body Now Checklist listed in this chapter—this ensures I can make healthy meals at any time. Next, I check my calendar while making a shopping list and plan my meals according to where I'll be and what I'm doing. For example, if I know I'll be driving kids to and from activities all weekend, I'll buy foods I can pack in the cooler or eat easily while on the go, such as wraps.

STOCK UP ON HEALTHY FAVORITES. My kitchen always has easy-to-prepare, smart nutritional choices, so even when I'm in a hurry I don't have to compromise my health. If you enjoy a crunch, choose almonds, soy chips and fresh-cut vegetables such as broccoli, carrots or cauliflower, and for a sweet tooth, try fresh berries and yogurt. When healthy foods are on hand, you're less likely to reach for junk food. I often use my juicer to whip up a batch of freshly prepared fruit and vegetable juice so I can boost nutrient intake.

KEEP HEALTHY OPTIONS WHEREVER YOU'RE GOING TO BE. At the office, in your gym bag, in your car—have simple on-the-go choices that keep your metabolism burning when you're not at home. These include fruit, nuts, homemade trail mix or granola.

PACK A COOLER. If you're on the go, don't rely on restaurants, office cafeterias or vending machines for healthy options—you won't find them. I pack a cooler with mini meals every day so I'm never far from good nutrition. Chicken breasts with steamed vegetables, salads and smoothies are easy to pack and carry. You'll need a small, soft-sided portable cooler, ice packs, plastic bags, water bottles and sealable glass containers to stick with the Best Body Now program no matter how hectic your schedule.

HAVE COOLER ITEMS READY THE NIGHT BEFORE. Even though I pack a fresh cooler each morning, I double-check that I have everything I need on hand the night before. My favorite easy-to pack foods include raw vegetables (cucumbers, carrots, green beans, radishes), cooked sweet potatoes, cooked oatmeal, applesauce, hard-boiled eggs, low-fat yogurt, cottage cheese and unsalted nuts.

A typical cooler pack for the day might include:

- ☐ Oatmeal with 1 cup nonfat milk or 1 cup rice, soy, almond or goat's milk
- ☐ Five 5-ounce servings of protein (chicken breast, canned tuna, egg whites, turkey)
- ☐ Four 1-cup servings of complex carbohydrates (apples, berries, mangoes)
- ☐ Five 1 ½ cup servings of raw vegetables
- ☐ 1 cup cooked brown rice
- ☐ 2 whole-grain wraps
- ☐ 1 piece whole-grain toast, dry
- ☐ ½ cup applesauce (to spread on toast)
- ☐ Steamed vegetables
- ☐ ½ cup unsalted nuts
- ☐ 2 tablespoons nut butter (to eat with fruit)

Even though you may feel like your body is strong and healthy, bone tissue begins to naturally become less dense in your thirties, and poor diet and lack of exercise can exacerbate the problem. This process will continue to speed up through your forties to the point where you're losing more bone cells than you're gaining. Loss of bone density can ultimately lead to osteoporosis and fractures. Fortunately, a nutritious diet can provide your body with nutrients, especially magnesium, that can stop and even reverse bone loss. One of the quickest ways to jump-start bone health is to stop eating sugar and processed foods—start *today*!

Many women in their thirties are dealing with health issues such as premenstrual syndrome (PMS) and high blood pressure, which can be prevented or lessened by eating nutritious, vitamin-rich foods that strengthen your immune system and help your body function better. For example, most women are only getting about half—600 mg—of their daily calcium needs from food. Studies show, however, that calcium deficiency is now being linked to PMS, high blood pressure and colon cancer.

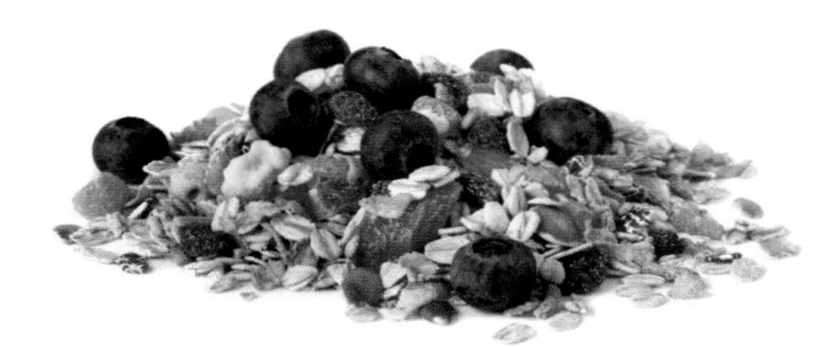

THE FIX? New Food Strategies for Your 30s:

1 PAIR PROTEIN AND COMPLEX CARBOHYDRATES AT EACH MEAL. Even if you're just eating a quick complex-carb snack, such as a banana or apple, remember to add protein, too, such as raw unsalted almonds or almond butter and unsweetened plain yogurt. You'll stabilize blood sugars, which means you avoid the carbohydrate crash that causes a slump in energy, curb cravings between meals and discourage overeating. Protein also aids in muscle repair post-workout, as well as general tissue repair.

2 BAN UNHEALTHY SNACKS. Foods such as candy, chips, cookies and ice cream that seem comforting or convenient in the moment will make you feel worse later. Seek other options to satisfy emotional eating, including apples for a sweet tooth, all-natural soy chips for crunch or avocado for a creamy texture. Keep Best Body Now options on hand, whether in your purse, at your desk or in the pantry, and the anti-foods out of the house. Even if your kids want it, they don't need the junk any more than you do.

3 EAT AWAY AT STRESS, RATHER THAN LETTING STRESS EAT AWAY AT YOU. Did you know that the vitamins and minerals found in healthy foods relieve stress naturally, just as they would help you fight a cold or boost your energy levels? For example, citrus fruits contain vitamin C, which studies published in *Pharmacology* and other scientific journals have shown reduces stress hormones, chemicals released by the brain in response to anxiety, and blood pressure at intakes of 3,000 mg a day. Omega-3 fatty acids, healthy fats found in flaxseed, fish, olive and walnut oils and nuts are linked to low cholesterol and better brain function. They also help regulate levels of cortisol, a hormone produced by the adrenal glands in response to stressful situations (cortisol is responsible for the fight-or-flight response). The prepackaged, processed foods found in vending machines, the frozen food section or the center grocery store aisles may make you feel better for the moment, but then your mood, energy levels and metabolism crash a few hours later, along with your blood sugar levels.

The vitamins and minerals found in healthy foods relieve stress naturally.

4 **LEARN TO PLAN *AND PREPARE* MEALS IN ADVANCE.** It might seem overwhelming at first to know that cooking healthy meals and having a kitchen stocked with fresh produce is essential to the Best Body Now eating plan. But it's actually easy when you plan your menus and prepare food for the week ahead of time. Planning ensures you can eat protein-carb combos and fresh produce six times a day, even when sitting in your office or driving the kids to soccer. Planning ahead also keeps you reaching for Best Body Now foods rather than something from a vending machine or the nearest drive-through. Even though it may take a bit more time to plan, you will save time in the long run, since you won't have to make any last-minute shopping trips or stress about meals. There is a great sense of comfort in knowing what you are going to eat and that it already exists in your kitchen.

5 **AVOID ALCOHOL AND CAFFEINE.** When you're overscheduled and overcommitted, you may reach for alcohol to calm your nerves or coffee to raise your energy levels. Unfortunately, these quick-fix energy boosters can interrupt your sleep cycle, causing you to gravitate toward unhealthy snacks the next day to battle residual fatigue from the night before. Alcohol also contains huge amounts of sugar and wasted calories, which detract from health and vitality. Coffee has many health benefits, so have a cup in the morning, but limit your intake in the afternoons, when consuming caffeine may keep you up at night. Instead of my midafternoon or postdinner coffee, I love hot herbal tea or hot water with lemon. Remember also that a cup of black coffee is very different from a caramel macchiato with whipped cream and sugar!

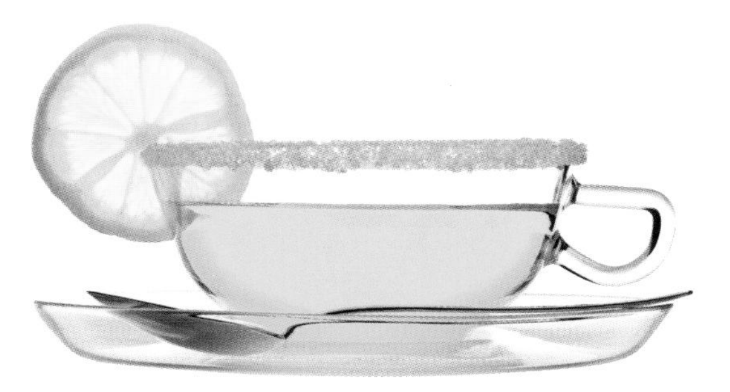

6 **GET SEVEN TO EIGHT HOURS OF SLEEP EACH NIGHT.** It may sound impossible to achieve, but countless studies show that getting enough sleep prevents you from reaching for empty carbohydrates to fuel your body. One study published in the *Annals of Internal Medicine* showed that getting less sleep caused people to feel hungrier and have a bigger appetite. That's because lack of sleep may cause fluctuations in the hormones that regulate your hunger. Refer to Chapter 6 for strategies to help you sleep better.

7 STEER CLEAR OF CANS AND BOXES. Convenience foods may be easier on your schedule, but they're almost always harder on your health and your wallet. For instance, the U.S. Food and Drug Administration (FDA) says the canning process reduces nutrient content by half for many antioxidants, including vitamins A and C and cell-strengthening riboflavin and thiamin, which helps turn blood sugar into energy. For each year a can of food is stored, nutrient levels can drop by as much as 20 percent. Many canned goods also contain preservatives, additives and artificial colorings and flavors—unwanted extras. Fresh and frozen fruits and veggies can be just as readily prepared without sacrificing nutrition. Because many diseases have a lead time of ten to twenty years, starting good habits now, even if it costs you a bit of extra time in the kitchen, will pay off in years added to your life.

8 INCREASE YOUR NATURAL SOURCES OF CALCIUM. Eating leafy greens, avocado, broccoli, soybeans, quinoa and other calcium-rich foods is one of the best ways to protect your heart from cardiovascular disease. A Boston University study showed that just eating from 300 to 1,110 mg of calcium a day cuts your risk of developing high blood pressure by 20 percent. Add leafy greens to your wraps or steam them with your favorite fatty fish for dinner. Avocados are a delicious addition to egg-white omelets and fresh salads because they deliver creaminess while providing an excellent source of natural calcium and flavor in this otherwise ordinary dish. A quick calcium fix I often use is to chop loads of fresh kale into a hearty soup.

9 DON'T FORGET YOUR MAGNESIUM. Many of us have never heard of magnesium or realized how extremely important it is in preventing disease and maintaining good health—I certainly didn't before I began Eating Clean. Research indicates as many as 90 percent of Americans aren't getting enough of this off-the-radar nutrient in their diets. However, more and more studies are showing it plays a significant role in numerous bodily functions, including relieving symptoms of PMS, building and maintaining strong bones, warding off cardiovascular disease, reducing the risk of colon cancer and alleviating stress. Studies also show that magnesium has relaxing effects—I often have a calcium/magnesium supplement at night so I can sleep better. Even though we might not think of magnesium often, the good news is you can easily get the Recommended Daily Allowance (RDA) of 320 mg by eating leafy greens, nuts, seeds and legumes, foods essential to your Best Body Now diet. For more on magnesium, see Chapter 6.

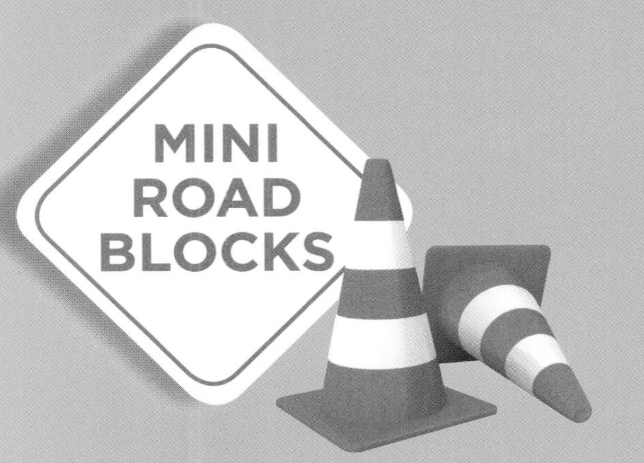

Over my years as a magazine columnist, I've had thousands of readers ask me what to do about issues such as curbing sugar cravings or eating healthy while on the go. Here are the top five obstacles you might be facing and proven tips for eliminating them. It's easier than you think.

1 I HAVE AN INSATIABLE SWEET TOOTH.

THE BEST BODY NOW FIX: Believe it or not, sugar cravings are not inevitable. Once you switch out processed sugars with healthier alternatives, your cravings subside. An easy way to start is to substitute fruits for candy, chocolates and cookies. It's easier than you think. Peaches, mangoes and bananas add amazing flavor to cereals and are much healthier than a donut or pastry. Or instead of a midday run to the vending machine, spread a tablespoon of nut butter over an apple or top low-fat plain yogurt with your favorite berries. Be patient—you'll need a few days to rid your body of its desire for sugar.

2 MY FAMILY IS ADDICTED TO JUNK FOOD.

THE BEST BODY NOW FIX: It's time for you to set an example for your family. I often give seminars at schools and find that kids get enthusiastic and excited about learning to eat well, especially once they see the benefits in their energy levels and brain power. Healthy foods don't have to taste like cardboard and can often look like the foods you already make. Vegetable-based spaghetti sauces with whole-wheat pasta can taste like standard versions made with ground meat and white pasta, but are much healthier.

3 WHO HAS TIME TO PREPARE HEALTHY FOOD?

THE BEST BODY NOW FIX: No one wants to be a slave to the kitchen, even if it means having a fabulous body. Make the most of your meal prep time by cooking several meals at once and dividing them into containers for the next few days or freezing them for easy options in the future. Many whole grains stay fresh for a week once cooked, so it makes good sense to depend on these for side dishes and lunches. Lunch foods such as wraps and pita sandwiches can be prepared in a flash if your kitchen is properly stocked (see "Tosca's Kitchen Makeover," page 60). Also, rely on fruits and vegetables as your new healthy "fast foods." Dip them in hummus or nut butters—it only takes a second. ▶

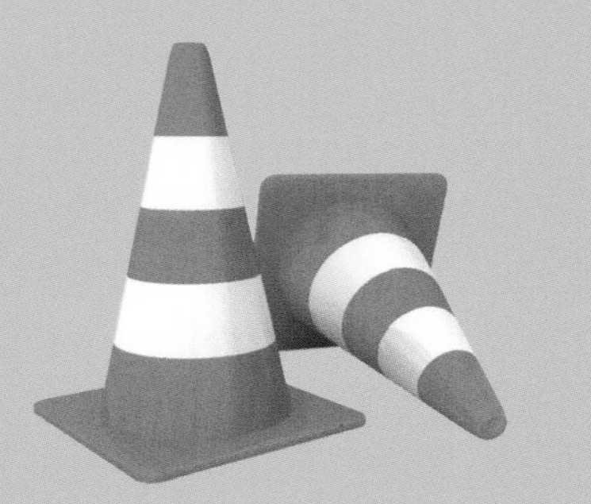

4 MY JOB REQUIRES THAT I EAT OUT A LOT.

THE BEST BODY NOW FIX: No matter where you're dining, from a gourmet restaurant to the corner take-out joint, you can eat smart. Set limitations; for example, I never eat bread, reserve desserts for celebrations and only occasionally drink wine. If you love one of these, consume it in moderation. If you have a goal of losing a certain amount of weight, then have that in your mind before you begin the meal. Keeping your goals firmly in front of you reminds you not to go crazy at the dinner table. When it comes to wine, I enjoy half a glass or a small taste shared with friends, which still allows me to enjoy but not overindulge. The key is to be faithful to the spirit of "just a taste" and not to use it as an excuse to fall off the wagon. Every sip and bite really does matter.

Next, befriend the server. With an advocate, it's easier to make sure your needs are met. Tell him how you'd like your meal prepared: no sauces, gravies, fats, oils or butter. If you're unclear on how something is prepared, ask. Don't assume it's healthy. Likely it's not. Get lean meats grilled or broiled. Appetizers are typically fat and calorie minefields. Opt for a salad if options are limited. Finally, if the portion sizes are massive, ask for a doggie bag when you order, or have a healthy appetizer as your entrée.

5 I'M NOT BIG ON BREAKFAST.

THE BEST BODY NOW FIX: For some people, breakfast is an acquired taste, especially when you don't have a lot of time. Make morning meals a no-brainer by having fast, easy options at your fingertips: drinkable low-fat yogurt with muesli, Ezekiel bread with nut butter, hardboiled egg whites with dry brown toast, oatmeal with two scoops of protein powder and berries, whole-grain cereal with low-fat soy milk and banana. If you're simply not hungry, start with a small protein smoothie with fruit just to get your metabolism fueled. Studies repeatedly show breakfast eaters to be slimmer than their non-breakfast-eating counterparts.

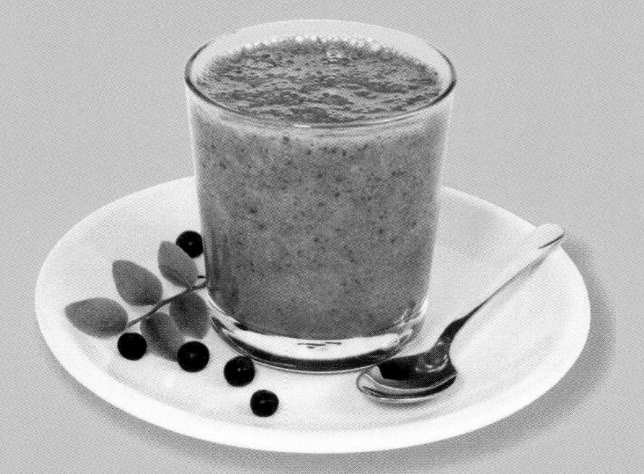

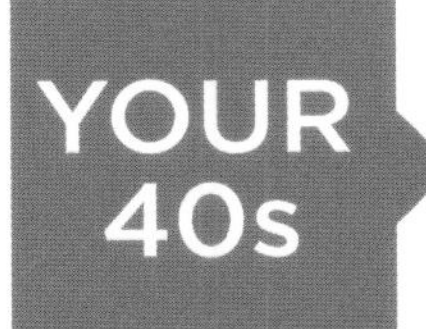

Protect Against So-Called Inevitable Health Issues

By the time I reached my forties, I was just beginning to embrace my new way of eating, yet seeing amazing changes in how I felt and looked. I realized my new plan was allowing me to combat and even offset much of what people think is the natural and inevitable aging process. Most doctors agree that many of the diseases we think are simply part of growing old are actually a result of your nutrition choices and thus are completely preventable or treatable, if not reversible. I discovered this miracle firsthand myself. Once I learned to make smarter decisions about how I fueled my body with high-quality food, the age-proofing began.

YOUR 40s

What's Happening in Your 40s That Impacts Your Nutrition Needs

Hormones are powerful substances in your body that control virtually all of your bodily functions, including regulating certain cells, organs and sexual functions. As early as your thirtieth birthday, you begin producing less and less of these vital hormones. For instance, estrogen and progesterone, the sex hormones produced by the ovaries, are responsible for developing and maintaining sexual characteristics and processes, including menstruation and pregnancy. Every year, you produce slightly less estrogen and progesterone, until you reach your forties and suddenly become aware of the effects of this slow tapering off. This time period is often referred to as "perimenopause." Hormone changes related to this stage of life are typically associated with hot flashes, night sweats, irritability, irregular periods and weight gain and mark the transition to actual menopause, the point at around age fifty when you haven't had a period for an entire year.

Heart disease risk and stroke risk in women increase with age. In fact, the American Heart Association reports that one woman dies from heart disease every two minutes in this country. Major risk factors include high cholesterol, diabetes, being overweight and excessive alcohol intake, all of which can be controlled or lessened through what we eat. Under age fifty, heart attacks are twice as likely to be fatal in women as in men.

Cancer risk increases with age. The average onset of the five most prevalent types of cancer in women—breast, lung, colorectal, uterine and ovarian—is in the forties. These diseases are all linked to high-fat diets and obesity, as well as other poor lifestyle habits, such as lack of exercise and high stress levels.

Aging can begin impacting your brain function as early as age forty, affecting such cognitive skills as memory, learning ability and attention span, according to a study published in *Nature* by researchers from Harvard and the Children's Hospital Boston.

▶ Because your metabolism begins slowing in your thirties at a shocking rate of about 2 to 5 percent every ten years, you consequently burn between 50 to 100 fewer calories a day. By the time you reach your forties, you're losing up to 8 percent of your muscle mass every decade. If you aren't proactive about this, weight gain is the natural outcome.

▶ While bone density begins to decrease in your thirties, it begins happening much more quickly in your forties, to the point where you lose more bone cells than you create. This suggests that you need to ensure you're getting a diet rich in natural sources of calcium—1,000 mg in your forties—and vitamin D, which helps maintain calcium and phosphorous levels in your bones so they stay strong. Certain elements of the average North American diet exacerbate bone loss, the most significant of which include overconsumption of sugar and refined foods as well as foods doused in chemicals. Be proactive by avoiding sugar and processed foods, both of which contribute to weakened bones.

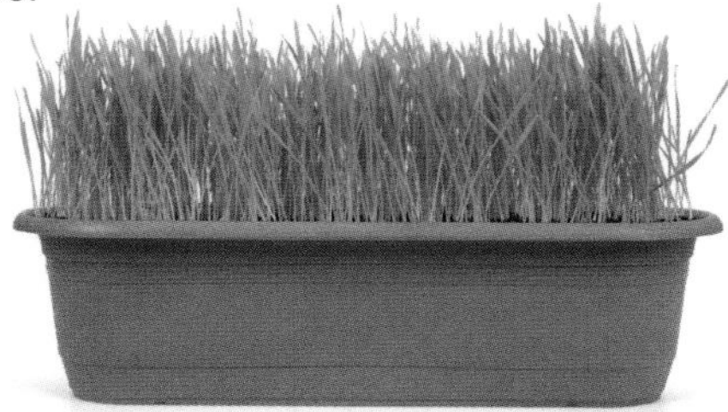

THE FIX? New Food Strategies for Your 40s:

1 IDENTIFY FOODS THAT CAUSE YOU TO GAIN WEIGHT AND ELIMINATE THEM. I don't eat bread, for example, particularly nutrient-void white varieties, because bread puts weight on me immediately. For me, eating as little as one slice of white bread will cause my belly to bloat and go into distress within an hour. While this food is a culprit for many women, many other kinds of foods can be your personal nemeses. By the time you are forty, you are more cognizant of which foods cause you to bloat or induce weight gain. I know I am not the only one when it comes to bread!

2 ADD A DAILY SHOT OF CANCER-FIGHTING WHEATGRASS TO YOUR DIET. Wheatgrass is a highly nutrient-dense type of young cereal grass that is often freshly juiced for its health benefits—I try to drink one glass of wheatgrass juice a day. You can buy the freshly juiced shots at health food stores or juice your own fresh wheatgrass at home. Studies show its nutrients, such as cell-strengthening folic acid (a type of B vitamin) and abundant chlorophyll, may boost energy, strengthen immunity and kill bacteria. Certain cancers, many with an average onset in your forties, shrink in the presence of this powerful health-boosting drink. For example, a study published in *Nutrition and Cancer* showed that breast cancer patients who drank wheatgrass juice had higher red and white blood cell counts, which lessened their need for immunity-boosting medications. Another important benefit of drinking wheatgrass juice and consuming plenty of greens is that this helps reduce acidity in the body and keep the pH neutral, which is the body's disease-free state. Try blending it with kale for additional antioxidants or into a smoothie at breakfast.

> Eating plant-based foods has a significant impact on the environment by reducing your carbon footprint.

3 START THE DAY WITH A GLASS OF HOT WATER MIXED WITH THE JUICE OF ONE LEMON—OR ANY FRUIT FILLED WITH VITAMIN C—TO DETOXIFY THE LIVER. In many Asian cultures starting the day with a glass of hot water and a shot of fresh lemon juice is the ultimate tonic. Taking a page from our Asian sisters, I have found that this refreshing beverage prevents me from drinking too much coffee while it helps me cleanse my liver. It doesn't hurt to help this workhorse organ because the liver performs all of the body's detoxifying tasks and some of its cleansing duties. When I don't know what to drink, I always juice a lemon and mix it with a cup of hot water.

4 BALANCE YOUR DIET WITH MORE PLANT-BASED PROTEIN SOURCES, INCLUDING SOY, LENTILS, LEGUMES, ALMONDS AND QUINOA, RATHER THAN STRICTLY MEAT. By embracing these plant-based proteins you will increase your vitamin and mineral intake, keep cholesterol levels down and reduce unhealthy saturated fat levels (fats that come from animal sources and are linked to high cholesterol). These factors can help offset the risk of heart disease as well as other conditions related to high cholesterol that naturally occur in your forties. Plus if you are keen on being "green," eating plant-based foods has a significant impact on the environment by reducing your carbon footprint.

5 GET YOUR DISEASE-FIGHTING FIBER REGULARLY. If you're on the Best Body Now eating plan, you are probably getting enough fiber from the multitude of fibrous foods recommended, including beans, oats, barley and citrus fruits, that form the backbone of this complex-carb-embracing eating plan. And that's a good thing for your health. Studies have shown that fiber-rich diets may protect against breast, ovarian and uterine cancers, all of which become risks in our forties, as well as diabetes, heart disease and kidney stones. For instance, the famous Nurses' Health Study, published in the *American Journal of Clinical*

Nutrition, shows that women who consume 25 grams or more of fiber daily reduced their risk of heart attack by 40 percent.

6 CONTINUE EATING A HEART-HEALTHY DIET RICH IN NATURAL SOURCES OF CALCIUM. Cardiovascular disease risk heightens in your forties, but you can lessen that risk through smart nutrition. By eating plenty of natural foods rich in calcium you not only protect your heart but also help your body stay lean. One study from the University of Tennessee showed that participants who consumed higher levels of calcium-containing foods lost an average of 11 pounds in a year. Natural sources include leafy greens (broccoli, spinach, bok choy, Swiss chard, collard greens and kale), nuts, sesame seeds, quinoa and calcium-fortified soy products (such as tofu, soy milks and soy cheeses). Try to eat 1,200 mg of calcium a day for maximum cardiovascular protection. It's more fun and tastier than you might imagine.

7 ADD HALIBUT TO YOUR MEAL PLAN FOR ADDITIONAL HEART HEALTH. Another incredible nutrient for heart protection is omega-3 fatty acids, found in fish such as halibut, Arctic char, salmon, tilapia and albacore tuna. For example, *Prevention* magazine reports that a 5-ounce serving of halibut contains your entire day's needs of heart-healthy omega-3 fatty acids, more per serving than other fish such as tilapia, to combat heart disease risk and high cholesterol. Fatty acids are also shown to reduce the decline of brain function associated with aging that starts as early as our forties, according to a Rush University study. Add at least one serving into your meal rotation each week to round out a nutritious diet designed for good heart health.

8 INCREASE YOUR INTAKE OF MAGNESIUM FOR MOOD AND HEART PROTECTION. For incredible mind and body benefits, try increasing your magnesium intake to 400–500 mg a day, just above the FDA recommendation. In a study published in the *American Journal of Cardiology*, researchers found that women who supplemented with 400 mg daily experienced an anticlogging effect on arteries and also exhibited a lowered risk of coronary heart disease. And a study published in the *Journal of Pediatric Gastroenterology and Nutrition* from researchers out of Tokyo's Showa University showed the mineral reduced cholesterol by as much as 20 percent. Other studies link the nutrient to a reduction in rates of depression and to stabilization in hormone levels. My favorite option: a handful of raw, unsalted pumpkin seeds. That amount contains 200 mg of magnesium and fits easily into my gym bag, car or purse.

9 ADD A HANDFUL OF NUTS TO REDUCE DIABETES RISK.

To combat a heightened risk of diabetes—a condition caused by high blood sugar levels—in our forties, add a serving of peanuts or natural peanut butter as one of your small snacks. A recent study from the Harvard School of Public Health shows that women who eat five servings a week decreased their risk of type 2 diabetes by 27 percent, thanks to the healthy fats and protein found in this delicious food.

> Eating fruits and vegetables is one of the smartest ways to keep your brain functioning at its best.

10 INCORPORATE MEMORY BOOSTERS TO IMPROVE BRAIN FUNCTION.

Eating fruits and vegetables is one of the smartest ways to keep your brain functioning at its best. A Harvard study showed eating more vegetables may slow the decline in brain function normally seen in aging, while other studies, such as one published in *Pharmacology*, have shown that essential brain-boosting nutrients found in certain produce, such as quercetin and anthocyanin, may reverse memory loss. These memory-enhancing foods happen to also be the powerhouses of my Best Body Now eating plan. They are found in:

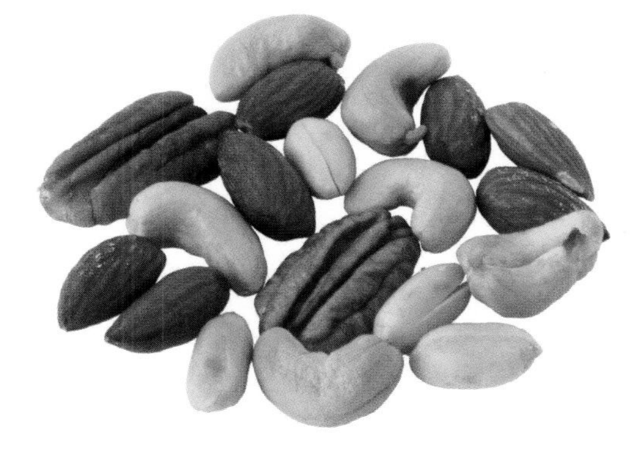

- Cruciferous vegetables (brussels sprouts, broccoli and cabbages)
- Leafy greens (kale, spinach and Swiss chard)
- Brightly colored produce (berries, red apples, eggplants and grapes)
- Onions, apricots, leeks and more

Many of these healthy foods, along with lentils, soybeans and fortified whole-grain cereals, also boast high levels of folic acid, which research has shown is directly linked to memory gains.

11 EAT MORE PUMPKIN FOR ALL-AROUND HEALTH.

This vegetable and its seeds contain significant amounts of antioxidants along with zinc, potassium and fiber. These nutrients have been shown to reduce hypertension, strengthen the immune system, prevent cancer and boost bone health. Incorporating them into your diet can be easy. I roast pumpkin with a medley of other vegetables as a side dish or add it to salads.

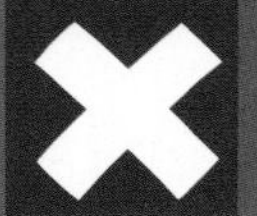

THE WORST NUTRITION HABITS

Some nutrition habits are unhealthy, and some are just awful. I've listed five of the worst foods you can put in your mouth, as well as easy ways to eliminate them from your current eating habits.

1 DIET SODA. Research tells us that diet soda isn't so diet-friendly after all. For example, a study in *Behavioral Neuroscience* has found that the artificial sweeteners in diet drinks can trigger overeating and cause you to crave even more sugary treats, as well as contribute to bone weakness. Flavor water with naturally sweet fruit slices (try oranges, limes or lemons) instead. If you don't enjoy sweet flavors, try cucumber and celery in your water.

2 COFFEE WITH "EXTRAS." Would you start your day with a caramel pie? Probably not, but if you enjoy flavored coffee shop extras, you may be consuming the nutritional equivalent of such a fattening dessert each and every morning. Aim to drink your coffee black. If you absolutely can't drink it black, a touch of skim milk is fine. Little extras, from cream to sugar to flavorings, can turn your morning coffee into a full-fledged high-calorie dessert and a Best Body Now sabotage.

3 PROCESSED OR DELI MEATS. Think processed or deli meats are an ideal source of protein? Think again. You're actually consuming a cocktail of chemicals including nitrates, other preservatives, sugars and sodium, all of which have been linked to diseases including cancer. It's better to roast a few extra chicken or turkey breasts and slice them up to enjoy between slices of hearty bread or in a wrap. And it's usually cheaper as well.

4 FRUIT JUICES AND FRUIT DRINKS. You may have been brought up to believe that orange, grapefruit or other juices are a healthy way to start the day. But consider this: drinking fruit juice—fruit without the important nutritional component of fiber—is the equivalent of dipping your spoon into a bag of sugar. One 12-ounce glass of orange juice contains a whopping 36 grams of sugar, which will send your blood sugar levels soaring, only to crash soon after. And what are labeled "fruit drinks" often have no real juice whatsoever, which means you may be drinking nothing more than sweetened, chemically altered water. If you want to enjoy the taste of fruit, eat a piece of in-season fresh fruit. If you're thirsty, have water. Or you can juice fruits and vegetables together to get the most of these important foods. When you juice the fruits yourself, you won't drink any added sugars or preservatives.

5 SUGARY BREAKFAST CEREALS. Navigating the cereal aisle can result in sensory overload—and you have to be a scientist to understand the nutrition labels. Know the other names for sugar—glucose, corn syrup, fructose, dextrose, sucrose, molasses, honey, artificial sweeteners, maltose and maple syrup—and look for them on labels. Switch to healthier options such as Kashi, shredded wheat, muesli, Ezekiel, Weetabix and All-Bran, as well as hot cereal products.

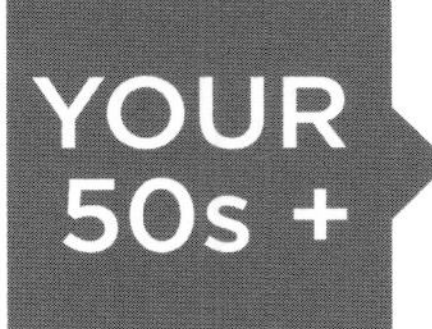

Strengthen Your Immune System

My nutritional approach for fifty is fundamentally similar to what I did in my forties. With a heightened awareness of how taking good care of myself nutritionally and physically rewards me with a lean physique and robust health, I continue to build on this proven platform. A healthier new mind-set toward eating combined with a diet abundant in unprocessed foods forms the backbone of my approach to handling my health and fitness in my fifties. I did incorporate several tweaks to deal with the natural and so-called natural changes happening to my body as it ages. The key is listening to my physiological signals about what needs to be different and discussing solutions with my doctor to get her okay before embarking on any changes.

YOUR 50s +

What's Happening in Your 50s That Impacts Your Nutrition Needs

- As you age, your metabolism naturally slows down due to both aging and lifestyle, making it more challenging to keep weight off, even if your nutrition is tip-top. By age sixty-five you have lost up to one-third of your muscle mass thanks to gradual declines in metabolic efficiency of 3 to 6 percent each decade.

- Drinking water becomes even more important as we get older. New research published in *Proceedings of the National Academy of Sciences* shows that as you age, you become more prone to dehydration for a variety of reasons, the most significant of these being that there is an increasing inability to recognize when we're thirsty. It also takes longer to understand that we require hydration, and the urgency to quench thirst drops in intensity. A more sedentary lifestyle also contributes to dehydration. This is why Your Best Body Now schedules water drinking into the program so there is never any doubt about how much and when to drink it.

- Hypertension, or high blood pressure, becomes an even more critical issue. Your body undergoes a steady increase in blood pressure with each advancing decade; however, after age fifty, blood pressure tends to rise even more steadily due to menopause. Although changing hormones are believed to be the cause, hypertension can be controlled and possibly prevented through eating foods rich in vitamins, antioxidants and other nutrients.

- Type 2 diabetes becomes more prevalent in your fifties. Your risk for developing type 2 diabetes increases as the body loses its ability to use glucose, a type of sugar found in the blood. This happens when your body becomes resistant to or doesn't produce enough insulin, the hormone responsible for regulating sugar in your cells, typically as a result of poor diet or lack of exercise.

- Heart health is more important than ever in your fifties. A Northwestern University study shows that your risk of cardiovascular disease increases by 50 percent if you reach fifty with two or more risk factors: high cholesterol, high blood pressure, obesity, being overweight, smoking or any disease that compromises your immune system or heart health.

- Doctors recommend screenings for colorectal cancer beginning at fifty for women, or earlier if you have a family history of the disease. The American Cancer Society reports that there is a strong connection between a low-fiber, high-fat diet and your risk for this particular type of cancer.

- Even if you think your memory is as sharp as it's ever been, now's the time to boost brain health with smart nutrition. Loss of brain function and the early start of dementia can occur by the fifth decade, with significant changes in memory, learning and attention span.

- Bone loss—caused by the depletion of minerals in bone tissue, which makes them weak and can lead to osteoporosis—continues. The National Osteoporosis Foundation reports that half of women over fifty will have at least one fracture from osteoporosis. Postmenopausal women are advised to adjust their calcium intake to 1,000 to 1,500 mg a day. After sixty-five, 1,500 mg daily is the recommendation. Not only is calcium deficiency the main cause of osteoporosis, but it's also believed to be linked to hypertension, high cholesterol and cancer. Once again, pay attention to your consumption of sugar and processed foods as these contribute to weakening bones.

THE FIX? New Food Strategies for Your 50s +:

1 STAY HYDRATED BY DRINKING TEN 8-OUNCE OR 250 ML GLASSES OF WATER A DAY. You'll see that water intake is programmed into the Best Body Now eating plan for all ages, but this is particularly important with advancing age and even more so if you're working out or live in a warmer climate. Why is hydration so critical? Water makes up about two-thirds of our body weight—muscles alone are 75 percent water. It regulates your appetite and your body temperature, keeps energy levels high, transports nutrients and flushes out wastes while ensuring that diminished thirst receptors—the parts of the brain that signal you to drink more—won't compromise your hydration.

2 WORK ALMONDS INTO YOUR DIET TO KEEP CHOLESTEROL DOWN. You may already know almonds are good for you, but you may not know they can be as effective as prescription medication in lowering cholesterol. Research has shown almonds can reduce unhealthy LDL cholesterol by nearly the same amount as doctor-prescribed, cholesterol-reducing statin meds. High cholesterol levels at age fifty increase risk for cardiovascular disease. Almond butter makes a quick snack when spread on a wrap and paired with a piece of fruit. My personal favorite is a whole-grain wrap spread with natural almond butter, sprinkled with ground flaxseed and then paired with a banana. Roll it up, eat and enjoy!

> Water regulates your appetite and your body temperature, keeps energy levels high, transports nutrients and flushes out wastes.

3 AVOID TABLE SALT TO REDUCE SODIUM INTAKE. Experts say women over fifty should cut sodium intake to 1,500 mg a day to help ward off heart disease. Instead, season foods with freshly ground spices or fresh herbs. They boost flavor without adding fat and may be linked to fighting certain health conditions, including cancer and heart disease. I've switched from regular table salt to sea salt—sea salt has eighty-two minerals and other elements, whereas table salt has just sodium chloride and a bit of sugar. You can also try Himalayan varieties because they're made from the purest, highest grade of natural salt, and help regulate and balance your body.

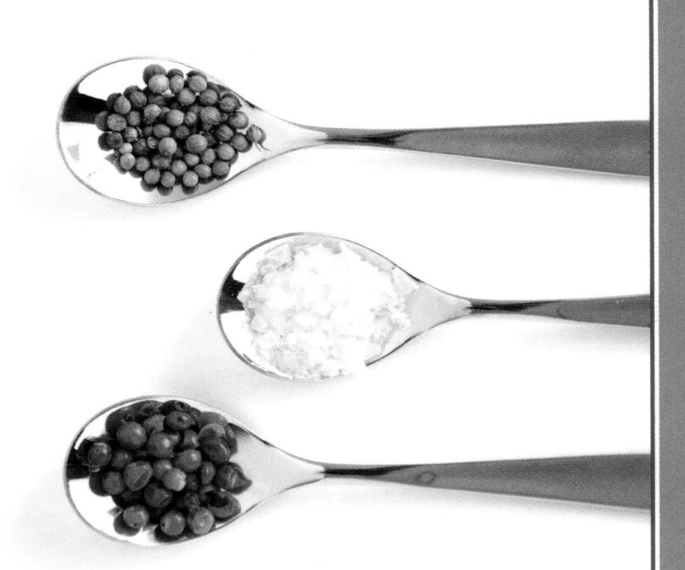

4 EAT MORE CANCER-FIGHTING PRODUCE. Combat the heightened risk of cancer in your fifties by eating a diet rich in leafy greens and cruciferous vegetables. In an eight-year study on colorectal cancer, people who ate large amounts of both types of vegetables significantly reduced their risk of this silent but deadly disease. For those already with the condition, cruciferous varieties such as brussels sprouts, broccoli and cabbage lessened the severity of the disease. A separate study published in *Gastroenterology* also showed that people who ate cruciferous vegetables cut their colorectal cancer risk almost in half. These vegetables are also filled with the disease-fighting antioxidant vitamin C, a nutrient said to improve your libido. Eat plenty of foods rich in vitamin C to boost your sex drive. One cup of steamed broccoli a day is your new green Viagra. (Definitely try this at home!)

5 SEASON FOOD WITH BRAIN BOOSTERS.

Even though experts say that memory typically declines in your fifties, it doesn't have to if you arm your body with the right nutrients. In addition to the memory-enhancing produce listed in the forties section, increase your daily servings of brain food by incorporating herbs and spices that are believed to elevate brain function, including turmeric, rosemary, sage, mint, ginger and black pepper. In fact, hormone specialist Dr. Uzzi Reiss, M.D., points to a UCLA study published in the *Journal of Alzheimer's Disease* that links Alzheimer's prevention to turmeric, a spice that contains 5 percent curcumin, a disease-fighting antioxidant. Study author Dr. Milan Fiala reported that half of patients saw an improvement in their immune cells' ability to clear out unhealthy amyloid plaques associated with the disease. Dr. Reiss also adds this healthy spice added to soups, stews, pilaf, sauces and more makes 2,500 genes work more efficiently and effectively. The key is cooking the spice rather than using it as a supplement. Study authors are looking into the potential disease-busting powers of ginger and rosemary because they have similar properties. Season creatively and you can improve your brain function at every meal.

Season creatively and you can improve your brain function at every meal.

6 SUPPLEMENT WITH FOODS THAT FIGHT DEPRESSION.

Healthy foods don't just fuel your body—they also can impact your mood and prevent or lessen depression caused by the changing hormone levels that occur with menopause. Be proactive by eating foods that contain magnesium, vitamins C and D and omega-3 fatty acids. These mood boosters trigger your brain's natural happiness regulators, the hormones known as serotonin and GABA. Bananas, brown rice, halibut, oranges, almonds, pumpkin, mangoes, oats, sunflower seeds, pumpkin seeds and grapefruit deliver these "happy nutrients."

7 INCREASE YOUR MAGNESIUM INTAKE FOR RELIEF OF MENOPAUSAL SYMPTOMS.

Post-menopausal women can find symptom relief by increasing their intake of this essential mineral and incredible nutrient to around 500 mg a day. In a study reported in the *Journal of the American Medical Association*, women in their fifties taking magnesium supplements were 60 percent less likely to develop colorectal cancer. This immunity booster has also been shown to lower blood pressure and cholesterol. In fact, several studies have shown that people who are magnesium deficient are twice as likely to develop coronary artery disease. Finally, in research published in the *Journal of the American Geriatrics Society*, high magnesium intake was shown to increase bone mass in older women and help prevent hip fractures. Pumpkin seeds are a valuable source of magnesium, with 150 mg per 1 ounce.

8 TAKE SOY FOR ADDITIONAL MENOPAUSE RELIEF. You may already know soybeans help you increase bone mass: 1 cup of soy milk contains 200 mg of calcium or 13 percent of your daily recommended intake from natural food sources. But studies, including one published in the *Journal of Endocrinological Investigation*, show it can also help reduce menopause symptoms, particularly hot flashes.

9 SUBSTITUTE IMMUNE-BOOSTING GREEN TEA FOR COFFEE. Studies show postmenopausal women who drink at least 3 cups of green tea a day experience numerous benefits including a robust immune system, and reduction in the risks of osteoporosis and breast cancer. For example, one study published in *Cancer Epidemiology Biomarkers and Prevention* found that green tea consumption reduced breast cancer risk by 37 percent. And research published in *Breast Cancer Research and Treatment* shows that consumption of green tea may also prevent breast cancer recurrence. Other studies have shown it contains the antioxidant power of red wine. I still love my morning cup of coffee, but I always drink at least three cups of green tea—a natural fat burner—every day.

10 EAT NATURAL APPETITE SUPPRESSANTS. It may be tougher to take off weight after menopause, but the Best Body Now eating plan makes it completely achievable. In addition to eliminating processed foods, add these dopamine-increasing natural appetite suppressants to your daily regimen: apples, spinach, unsalted almonds, egg whites and carrots.

11 ADD MORE HEART-HEALTHY, CALCIUM-RICH FOODS TO YOUR DIET. For maximum cardiovascular health, try to eat 1,500 mg of calcium a day from food sources. Nuts are one of the easiest snacks to pack, and a few types are filled with this cardio booster—particularly pecans (79 mg per ounce), Brazil nuts (45 mg per ounce) and almonds (70 mg per ounce). Studies, such as one published in the *British Medical Journal*, show that less than an ounce a day, about 5 ounces weekly, can reduce heart disease risk by 25 percent. I'll mix mine into a trail mix or muesli for variety. I also lean heavily on quinoa, a grain rich in easily absorbable calcium.

12 EAT OMEGA-3 FATTY ACIDS FOR ADDITIONAL CARDIOVASCULAR PROTECTION. In the years when your heart disease risk is likely to increase, lower your odds by eating good fats, such as those prevalent in fatty fish, fish oil, flaxseed, flaxseed oil, extra-virgin olive oil and soy products, including soybeans, tempeh, miso and tofu. The American Heart Association recommends at least two servings of mackerel, herrings, sardines, albacore tuna or lake trout each week for heart-healthy omega-3 fats.

13 INCREASE YOUR BERRY INTAKE. Berries are one of the most powerful foods you can add to your diet. They've got the highest levels of antioxidants and vitamins of any fruits. Not only do they help prevent cancer and heart disease, as well as strengthen the immune system, but studies published in *Neurology* show they may also improve brain function. Blueberries, cranberries and goji berries are some of my favorites—the dried varieties are easy to pack as a snack. Another simple way to incorporate berries is to blend them into smoothies. I always keep a variety of frozen options, such as cherries, strawberries and blackberries, in the freezer. I also add fresh pomegranates to my diet whenever I can.

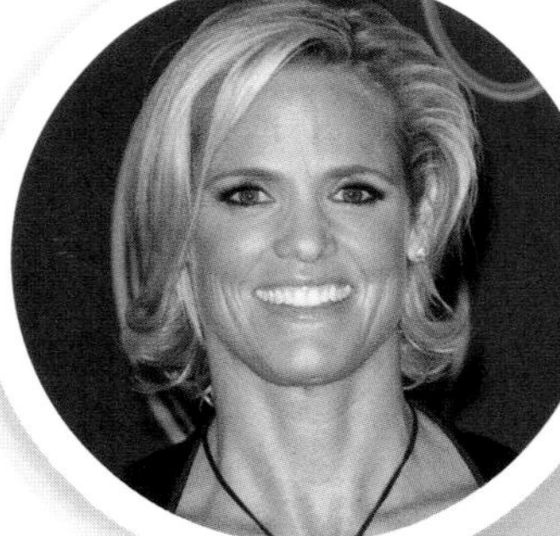

The "H" Factor: A-List Proof That Life Gets Better at 40

Every woman I know was on the edge of her seat when Dara Torres hit the water during the 2008 Summer Olympics. Sure, this Olympic swimming favorite was long considered a strong athlete—she's competed in five Olympics and is set to compete again in 2012—but it wasn't until the birth of her daughter and her fortieth birthday that she became a household name and a worldwide inspiration by breaking world records and making history. Today she easily leaves younger swimmers in her wake and says; "Everyone assumes that as you age, those feelings of competitiveness dissipate, but they don't. People my age and older have been telling me they are going to do something they have never done before. I love that."

MY BEST BODY NOW

Triumph of the Not-So-Average Jane
Shelley Johnson's Journey

THEN
5'7", AGE 35
218 POUNDS

NOW
AGE 37
128 POUNDS

At my turning point, I was wearing the same size 20 jeans and XXL gray sweatshirt every day. I was depressed, rarely leaving the house. Hormone fluctuations from a hysterectomy the year before wreaked havoc on my physical and mental health. My lowest point came during a meal out with a friend when I ate too much and to my horror found that I couldn't breathe—not only were my jeans making a huge indentation into my fat, they were actually cutting off my circulation and bruising me.

I realized that if I didn't make a change, I was seriously jeopardizing my life. An upcoming family trip to Hawaii was the goal I needed to implement healthy changes. I started Eating Clean, as well as doing weight training and incorporating motivational tips to keep me on track. The results? Greater energy, more sleep, more sex with my husband and a fresh new outlook on life. My health has improved, too: my resting heart rate has dropped drastically, from 90 beats per minute to 60, and my depression is gone. I really am different now, not just physically but in all sorts of good ways. I enjoy life. Mentally and emotionally, I'm strong. I don't care what people think of me—I'm such a confident person now that I don't rely on any one person's opinion of me to define who I am.

It took one year and nine months to drop from a size 20 to a 4, and I've maintained my new weight for nearly two years. I love my body and my life. I told my mom that I never knew I had a hot body—if I had known that, I would've done this years ago. Some days I even wake up forgetting that I'm not fat anymore. Suddenly I realize, "Oh yeah, I'm lean." I jump out of bed to arise to my day with excitement and vigor, as though a dream has come true. And it has.

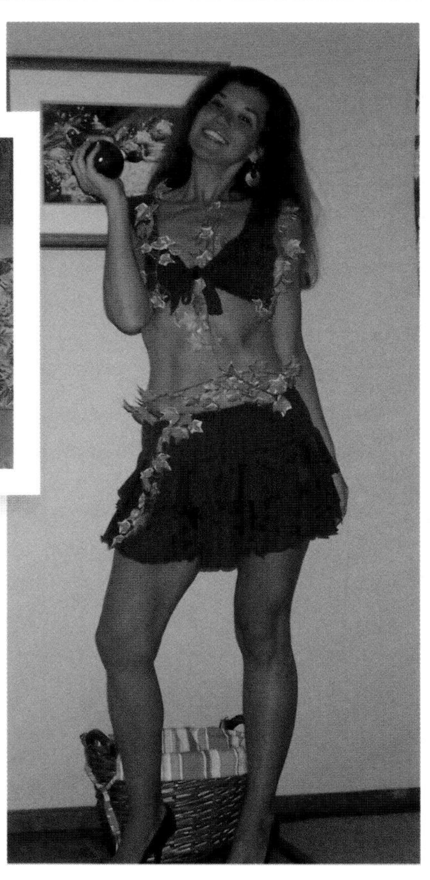

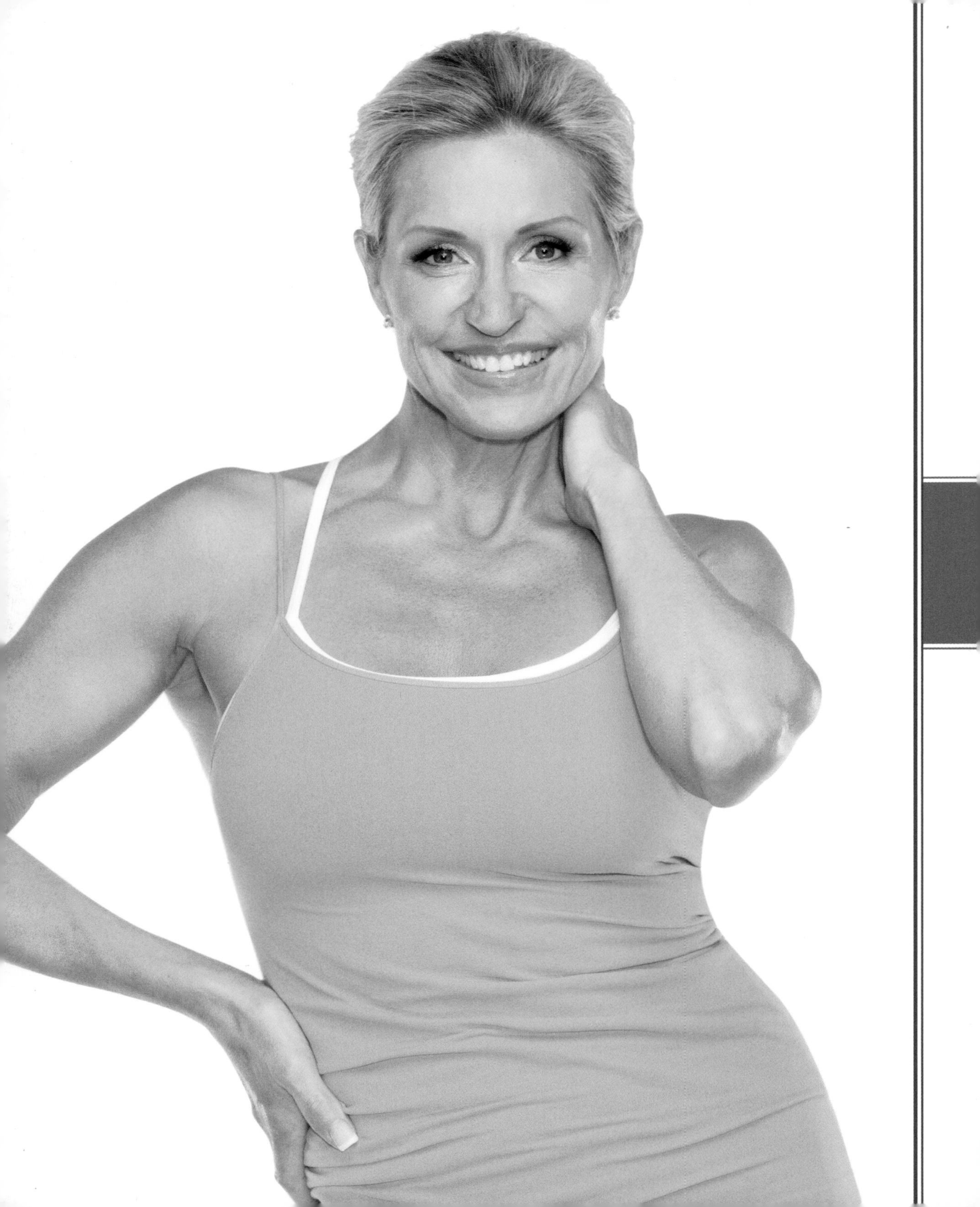

5 Best Body Now Fitness

WHEN I FIRST BEGAN WORKING OUT, I FOCUSED MAINLY ON cardiovascular exercise, using the treadmill, the elliptical machine and the rowing machine at least three days a week. They helped me shed the initial pounds, which gave me the confidence to move to other areas of the gym. Unfortunately, the treadmill only took me so far. You can do as much cardiovascular work as you like, but to get gorgeous, hard-body results—sexy, shapely curves and lean, toned muscles—you need weights. For me, exercise has been a fountain of youth, and with this Best Body Now program, it can be yours, too.

New Moves for Muscles Fighting Against Gravity

LIKE MY NUTRITION PROGRAM, MY BEST Body Now fitness strategies are similar to those used by professional weight lifters to get amazing, and clearly visible, results. The entire Best Body Now philosophy is based on the very simple notion that muscle burns more calories than fat. Muscle also takes up less space than fat—that's why a muscular person can weigh more but wear a smaller size. And once you begin to build strong muscles, the excess weight melts off, revealing the sexy, gorgeous you underneath. These results have been proven time and time again, not just by the pros, but by me and thousands of women and men who follow the Best Body Now fitness plan.

> Muscle burns more calories than fat.
>
> Once you begin to build strong muscles, the excess weight melts off, revealing the sexy, gorgeous you underneath.

If you do these moves regularly, combined with Eating Clean, your body absolutely *must* respond. Why? Because weight training helps counter nearly every challenge or issue your body faces due to aging, changing hormones, lifestyle shifts and more.

HOW DO THESE BEST BODY NOW RESULTS SOUND?
Lower body fat due to greater muscle mass
Stronger bones to fight osteoporosis
Reduced blood pressure
Lessened risk of cardiovascular disease
Higher energy levels
Better sleep
Happier mood, less anxiety and depression
Greater confidence and self-esteem
Heightened stamina, endurance and physical strength
Fewer injuries thanks to stronger bones and muscle, as well as greater flexibility
Boosted immune system
Improved flexibility and balance
Heightened sex drive
More radiant skin
Fewer illnesses

The building blocks of my regimen can be summed up in four words: pick up the weights. That's it—that's the secret. No magic potions, no living at the gym, no extraordinary genetics required. Anyone, any age, anytime will be stronger, fitter, healthier, more energetic—yes, this means *you*—from this plan.

WARM UP BEFORE YOU SWEAT AND COOL DOWN WHEN FINISHED. Five to ten minutes of light cardio and stretching is a great way to increase your circulation and heart rate and prepare your body for exercise. Start by walking, jogging at a slow pace or jumping rope for a few minutes. Once your body is warm, perform light stretches to get your muscles ready and raise your body temperature, which helps prevent injury and improve performance. When stretching, it's important not to bounce or you risk tearing or pulling a muscle. Instead, simply stretch the muscle and hold for ten to thirty seconds. Finish your workout with five to ten minutes of cool-down, which allows your heart rate to return to normal. Start by walking for a few minutes until you feel your heart rate come down, then stretch the muscles you worked.

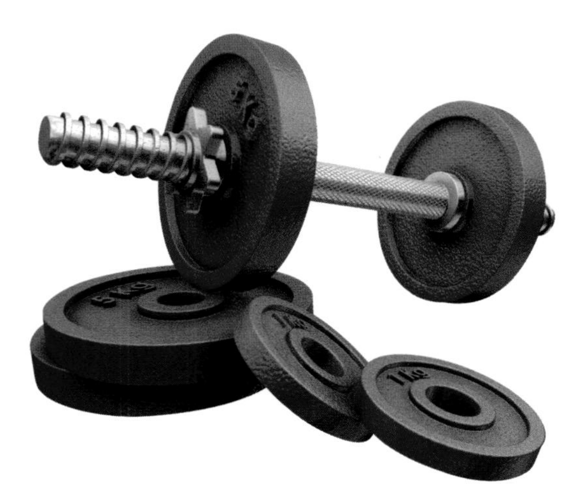

USE RESISTANCE OR WEIGHTS YOU ENJOY. Strength training can be done with free weights or dumbbells, machines, resistance bands, the ball and even your own body weight, whether you're at the gym or at home. Start by using the weights you think you'll enjoy the most, which will help you create a habit, then branch out into other areas later to challenge your body and avoid boredom.

STOCK YOUR SPACE WITH FITNESS GEAR. If you're exercising at home, be sure it's stocked with the essentials:

- A set of 3-, 5-, and 8-pound dumbbells for beginners, and 10- or 12-pounders for intermediate and advanced levels
- A bench, preferably an adjustable incline style
- A barbell set that contains 110 pounds of weights total in sets of 5-pound, 10-pound, 15-pound and 20-pound dumbbells initially

Even if you have a gym membership, it's good to create a backup space at home in case there are times you can't get there to do your workout.

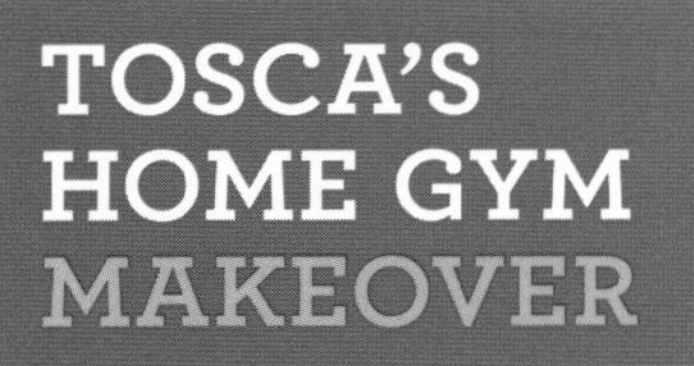

TOSCA'S HOME GYM MAKEOVER

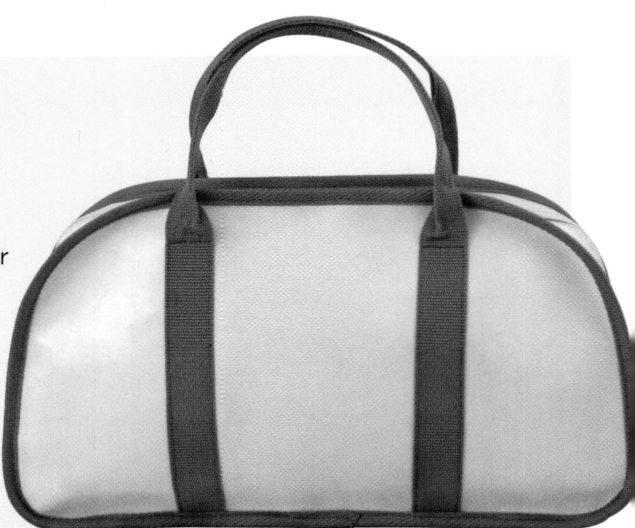

Renovate your fitness space and gym bag for success.

Even though I love how exercise makes me feel, I've created a zone in my home and gym so it's always easy to say yes to workouts. Everything is ready for me at any time, so all I need to bring is my best effort. Here are my workout tools that have given me my Best Body Now—they can do the same for you.

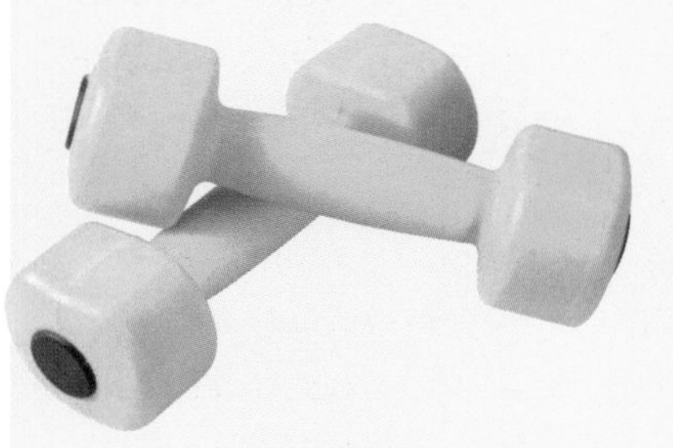

A BENCH for inclines, bench press and countless exercises.

A SET OF DUMBBELLS ranging from 5 to 40 pounds. If you're a beginner, you can begin with 2 to 3 pounds for arm exercises.

MEDICINE BALLS are perfect for abdominal moves. I have them in various sizes.

RESISTANCE BANDS are smart for travel.

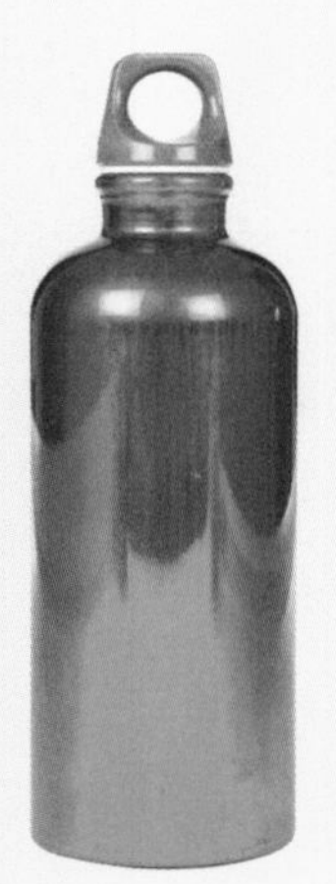

A MAT inspires me to do my yoga moves, stretches and floor work.

WATER BOTTLES are always in my gym bag, tote and workout area.

MUSIC. Nothing can get your game on faster than energetic, heart-pumping songs.

DREAMBOARD. This is a collage that represents your personal goals. One hangs in my space to remind me of my goals.

MOTIVATIONAL MANTRAS. Keep a few posted in full view so I can be inspired by them at a glance.

WORK OUT THREE TO FOUR TIMES A WEEK AT MINIMUM. If you start resistance training right now, in just thirty minutes of strength training per session, you'll see improved definition and tone in just two to three weeks, which is a small investment with a big payoff in your health.

PERFORM THREE SETS OF TWELVE REPS. This is the program I follow. You can either run through each move one time, then repeat the sequence three times, or do three sets of one move before performing the next—mix it up to keep muscles challenged. Between each set, rest approximately twenty to thirty seconds. When you can do 12 reps easily, increase your weights by 2 to 5 pounds, depending on the body part you're working. Keep in mind the larger the muscle, the bigger the weight increase you'll need.

The only exception is abdominals. For abs, increase the reps to 50 or more once you are comfortable doing so, performing three sets of three different moves. That's because the abs are made up of a complex network of muscles, so it takes more time and focus to hit them all. I also like to consider the first set of virtually all resistance as a warm-up or throwaway, a transition set where you now focus on training that particular body part and get into the groove. Your first set should always be moderately light and an opportunity to practice good form before you go on to the next sets.

Remember that breathing correctly will allow you to perform each move more effectively and efficiently. Inhale prior to starting the move, then exhale slowly as you perform the exertion, such as lifting or pushing a weight.

DO EARLY-MORNING CARDIO. Exercising on an empty stomach is an incredible way to reduce fat. Why? Blood sugar levels are low in the morning because you fasted while you slept the night before, so your body looks to fat, rather than glucose, for the energy it needs to work out. Personally, I like cardiovascular exercise of all kinds, including running, cross-country skiing, snowshoeing, swimming, skipping rope and cycling. I aim for at least three good sessions of about thirty-five minutes each per week. But remember I don't rely on this form of exercise to shape my physique or chase away the evils of poor eating habits. That is pure folly and an exercise in frustration. It just doesn't work that way.

TOSCA TIDBIT

When lifting, think of each muscle contracting as it works. Sometimes it helps to put your hand on the area working to make sure you're flexing enough. And always, always, always keep your abs tight when training.

CHALLENGE YOURSELF TO FATIGUE. When you work your muscles sufficiently, it's natural to feel tired or sore the next couple of days. This temporary soreness is called delayed-onset muscle soreness and occurs because you're breaking down muscle fibers, then rebuilding muscle mass. This is quite different from pain due to injury. If you feel serious discomfort, check in with your doctor, and avoid any moves that cause you pain.

DEDICATE YOUR ENTIRE FOCUS TO THE SWEAT SESSION. This means turning your attention to the muscle you are exercising so that you maximize your results. Look at the muscle, watch it in the mirror, and think about it contracting. You can get more done in a half hour when you're engaged than in three hours if you're talking, reading the paper or answering the cell phone while lifting. (These are all no-no's!)

> Depend on that important day of rest to let the body heal and to recharge your batteries.

DON'T FORGET YOUR REST DAYS. Muscles need time to rebuild. Typically, I shoot for two days of training, followed by one day of rest. And I never train the same body part on back-to-back days. It can lead to injury and give your muscles a stringy look because you have not let them properly recuperate. Overtraining yourself because you want to lose weight and tighten up faster will actually cause you to break muscle down, which is opposite to the result you are looking for. A healthy full muscle has a ferocious appetite that fires up the metabolism, thus burning more fuel. Resist the urge to overtrain. Depend on that important day of rest to let the body heal and to recharge your batteries.

DRINK WATER BEFORE, DURING AND AFTER EXERCISE. Staying hydrated is critical to fueling exercising and repairing muscle that's used during strength training. Strive to drink at least 8 ounces before and after your workout for best results. If you are involved in endurance cardiovascular exercise or training in a hot area you must listen to the body's natural signals to drink more water. If you are thirsty while exercising, drink water! It's that simple.

STAY DEDICATED TO YOUR PLAN. If I skip a week's worth of training, I begin to notice a difference in my muscle definition, so I'm not casual about workouts. It's harder to get away with skipping a workout as you get older. If you need a few days' downtime then take that time off, but do come back recharged and eager to get back on the plan. Every little bit of exercise counts, and yes, we all have speed bumps. It's normal and, more important, it won't stop you from your long-term goal if you recommit yourself right away.

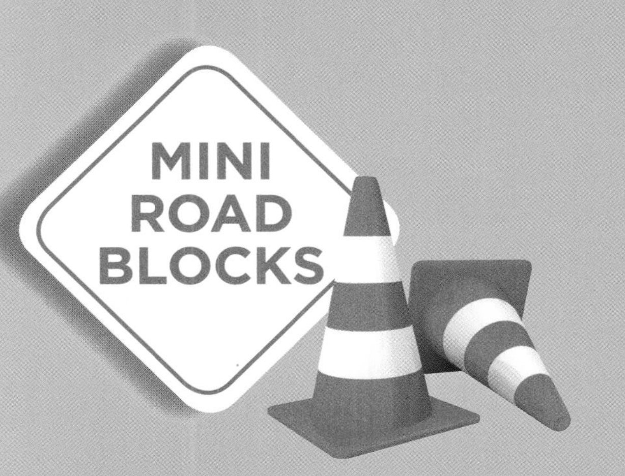

On the quest for your Best Body Now, life can seem to get in the way, but only if you let it. Here are the top obstacles you might be facing and proven tips for knocking them down. I've been through many of these same challenges and hurdled them all.

1 I DON'T HAVE TIME TO WORK OUT.

THE BEST BODY NOW FIX: I was there once, too, putting everyone else's needs ahead of my own. My new philosophy is that you can only be the best mother, wife, sister, friend and amazing woman you are when you are your healthiest, strongest, most empowered self. This means you become the number one priority. Does this mean neglecting your family, your job, your life? Absolutely not. It simply means that you are committing to excellent health and in doing so, need to make a few lifestyle changes. Evaluate your schedule and find areas that can be tweaked or eliminated. Perhaps you delegate more at work, arrange ride sharing with other parents for your kids, redistribute household chores with your husband or even simply choose to not work through lunch. When you put yourself on the schedule first, everything else will fall into place.

2 I DON'T LIKE TO WORK OUT.

THE BEST BODY NOW FIX: Maybe you're not so hot for lunges and squats, but I know you'll love what they do for your body. The upside to my program is that it's completely modifiable, so you can work using the machines and moves you like. And half the fun of working out is trying new exercises until you find the ones that work best for you. I suggest test-driving the options your gym provides, as well as those listed in women's health and fitness magazines each month. Once you begin to see results and notice how much healthier you feel, you'll associate working out with feelings of success and empowerment. If you have children, you're also setting the best example for them. Help them learn what an active lifestyle looks like by doing family activities, including bike riding, jumping on the trampoline, gardening or doing charity walks/runs. ▶

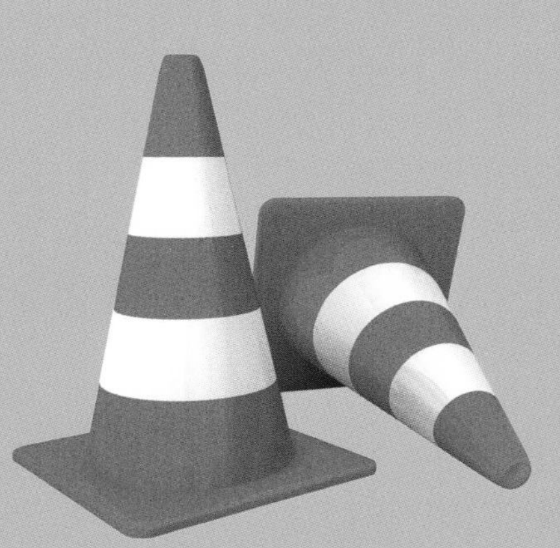

3 I CAN'T AFFORD A GYM.

THE BEST BODY NOW FIX: This program will give you a gorgeous toned body, even if you don't have a membership. If you're a beginner, there are many exercises you can do with just the resistance of your body weight such as lunges, squats and push-ups. As you advance, you'll simply need a set of barbells and dumbbells, along with an adjustable bench. For a small initial investment, you can do every single move I do on a daily basis. And you don't need a gym membership to hit the pavement, so you can commit to walking or running, or even biking, without straining your budget.

4 I DON'T MOTIVATE MYSELF ENOUGH AT HOME OR AM TOO DISTRACTED.

THE BEST BODY NOW FIX: If you're easily distracted at home, seek help from your family. Ask that they respect your training time and interrupt only if it's an emergency. If you've got household duties on your mind, see if you can delegate those to your husband or older children for an hour. Also, the best workout space is one with a door. Close it, turn up the music and lose yourself in the program—it's just a half hour to an hour a day. You've got another twenty-three hours to spend with loved ones. Finally, if it's just a matter of getting into the zone, load your MP3 player or CD player with music that gets your heart pumping and feet tapping. Then use that instant spurt of energy to fuel your workout.

5 I DON'T KNOW HOW TO EXERCISE.

THE BEST BODY NOW FIX: When I stepped into the weight room the very first time, I had no clue what to do with the equipment. It was extremely intimidating, but what I quickly realized is that the only one focused on you is you. Everyone else concentrates on his or her own workout. The specific moves in this program are simple and require absolutely no previous experience. The secret to success is not how difficult the actual move is; rather, it's how much you challenge your muscle in the move. This could be something as simple as a biceps curl if you've got correct form and use enough weight.

A TYPICAL BEST BODY NOW WORKOUT

You don't have to spend hours a day at the gym to get amazing results. Instead, I train three body parts in thirty minutes, with two days on, then one day of rest. Just thirty minutes four to five days a week is all you need to create your Best Body Now. This is the same workout I began ten years ago, at forty, and the same fundamental formula I'm using in my fifties. Why? Because it works, no matter what your age.

Just thirty minutes four to five days a week is all you need to create your Best Body Now.

Your Best Body Now Muscle Makeover:

Day 1	Day 2	Day 3	Day 4	Day 5	Day 6	Day 7
Calves, shoulders, upper back and abdominals	Biceps and triceps	Rest day	Back and chest	Glutes, abs and shoulders	Rest day	Upper and lower legs plus bonus round of glutes or abs

This routine will give you maximum Best Body Now results. It is also not so over-zealous as to be intimidating. Once you see the initial results you will want to come back for more. If you're also adding in cardio, get your sessions in when you can. Ideally, you should aim for every other day, but back-to-back cardio sessions are fine, too.

For stubborn areas such as the butt and abs, I'll tack on an extra round of focused training so that I get two or three workouts a week where I specifically work those spots. Perhaps as I get older I will be tacking on extra workout sessions for every body part as it slowly heads south! Who knows? I will keep you posted.

START YOUR BEST BODY NOW

SMALL STEPS LEAD TO BIG RESULTS. Working too hard and too fast can lead to burnout or injury, especially if you're new to training. What worked for me? Weekly strength-training goals that were manageable and allowed me to celebrate my achievements regularly. Try these easy steps that guarantee success—no matter where you're at today. You can do this!

1 CHECK IN WITH YOUR DOCTOR. Have your physician give you a stress test and a complete physical before you embark on a weight-loss plan. This will be an excellent baseline for you to evaluate if you are healthy enough for exercise and diet adjustments. If you plan a follow-up physical exam after a few months of following the Best Body Now program this will give you a chance to assess your progress. Your physician can be one of your strongest supporters, as mine was in my early days of embarking on my physique renovation.

2 CREATE A WORKOUT SANCTUARY. Constant visual reminders serve as instant motivators for training. If you've dedicated a space in your home to exercise, be sure it's always stocked with equipment, water, towels and so on, so when it's time to work out you have no excuses. I have also posted motivational sayings on the wall so I can remind myself to keep going even when it gets difficult. The same strategy is true if you belong to a gym: keep your gym bag clean, packed with gear and handy, so when the mood strikes, you can exercise. My trick? I keep extra clothes and sneakers in my car and office, so if space opens in my schedule I'm ready for extra gym time.

3 CONSULT A PERSONAL TRAINER. I had anxiety when I first started the gym with 70 pounds of excess fat, and you may be intimidated, too—it's natural and it's okay. Trust that you belong there, alongside the hardbodies who will eventually be admiring you. In the meantime, if you want the security of knowing how to use complicated-looking gym equipment, see if your gym offers one or two personal training sessions to help you become familiar with the equipment. Or if you're working out at home, have a gym rat friend or trainer come to your home to make sure your technique is spot-on. You'll immediately boost your confidence if you feel comfortable moving around the equipment and the space. I've always referred to fitness magazines to help me with training routines and correct form.

4 CREATE MANAGEABLE GOALS. Start small. If you're not a runner, for example, don't think you need to start your program by logging five miles a day. Instead, start by walking around the block and build up to a jog, increasing distance gradually. Or, if you're afraid to strength-train, strap weights to your ankles to get comfortable with the idea, then move to dumbbells when you're ready. Set yourself up for success by choosing what works for your level. Studies repeatedly show that setting smaller goals and achieving them contributes to success more reliably than trying to run a marathon on your first day of training.

5 RECORD PROGRESS IN A JOURNAL. This is my favorite trick because it's so effective. I list all of my workouts, including the exercise, number of sets and reps, and the weight. Not only does this record your progress, it also inspires you to keep the momentum—it's the story of your new fitness life.

6 DO A PHOTO SHOOT. Take some digital photos of yourself at varying angles and hang them in your workout space or tuck them into your gym bag. These images will serve as your ideal inspiration for challenging workouts when you're slow to start, and they will also help you monitor your progress.

7 BUY NEW TRAINING SHOES. Good trainers are essential for workouts, especially cardio. Pounding on the treadmill with unsupportive or ill-fitting shoes can cause shin splits and other injuries. I also happen to think that lacing up a quality pair of sneakers is like arming yourself for the tough workout you're about to begin—it's the perfect ritual for getting yourself mentally prepared and inspired. When I find a pair of shoes I really love I buy another pair right away!

8 START EATING CLEAN. One of the biggest mistakes people make is thinking that increasing their exercise levels means they can eat whatever they want. Sure, you'll still build muscle just by strength training, but to truly take your body to sexy new heights, you've got to incorporate the principles of Eating Clean. The good news is that when you combine the two strategies, the fat melts off and your Best Body Now emerges.

9 BANISH THE BATHROOM SCALE. Muscle weighs more than fat, so depending on your starting point, you may be slow to lose actual pounds, even though you're shedding inches. Scales can be deceiving and disempowering, so the rule in our house is no scales. Muscle, however, takes up less room than fat, so you'll see the results in how you look and feel. Instead of tracking progress on the scale, track it with a tape measure—you will see the results.

BEST BODY NOW MOVES

HERE ARE SOME OF MY FAVORITE exercises that truly challenge your muscles—they're a perfect way to start working toward your Best Body Now. Just pick three per section for your first workout routine, then mix them up after three weeks to keep challenging your muscles. Bonus: you can do most of these moves at home. I've also listed some exercises that require a bench or machine in each section, in case you're working out at the gym.

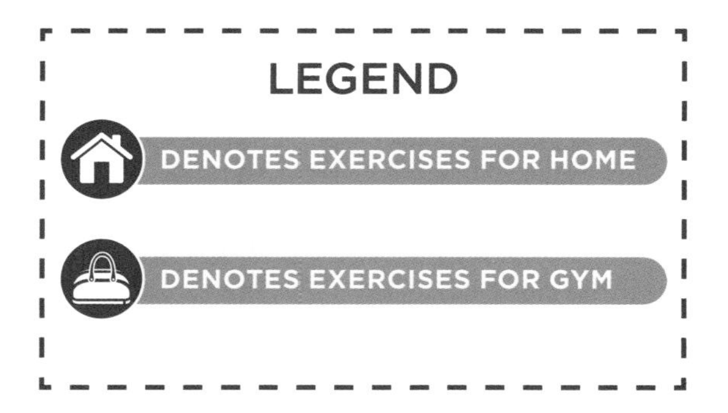

REVERSE BENCH CRUNCH

Ⓐ Lie on your back on a flat bench with your legs together and your knees bent over the end of the bench so that your toes touch the ground. Ⓑ Keeping your knees bent, lift your legs from the ground until your butt rises slightly off the bench. The feet will end up high over your head after the butt lifts from the bench. Lower and repeat. Do not swing legs. Use controlled movements, keeping spine flat on bench for maximum abdominal effect. For a tougher challenge, try this move while wearing ankle weights.

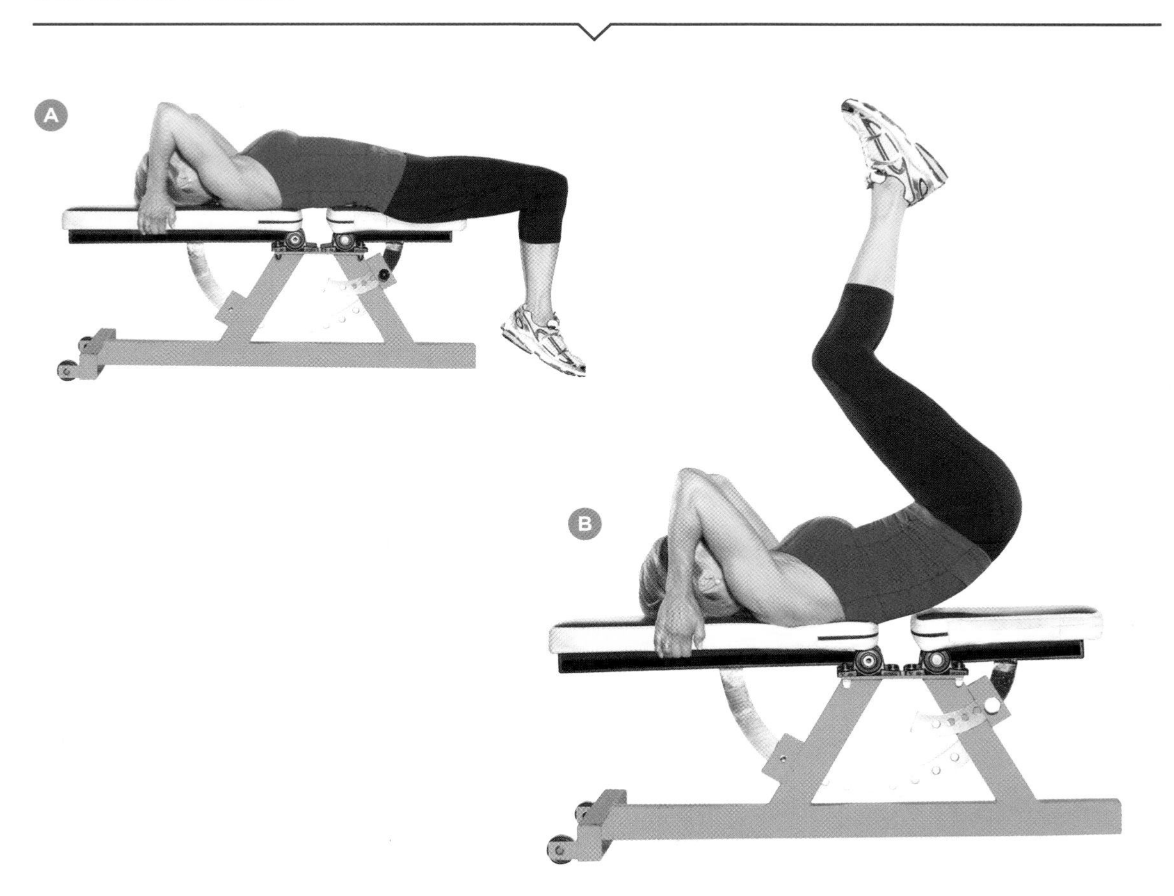

OBLIQUE CRUNCH

Stand with your feet shoulder-width apart and your hands down by your sides. Bend at the waist to the left, reaching your hand toward the floor, using the oblique muscles to pull you down, and then repeat on the right side. Maintain a steady rhythm for the entire set. I like to do this to music to keep steady movement. I can hear the Black-Eyed Peas singing "Boom Boom Pow" right now!

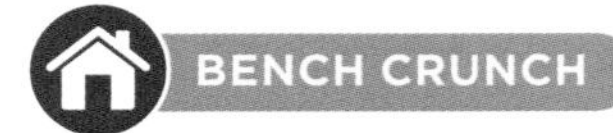

BENCH CRUNCH

(A) Lie on your back on the floor with your knees bent at a 90-degree angle so that your lower legs rest horizontally on a flat bench. Tuck your chin to your chest. (B) Raise your head, neck and shoulders until lifted off the ground. Do not rise all the way up. Lower and repeat.

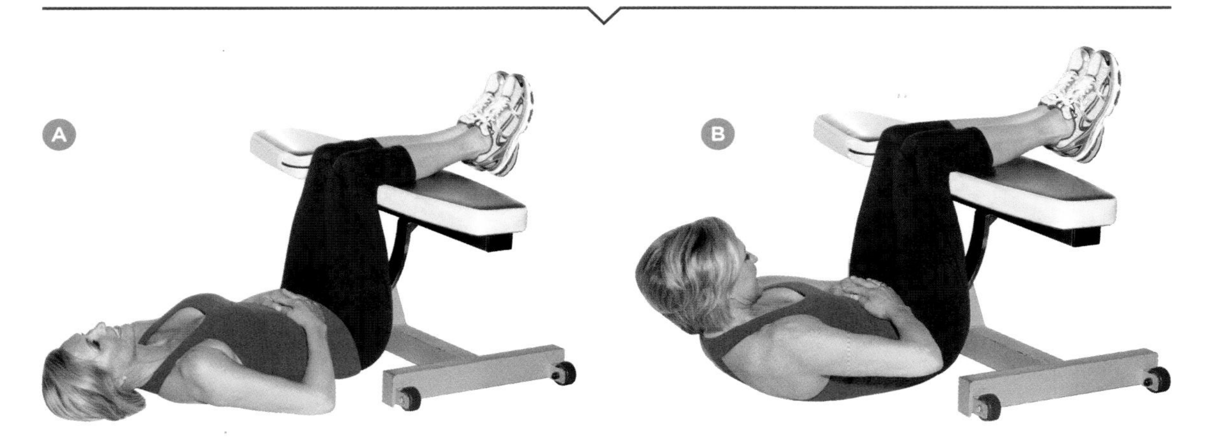

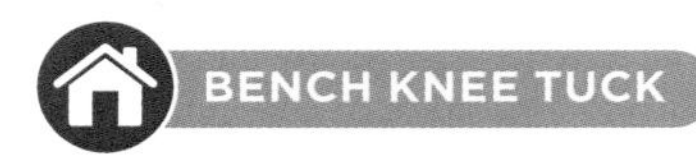

BENCH KNEE TUCK

(A) Sit on a flat bench with your legs stretched out in front of you. With your hands gripping the edge of the bench on either side of you, lean back and hold on to the side of the bench for balance. (B) Bring your knees in to your chest and return to the start position. Repeat for your chosen number of repetitions.

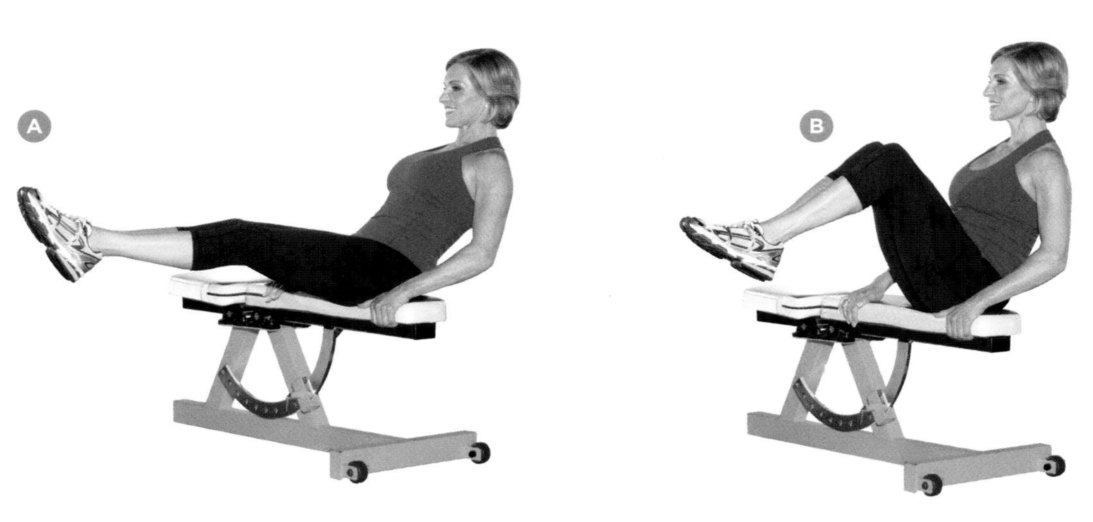

ROMAN CHAIR SIT-UP

Ⓐ Climb into a Roman chair apparatus where your legs are secured under a pad and the torso is free to move up and down. You should be sitting up and facing forward. Ⓑ Lower your torso slowly, using your abdominal muscles to control the movement. At the bottom of the movement, again using full abdominal contraction, raise your body back to the start or sitting up position. Repeat.

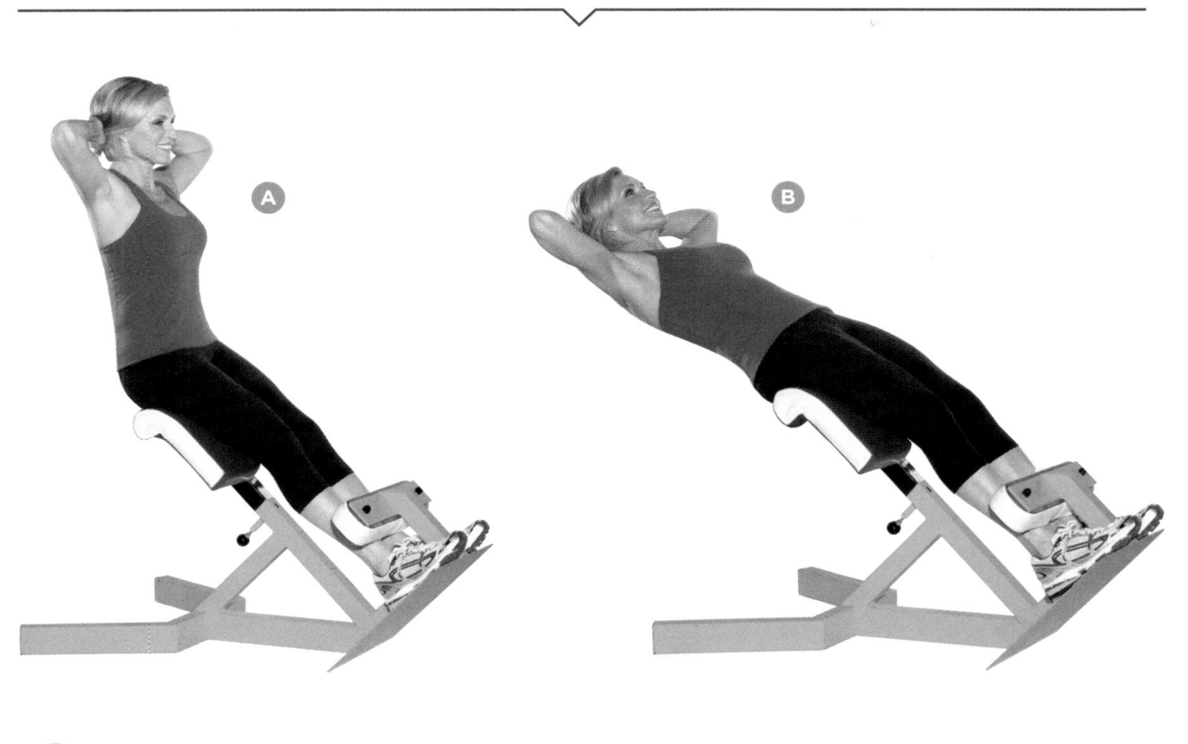

TWIST

Stand with your feet shoulder-width apart, keeping your knees soft. Fold your arms in front of your torso and keep them at chest height. Twist from the waist, moving from side to side, keeping hips facing forward and square over the feet.

HANGING LEG RAISE WITH TWIST

Grip a horizontal chin bar with your hands just wider than your shoulders. Bend your knees to your chest and lift your legs up and out to the right. Lower and repeat, alternating between your left and right sides. The goal is not to extend the legs so they are parallel to the floor. The focus must be on contracting the lower abdominals.

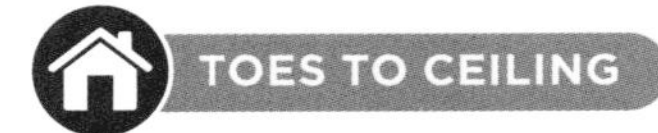

TOES TO CEILING

(A) Lie on a flat bench or on the floor. Position your legs vertically with your arms resting on the floor by your sides or gripping the bench by your ears. Point your toes toward the ceiling. (B) Lift your butt off the floor or bench, making sure that as you raise your legs they maintain the vertical position throughout. Lower and repeat.

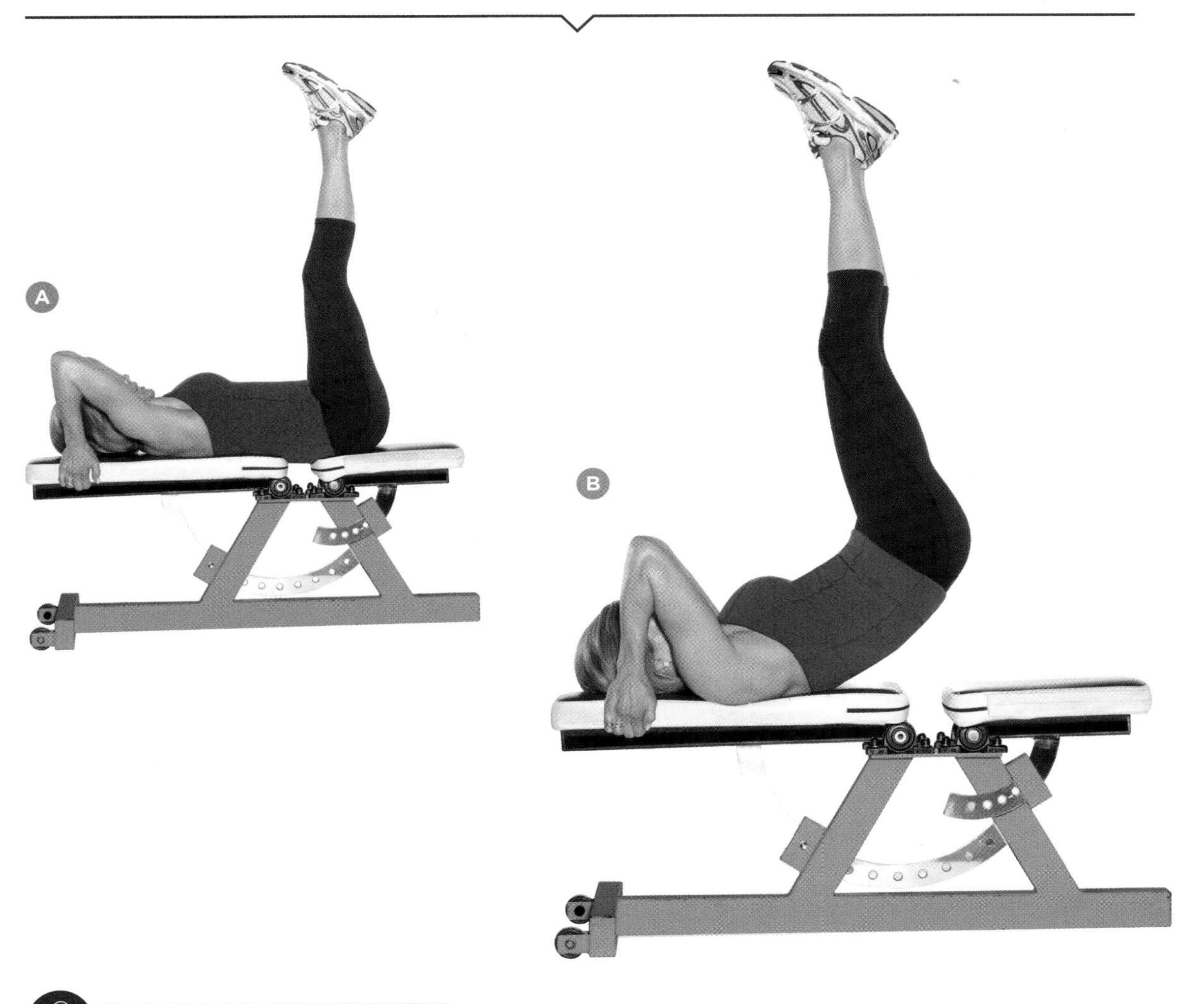

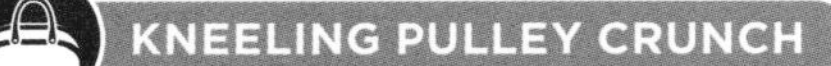

KNEELING PULLEY CRUNCH

Select a desired weight on the weight stack of a pulley machine. Kneeling on the floor in front of the weight stack, grab the pulley cable handle or straight bar. Start by kneeling upright, then bend at the waist and curl forward so that your head is close to the floor. Use your abdominal muscles to maintain control as you resume an upright position and repeat.

DUMBBELL PRESS

Stand with your feet shoulder-width apart holding a dumbbell in each hand. Begin the press with your arms bent and your hands holding dumbbells at shoulder height, palms facing forward. Raise or press dumbbells directly over shoulders until arms are fully extended. Lower and repeat. Do not bounce weights on shoulders. Some people drop the weights down to the shoulders quickly, which defeats the purpose of the exercise. There must be a degree of tension in the muscles at all times. Bouncing can also cause injury.

BENT-OVER LATERAL RAISE

Ⓐ Sit on the end of a flat bench with your knees and feet together and a dumbbell in each hand. Bend forward at the waist, keeping your feet firmly on the ground. Hold your head up. Ⓑ Raise your arms, keeping them slightly unlocked, out to the side. Rotate your hands so that your palms face back and your thumbs down. The idea is to have the elbows slightly higher than the hands for correct form. Lower and repeat.

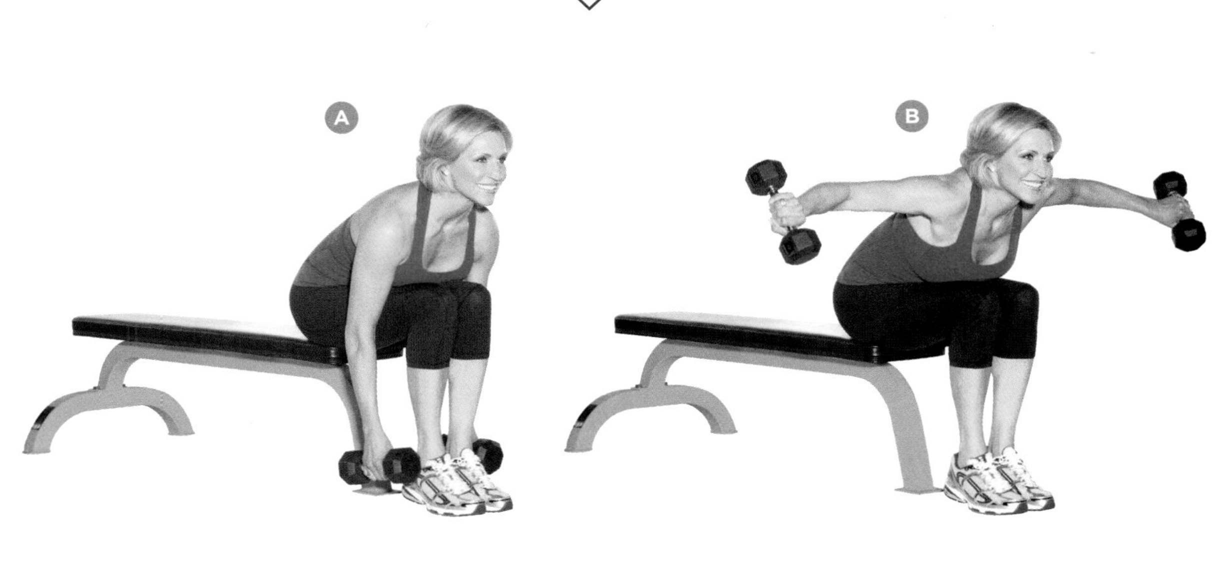

FACEDOWN INCLINE LATERAL RAISE

Set an incline bench at a 45-degree angle. Lie facedown on the bench, feet flat on the floor. Holding a dumbbell in each hand at arm's length, raise the arms straight out to the side as high as you can. Lower and repeat.

INCLINE LATERAL DUMBBELL RAISE

Ⓐ Lie with your chest against an incline bench set at approximately 40 degrees. Hold a light dumbbell in each hand in the arms-straight-down position. Ⓑ Raise both weights together out to the side, no higher than your shoulders, keeping the arms in line with each other. Lower and repeat.

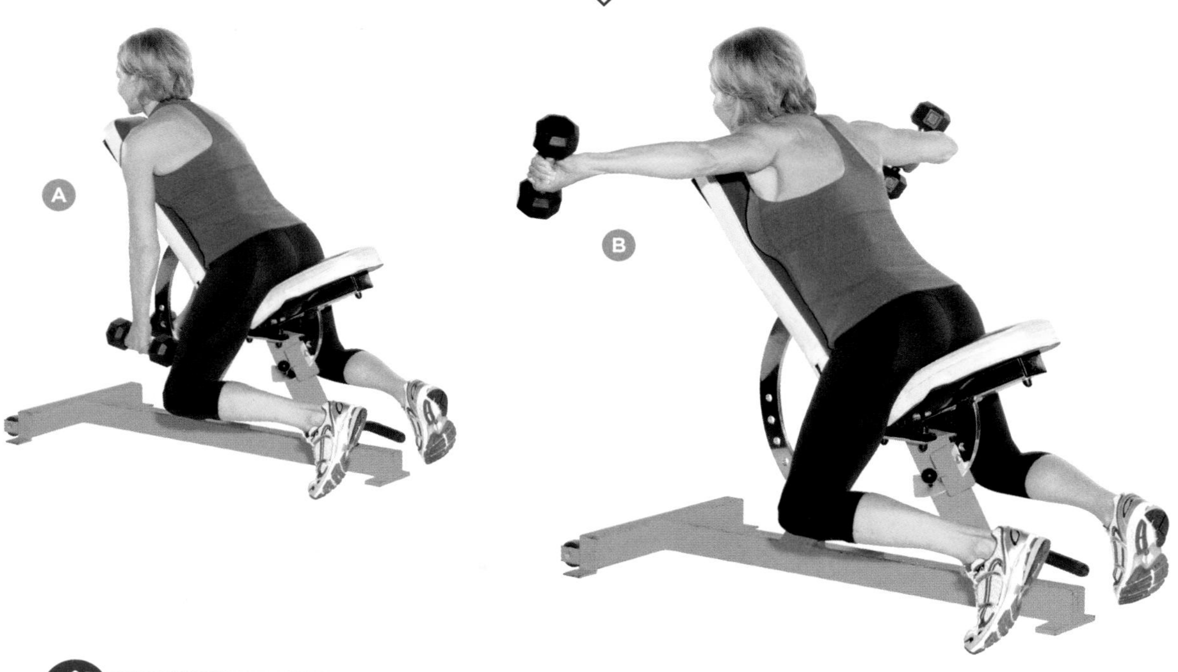

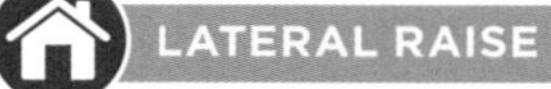

LATERAL RAISE

Stand with your feet shoulder-width apart. Hold a dumbbell in each hand and let your arms hang down by your sides, keeping the elbows slightly unlocked and your palms facing in. Raise your arms out to the side in a slow, controlled motion. The elbows are always slightly higher than the hands for correct form. Lower and repeat. Do not swing your arms wildly—this can lead to injury and doesn't work your muscles effectively.

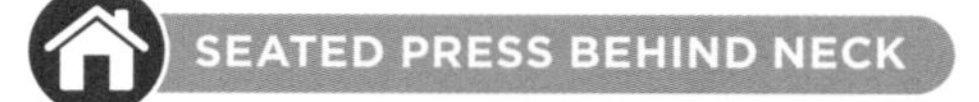

SEATED PRESS BEHIND NECK

Sit at the end of a flat bench, feet flat on the ground. Hold a loaded barbell on your shoulders behind your neck with your palms face out. Your grip should be somewhat wider than your shoulders. Press the barbell overhead until your arms are fully extended, making sure your elbows are held back. Lower and repeat, being careful not to hit your head when returning to the start position.

LYING DUMBBELL SIDE RAISE

Ⓐ Lie on a flat bench on your left side with your left arm tucked under your head or extended straight out to the left of you. Your right arm, gripping the dumbbell, should rest right in front of you. Ⓑ Lift the right arm and dumbbell until it is in the vertical position. Lower slowly and repeat. Work the left shoulder by lying on your right side and holding the dumbbell in your left hand.

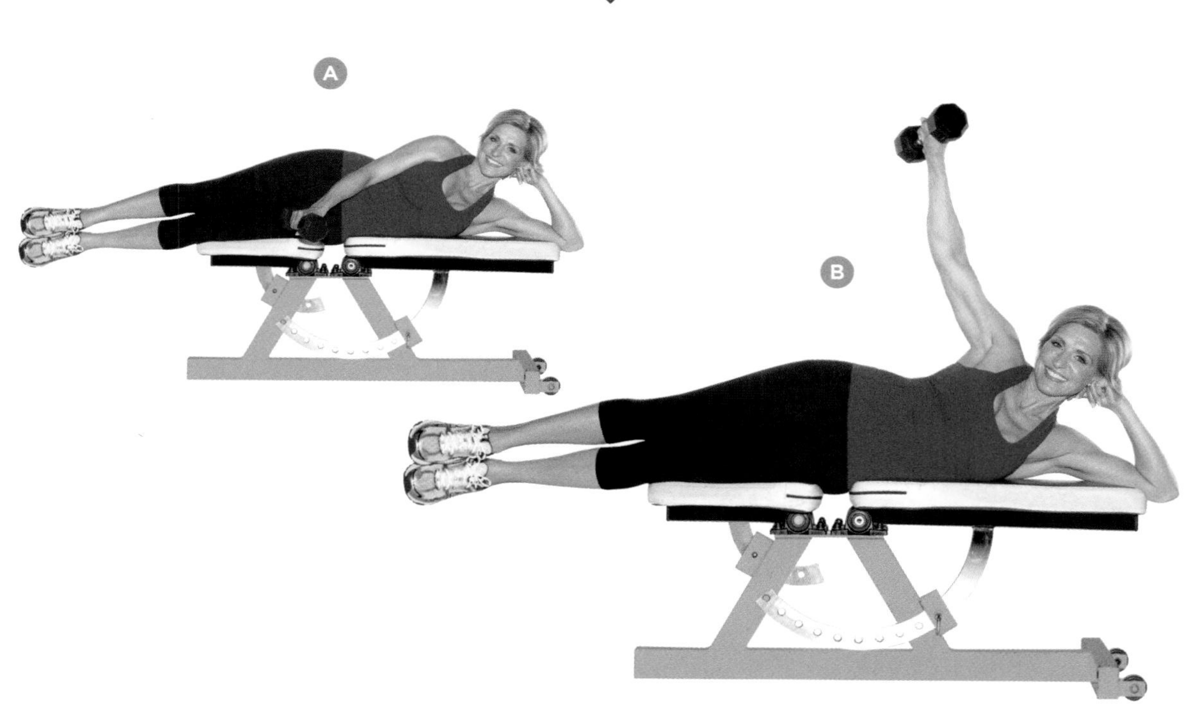

STANDING BARBELL UPRIGHT ROW

Stand with feet comfortably apart, holding a barbell in the arms-down position, with palms facing in. Grip spacing should be about 8 to 14 inches apart. Keeping the elbows up, raise the bar until the hands are just under the chin. Keep the bar parallel to the floor for the entire movement. Lower and repeat.

SEATED BARBELL PRESS

Sit at the end of a flat bench holding a loaded barbell at your shoulders with your palms facing out. Grip spacing should be about 8 to 14 inches apart. Keep the back straight, press the barbell to full extension above the head. Lower and repeat.

REGULAR DEADLIFT

Ⓐ Stand with feet shoulder-width apart and knees slightly bent. Place a barbell on the floor in front of you. Bend over and take a grip slightly wider than shoulder-width. Ⓑ Squat down, keeping your head up, back flat and butt out. Breathe in as you lift the bar off the floor to your upper thighs with leg power, keeping the back flat at all times. Exhale deeply and lower the bar back to your start position but do not let the barbell touch the floor between reps.

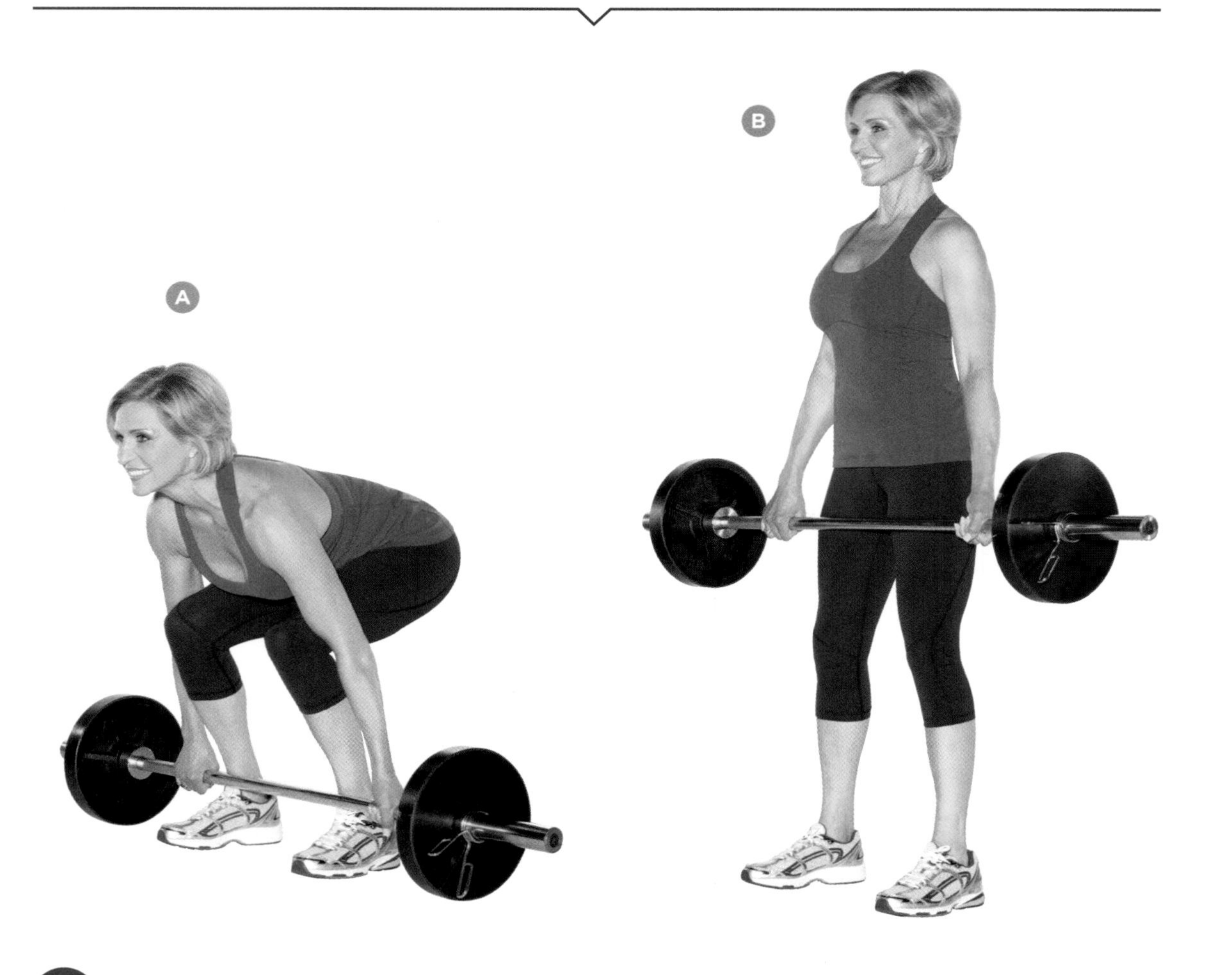

BENT-OVER DUMBBELL ROW

Stand with your feet together and a dumbbell placed beside each foot. When ready bend over and take hold of the dumbbells. Hold your head up and keep the back flat. Raise the dumbbells to either side of your chest. Lower and repeat. Don't let the dumbbells touch the floor until you have completed the set.

ALTERNATE DUMBBELL ROW

Stand with feet shoulder-width apart. Holding a dumbbell in each hand, bend over at the waist until the dumbbells are almost touching the floor. This is your start position. Raise the left dumbbell to the side of the waist and lower. Repeat with the right dumbbell. Alternate raising the dumbbells to the side of the midsection until the set is complete.

SINGLE DUMBBELL PULLOVER ON BENCH

Position a flat bench near you. Stand a dumbbell on its end at one end of the bench. Lie down on your back on the bench with your head hanging over the end where the dumbbell has been positioned. Plant feet squarely on either side of the bench. Reach behind you and grasp the dumbbell in your left hand. Rest your right hand across your abdomen. Lift the dumbbell that is at your chest. Breathe in and lift the dumbbell off your chest until your left hand is fully extended, keeping the elbow soft. Lower the dumbbell behind your head, keeping your arm as straight as possible. Exhale and raise the dumbbell back to the start position. Complete sets and reps and work the right arm similarly.

SINGLE-ARM DUMBBELL ROW

Position a flat bench in front of you and place a dumbbell to the left of the bench. Stand to the left of the bench and place the right knee on the bench. Lean forward at the waist, keeping your back flat, and position your right hand on the bench for support. Grasp the dumbbell in your left hand, palm facing in. Breathe in and, bending at the elbow, raise the dumbbell to your waist. Breathe out and lower the dumbbell to just above but not touching the floor. Complete your reps and sets for this side and work the right side.

WEIGHT-ASSISTED PULL-UP

Take the position on the weight-assisted pull-up machine as directed. Use a weight selection that will allow you to perform 10 to 12 good repetitions. Pull yourself up as high as you can go. Lower and repeat.

WIDE-GRIP CHIN-UPS

Grasp a chin bar with hands shoulder-width apart and palms facing away from you. Bend knees behind you. This leaves you hanging from the chin bar. Inhale and pull your body up until your chin is above the bar. Lower and repeat.

SEATED LOW PULLEY ROW

Ⓐ Attach a V-handle to the low cable pulley machine. Seat yourself so that you are facing the weight stack and your feet are shoulder-width apart on the footpads. With knees bent, lean forward and grasp the V-handle with palms facing in. Use your legs to push you a bit further back on the seat so that your knees are just slightly bent. Ⓑ Lean back so that your abdomen is upright. Keep the torso upright and inhale as you pull the cable back into your waist. Use control. Exhale and return to start position. Repeat.

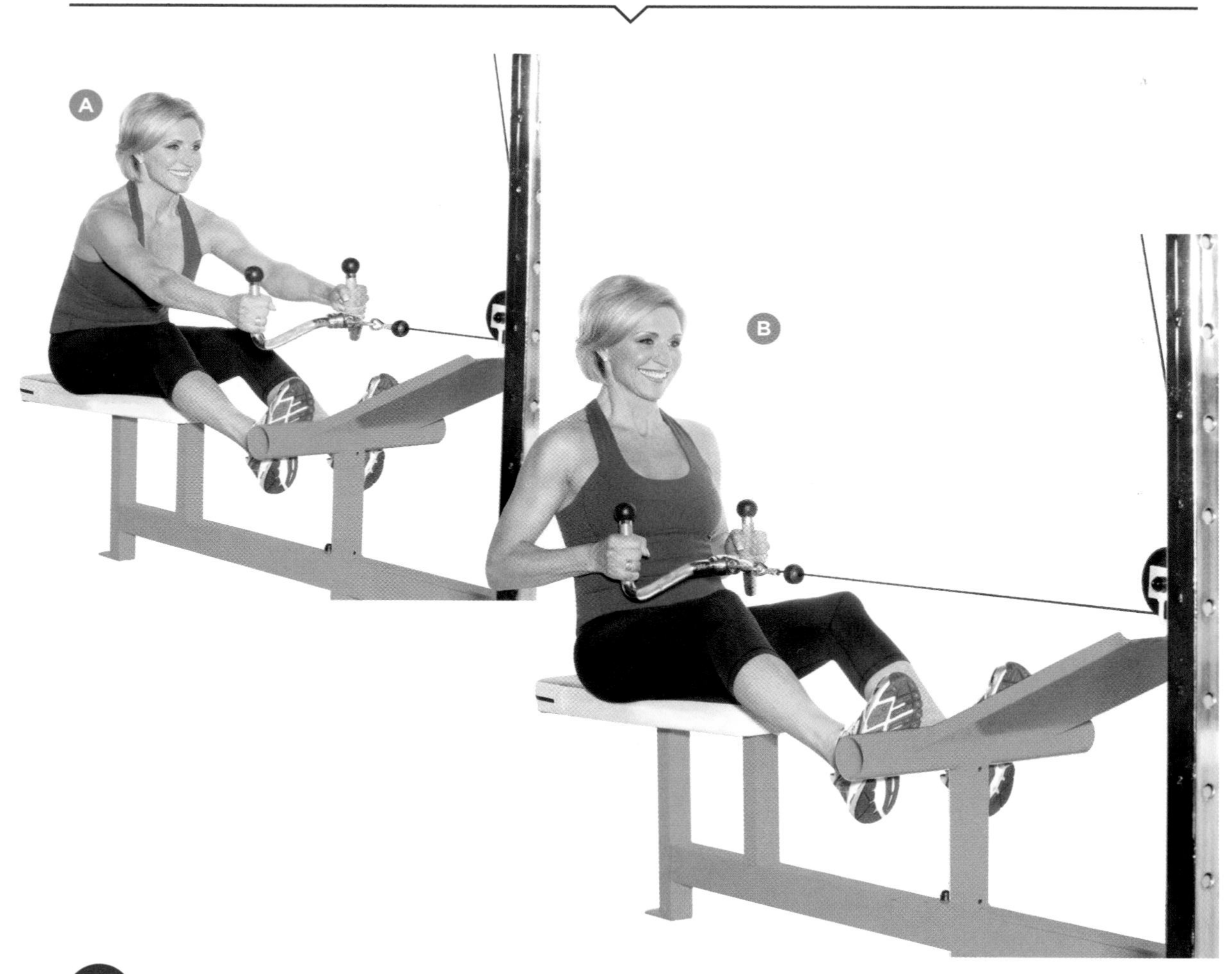

BENT-OVER BARBELL ROW

Place a barbell on the floor in front of you. Feet should be shoulder-width apart. Bend over, making sure your back is flat and your knees are soft. Grasp the barbell in an overhand grip so palms face your legs. Breathe in and lift the barbell into your waist, then lower. Repeat.

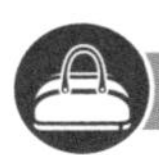

LAT MACHINE PULL-DOWNS

Ⓐ Place a straight bar on an overhead cable. Reach up to grasp the bar, hands shoulder-width apart, palms facing away from you and body facing the weight stack. Your arms should be fully extended over your head. Securely tuck your legs under the kneepads in the machine. Ⓑ Breathe in as you slowly pull the bar down in front of you to just above your chest. Exhale and let the bar return to the start position with control. Repeat.

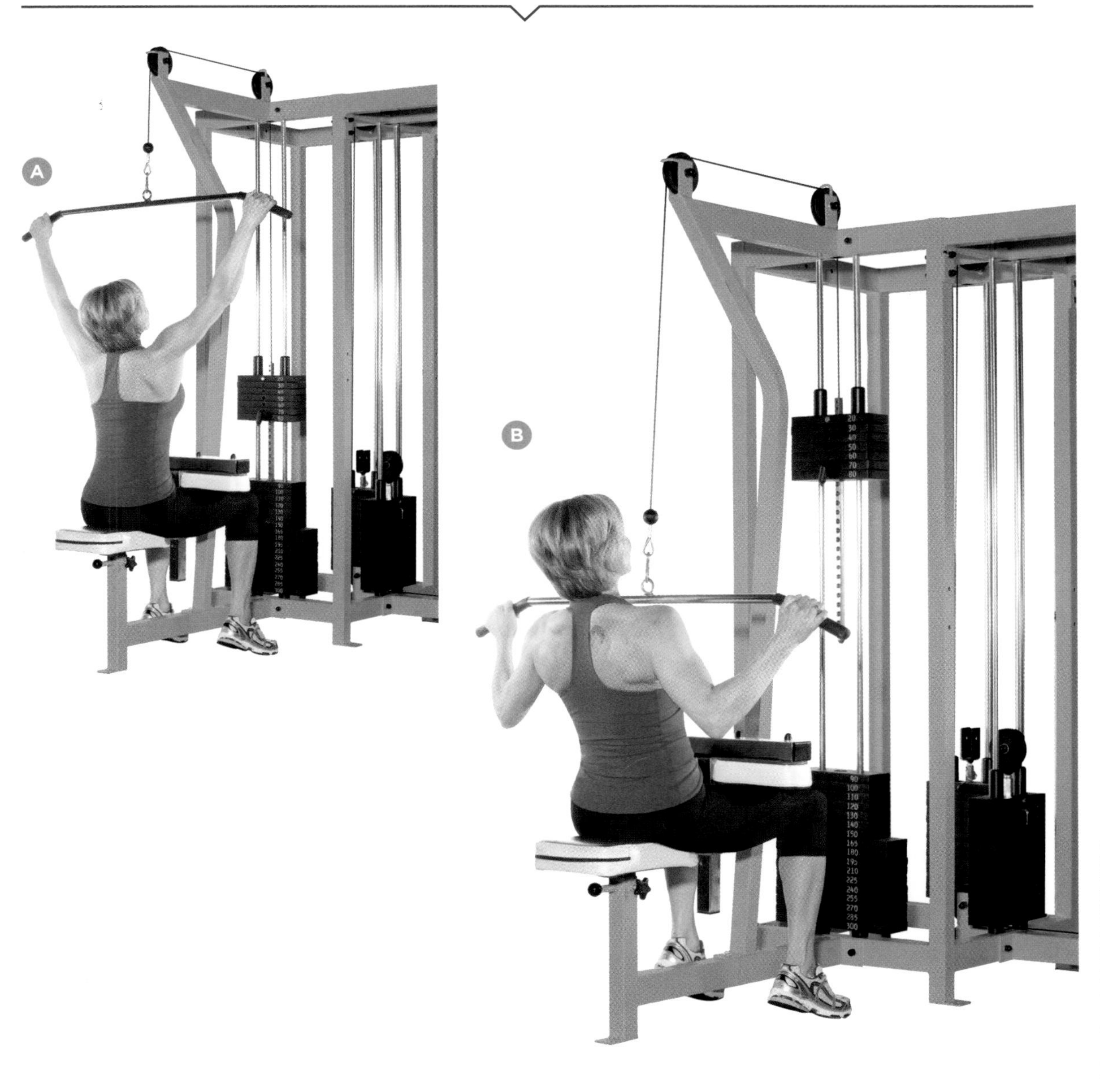

TRICEPS REVERSE DIP

Ⓐ Place two benches parallel and close to each other—this distance varies depending on the length of your legs, but it is about two-thirds the length of your legs. Sit on the long side of one bench so you are facing the other bench. Grip the edge of the bench quite close to your butt. Place your feet on the other bench. With your weight fully resting on your arms, lift your butt off the bench and edge forward so that you can lower yourself below the bench. Ⓑ Inhale as you lower your torso using arm strength until you can't drop any more. Exhale and lift yourself up again. Repeat.

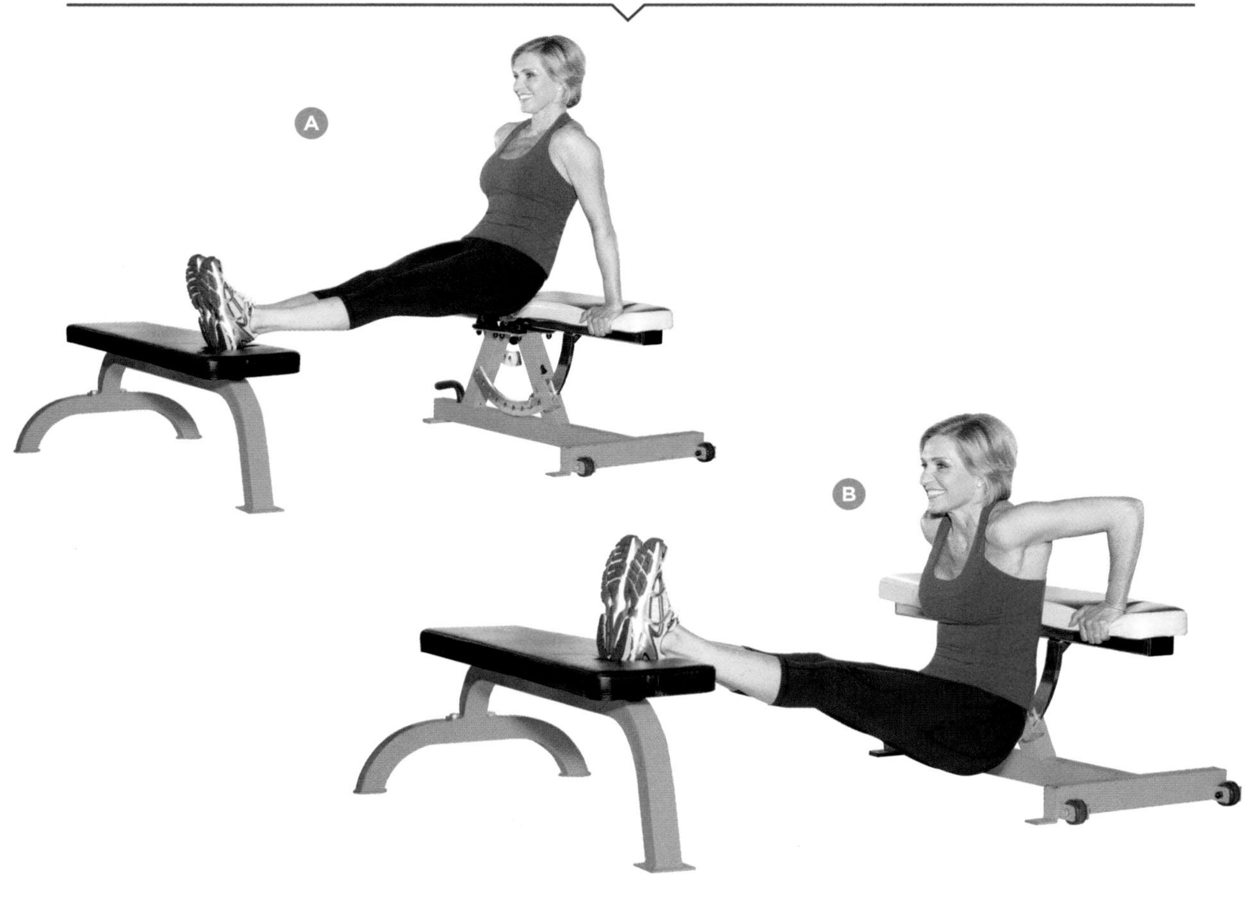

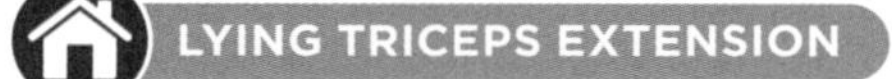

LYING TRICEPS EXTENSION

Lie faceup on a flat bench, feet planted squarely on either side of the bench, and hold a dumbbell in each hand, arms fully extended vertically above the body. Lower both dumbbells to the sides of the head while keeping the upper arms vertical. Still keeping the upper arms vertical, raise the dumbbells to the start position. Imagine a hinging action taking place at the elbows. Repeat.

SUPINE SINGLE ARM ACROSS CHEST TRICEPS EXTENSION

Ⓐ Lie faceup on a flat bench with feet planted securely on either side of the bench. Hold a dumbbell in your right hand with your arm held vertically above your body and the dumbbell pointing up. Your left hand is down by your left side, or you can gently stabilize your lower right arm by holding it with your left hand. Ⓑ Lower the dumbbell to the left side of the chest while keeping the right upper arm vertical. Straighten and repeat. Work the left arm in the same manner.

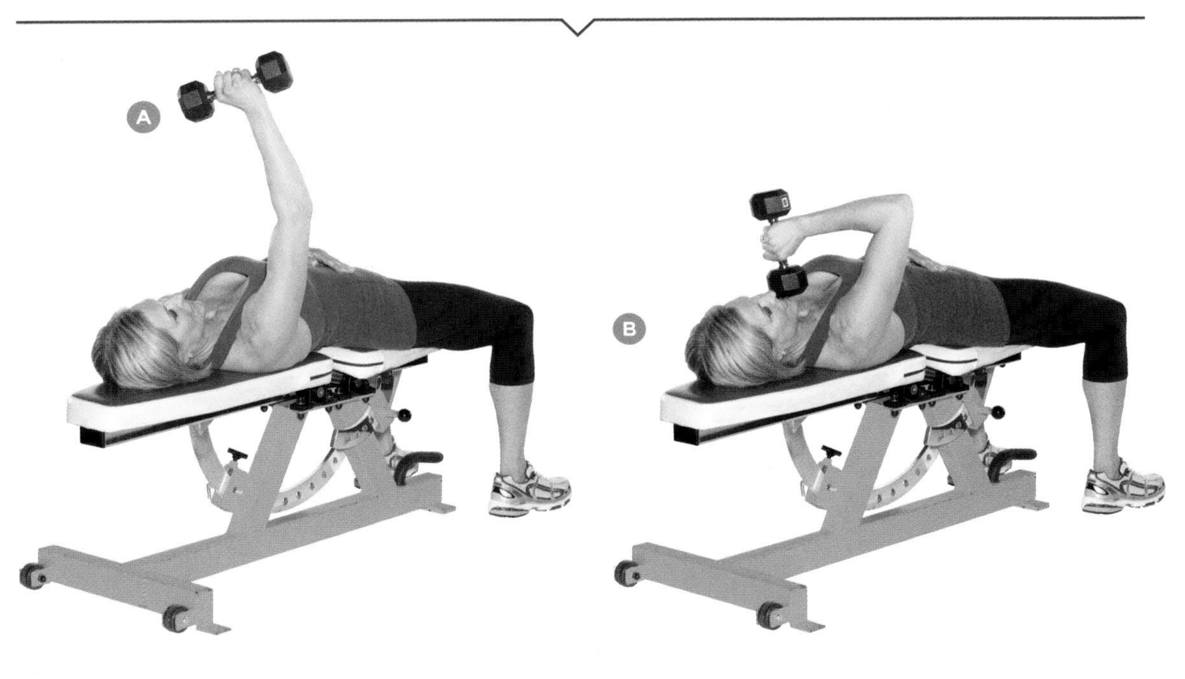

SINGLE ARM TRICEPS EXTENSION

Sit on the long side of a flat bench, holding a dumbbell in your right hand and with your left arm tucked into your side. Lift the dumbbell so the arm is fully extended above your head. Keeping the arm pointing upward, bend your elbow and lower the dumbbell until it is behind your head. Your right elbow remains near your right ear. Raise the dumbbell and repeat until all reps and sets are complete. Now train the left arm.

STANDING SINGLE DUMBBELL TRICEPS EXTENSION

Stand or sit so your feet are shoulder-width apart and square. Keep knees soft. Grasp a dumbbell in your left hand, letting your right hand hang by your side. Lift the dumbbell straight up so your left arm is fully extended overhead. With dumbbell pointing up, breathe and lower the dumbbell behind your head. Breathe out as you raise the dumbbell to the start position. Repeat.

STAY ON TRACK

ANY SORT OF CHANGE CAN BE TOUGH TO IMPLEMENT, BUT ONCE YOU see your body take on a fabulous new shape, you'll love the Best Body Now workout plan. Ensure that you stay committed and motivated by trying some of my tricks below.

1 CREATE GOALS. It's easier to stay focused when you write down your goals. Identify your big dreams, those very specific long-term goals that may take some time—such as lose 10 pounds, trim 2 inches from your waist—then list interim targets that will help you get there. For example, "I'll strength-train three days out of the next five," or "I'll prepare Eating Clean menus for the week in advance." When you cross your interim targets off your calendar, you see your accomplishments come to life before your eyes. I'll also post little notes for myself on the bathroom mirror or on the fridge to remind myself that I'm working toward something special and the end game is worth the work it takes to get there.

2 CRAFT A SCHEDULE. Making the gym a daily habit may feel a little too strict at first, especially if you're juggling kids or a hectic life. One trick is to put workouts on your calendar as a date with you and your weights. I like to map out my sessions on Sunday nights before the week begins. Mark them as meetings on your work calendar, so others won't plan conflicting appointments, and let family know that your "me time" is set in stone.

3 ARM YOURSELF WITH A PLAN B. No matter how disciplined and motivated you are to get back into shape, invariably life will throw you a curveball. If your daily to-do list gets changed by a last-minute work emergency or a sick child, always have another option for working out—have several workout DVDs on hand if you miss your favorite class, go for a brisk walk at lunch, run stairs at home or the park after work. This way, healthy habits and strong momentum remain on track. Remember also that sometimes a day off has a silver lining, since a much-needed rest is as important to your Best Body Now progress as training.

4 HAVE A SNACK. Nutrition can fuel a butt-busting workout and keep hunger pangs at bay if you're near dinnertime. My favorite snack? An apple with natural nut butter. It's the perfect carb-protein combination.

5 DON'T QUIT UNTIL YOU'VE REACHED YOUR CHECKPOINT. If you're the type who's easily talked out of exercising or has trouble staying motivated, make a pact that you won't quit until after you've gotten dressed or swiped your membership card at the gym. By the time you tie your cross trainers or enter the locker room, you'll be more than halfway there. It will take just as much effort to pack up your things and quit as it will to work out.

6 COMMIT TO A GROUP OF FELLOW EXERCISERS. I love when my friends and I keep each other motivated and dedicated, and I have a legion of men and women who help me this way. Enlist friends who also want to get fit and arrange weekly check-ins, plan weekend walks or hikes, talk about your challenges and successes and encourage each other through hurdles. When others are in your corner, working hard to achieve similar goals, you become more accountable to each other and ultimately feel more conscientious about staying the course.

7 REMEMBER THAT THIS IS A LIFESTYLE CHANGE. Your ultimate goal is to incorporate fitness into your life so that it becomes part of who you are and what you love to do. This means if you have a day where you take it easy at the gym or you skip a workout to have dinner with a friend, don't be too hard on yourself. You're creating lasting changes, and it's normal to fall off the wagon. The next day, do some extra reps or add a cardio segment to your workout—it will boost your confidence and erase any guilt you might feel from skipping exercise the day before.

8 KEEP UP-TO-DATE. Read books on nutrition and exercise to keep up with trends. Subscribe to magazines dedicated to women's health and fitness to keep motivated and well informed.

TRICEPS

TRICEPS KICKBACK

Ⓐ Position a flat bench in front of you. Place a dumbbell on the right side of the flat bench. Stand on the left side of the flat bench and place your right knee on the bench with your right hand in front of you for support. Your back should be flat and your head up. Grasp the dumbbell in your left hand, palm facing in. Lift the weight so that the upper arm is parallel to the floor and the elbow is tight to your side. Ⓑ Extend your arm so that the dumbbell is pointing straight behind you. With control, return to the start position and repeat.

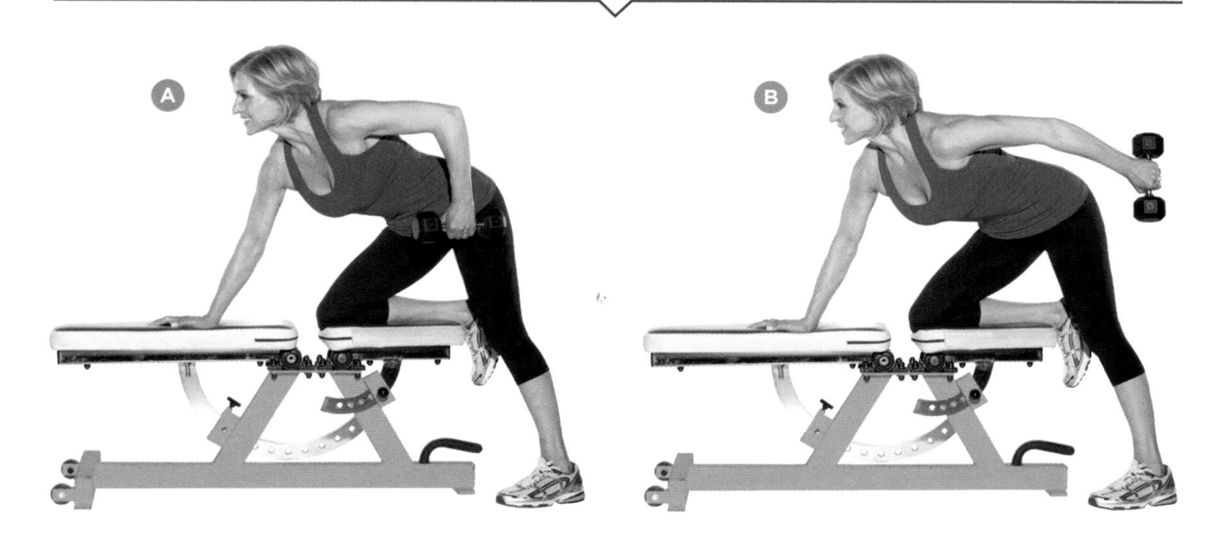

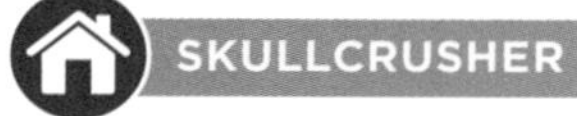

SKULLCRUSHER

Balance a barbell with appropriate weight on the very end of a flat bench. Lie faceup on the same flat bench, feet on the floor on either side, and your head almost touching the barbell. Raise your hands over your head, keeping elbows pointing up, and grasp the bar, palms facing up and hands shoulder-width apart. Moving only the forearms, slowly raise the barbell up until your elbows are locked. Exhale and lower the bar to just behind the head while keeping the upper arms as vertical as possible. Return to start position and repeat. For beginners, a spotter is recommended.

TRICEPS PRESS-DOWN

Attach a straight bar to a high cable on a weight stack. Stand upright, feet shoulder-width apart and knees soft, facing the press-down bar. Place both hands, palms down, on the bar about 6 to 8 inches apart. Keeping the upper arms close to your body, press the bar downward until both arms are straight. This exercise is most effective if you keep the upper arms tight against your body and move only your forearms. Return to start position and repeat.

BICEPS

INCLINE DUMBBELL CURL

Ⓐ Set the angle of your incline bench at approximately 40 degrees. Take a dumbbell in each hand, allowing the arms to hang down at the sides. Ⓑ Start by curling with the thumbs-up position, but as the curl proceeds rotate the wrists until the palms are facing upward, being careful not to bend your wrists. Lower and repeat.

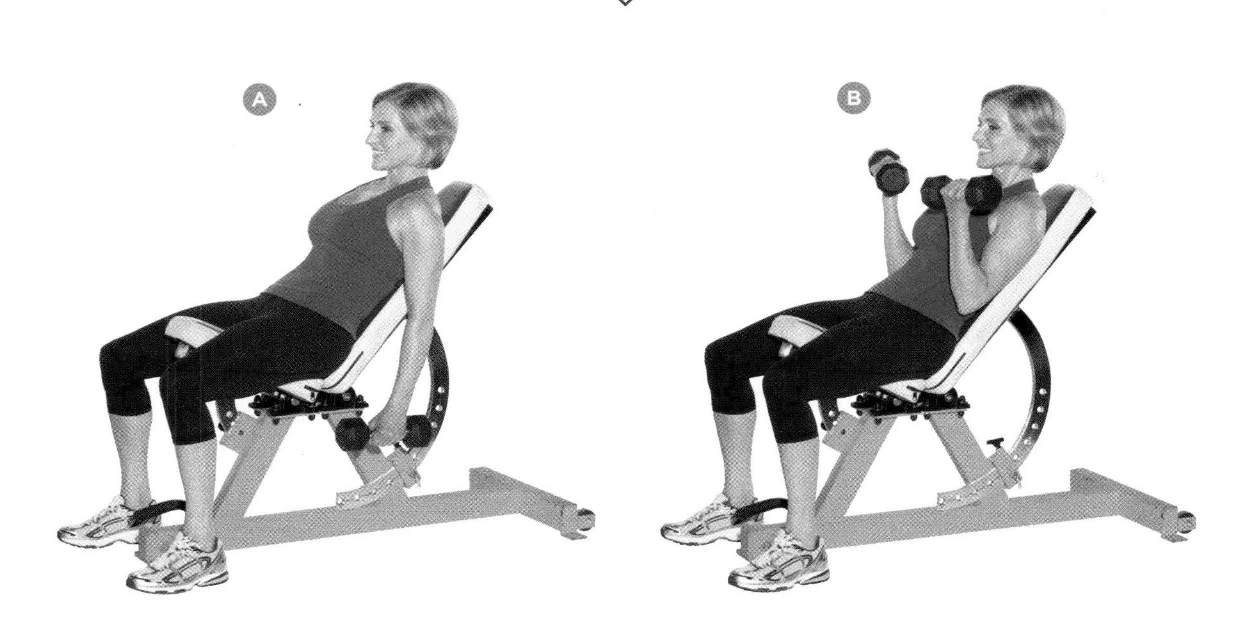

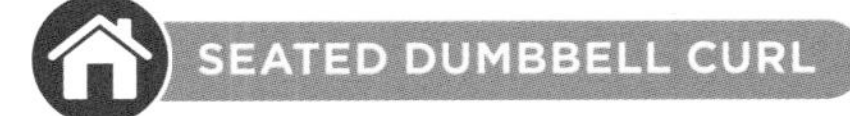

SEATED DUMBBELL CURL

Sit at the end of a flat bench holding a dumbbell in each hand. Keep your back straight, your head up and your feet flat on the floor. Dumbbells should be hanging down by your side. Inhale and curl the weights up to the shoulder, keeping palms up. Don't curl your wrists. Exhale and slowly lower. Repeat.

STANDING DUMBBELL CURL

Stand with feet shoulder-width apart and knees soft, holding a dumbbell in each hand. Dumbbells should be hanging down by your side. Inhale and curl both dumbbells up to the shoulders, making sure that the palms are facing upward during the curling action. Lower and repeat.

PREACHER BENCH CURL

Ⓐ Set the preacher bench pad at approximately 45 degrees. Sit in or lean against the preacher bench and grasp a barbell with both hands, palms facing up and hands shoulder-width apart. Keep the forearms resting tightly against the inclined pad. Ⓑ Breathe in and curl the barbell up until it comes close to your chin. Lower the weight with control to the start position and repeat.

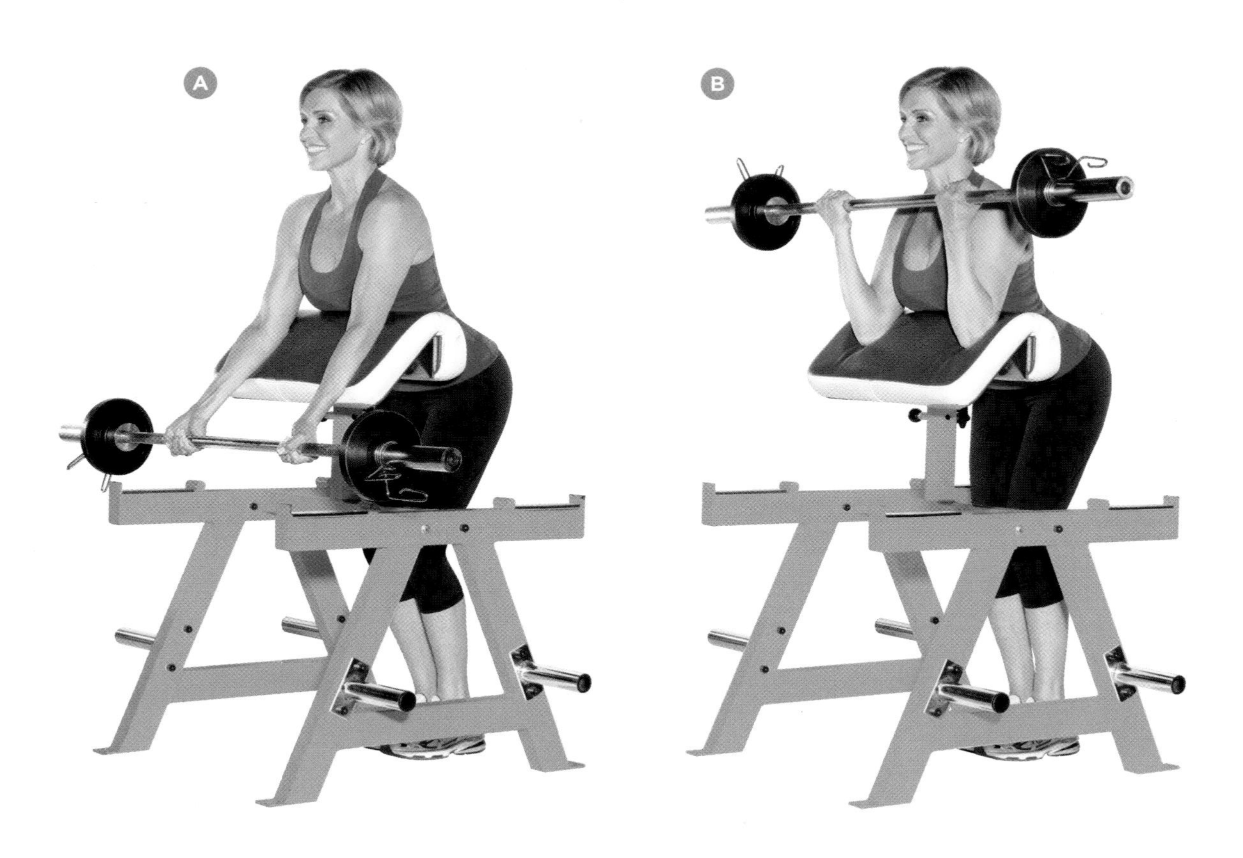

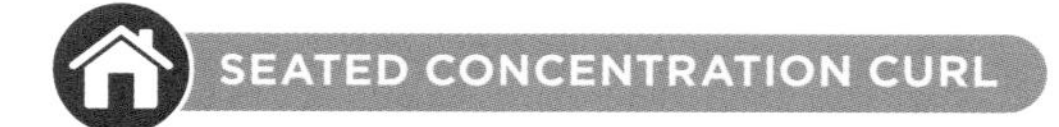

SEATED CONCENTRATION CURL

Sit at the end of a flat bench with your feet well apart. Place the elbow of your right arm against the inside of your thigh. In this leaning-forward position the dumbbell is in your right hand and resting on the floor. Curl the dumbbell up while locking the upper arm in place with the stability of the right leg. Palms are facing up. Lower and repeat. Work both arms with the same weight and number of sets and repetitions.

STANDING HAMMER CURL

Stand with your feet shoulder-width apart and knees soft, holding a dumbbell in each hand. Dumbbells should be hanging down by your side with the palms facing each other and thumbs uppermost. Curl the weights up, maintaining the thumbs-up position at all times. Lower the weights and repeat.

STANDING BARBELL CURL

Begin by standing with feet shoulder-width apart. Grasp a barbell so hands are also shoulder-width apart and palms are facing upward. The barbell should be hanging down by your upper thighs in the start position. Breathe in and curl the barbell up to your shoulders. Keep your back straight and legs and hips planted firmly for support. Lower the barbell to the start position and repeat.

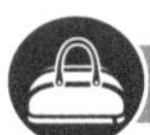

SINGLE-ARM LOW PULLEY CURL

Attach a handle to the lower pulley on a cable. Stand 1 ½ feet from the weight stack with feet shoulder-width apart and knees soft. Pick up the handle in your left hand, palm facing away. Stand and raise the weight until it comes to your upper thigh. Your right hand supports your left lower back. Curl the weight slowly toward your chest until the biceps is fully contracted. Lower with control to the start position and repeat.

WIDE-GRIP BARBELL CURL

Begin by standing with feet shoulder-width apart. Grasp a barbell so hands are as far apart as possible with palms facing upward. The barbell should be hanging down by your upper thighs in the start position. Breathe in and curl the barbell up to your shoulders. Keep your back straight and legs and hips planted firmly for support. Lower the barbell to the start position and repeat.

BENT-OVER CLOSE-GRIP BARBELL CURL

Begin by standing with feet shoulder-width apart. Grasp a barbell so hands are also shoulder-width apart and palms are facing upward. The barbell should be hanging down by your upper thighs in the start position. Bend over, keeping back flat and head up. Breathe in and curl the barbell up to your shoulders. Keep your back straight and legs and hips planted firmly for support. Lower the barbell to the start position and repeat.

STANDING MACHINE CALF RAISE

Ⓐ Stand in front of a standing calf machine. Place your shoulders underneath the shoulder pads of the machine and put your hands on the handles. Now step onto the foot plate with the balls of your feet and nothing else touching the plate. Your heels are hanging over the edge. Feet are shoulder-width apart and toes point forward. Ⓑ Lift the shoulder pads/weight by straightening up and then rising up on your toes using calf strength only. Lift your heels as high as you can. Lower until heels are pointing down as far as you can go. Return to start position and repeat.

A

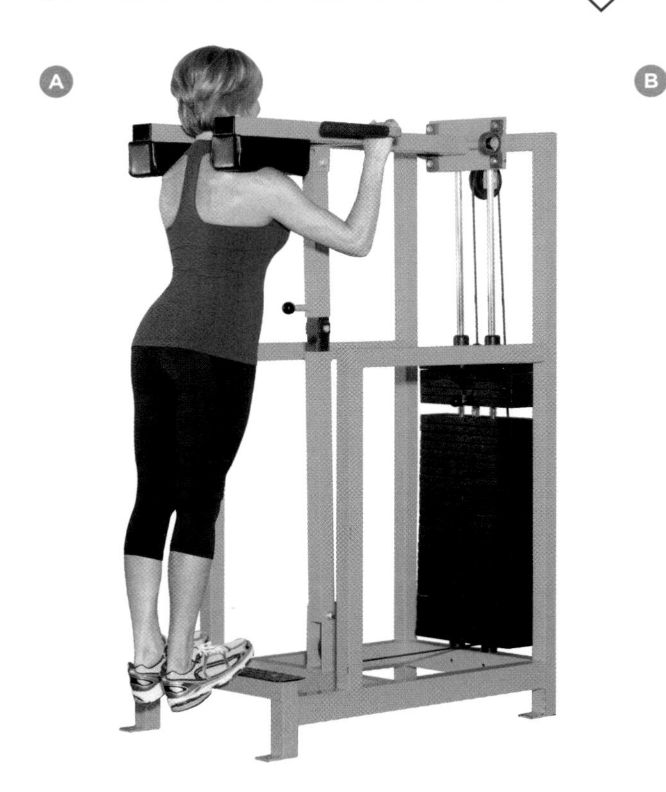

B

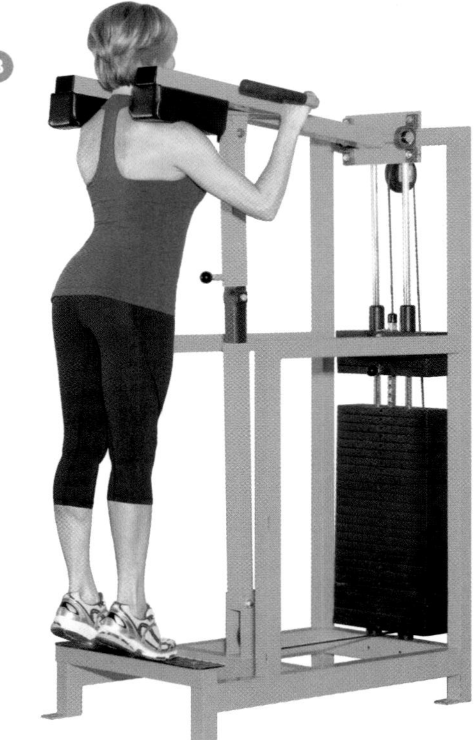

SINGLE-LEG CALF RAISE

Stand on the bottom step of a staircase holding on to the rail for support. Only the toes of your right foot should be on the step. Place your left foot behind your right ankle. Using calf strength only, raise yourself up until you are fully extended on your right foot. Lower yourself to the start position and repeat. Repeat the entire set of instructions for your left calf.

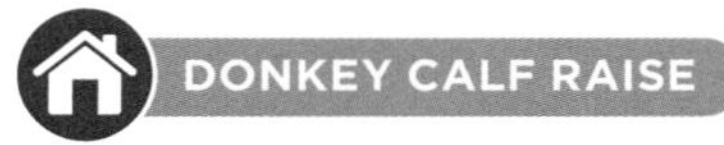

DONKEY CALF RAISE

Stand near a sturdy table or bench. Bend over at the waist, supporting your torso by placing your hands on the supporting surface you have chosen. Have a partner sit on your lower back. (Be sure the partner isn't too heavy for you.) Rise up on your toes, using calf strength to do so, until you are fully extended. Then lower yourself to start position and repeat.

STANDING CALF RAISE WITH DUMBBELL

Stand on the bottom step of a staircase holding on to the rail for support. The toes of both feet should be on the step. Grasp a dumbbell in your free hand and let it hang down by your side. Place your left foot behind your right ankle. Using calf strength only, raise yourself up until you are fully extended on both feet. Lower yourself to the start position and repeat. As an alternative, work each leg seperately, alternating sets on your right and left.

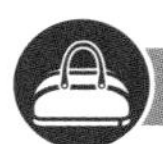

SEATED CALF RAISE

Ⓐ Sit up straight on the seated calf raise machine and tuck your knees securely under the kneepads. Place the balls of both feet on the footplate. Lift the kneepads/weight off the rest and into the start position. Ⓑ Release the weight resistance handle. Press up from the balls of your feet, your toes lifting your heels as high as they will go above the footplate. Breathe out and lower your heels below the footplate as far as you can. Repeat.

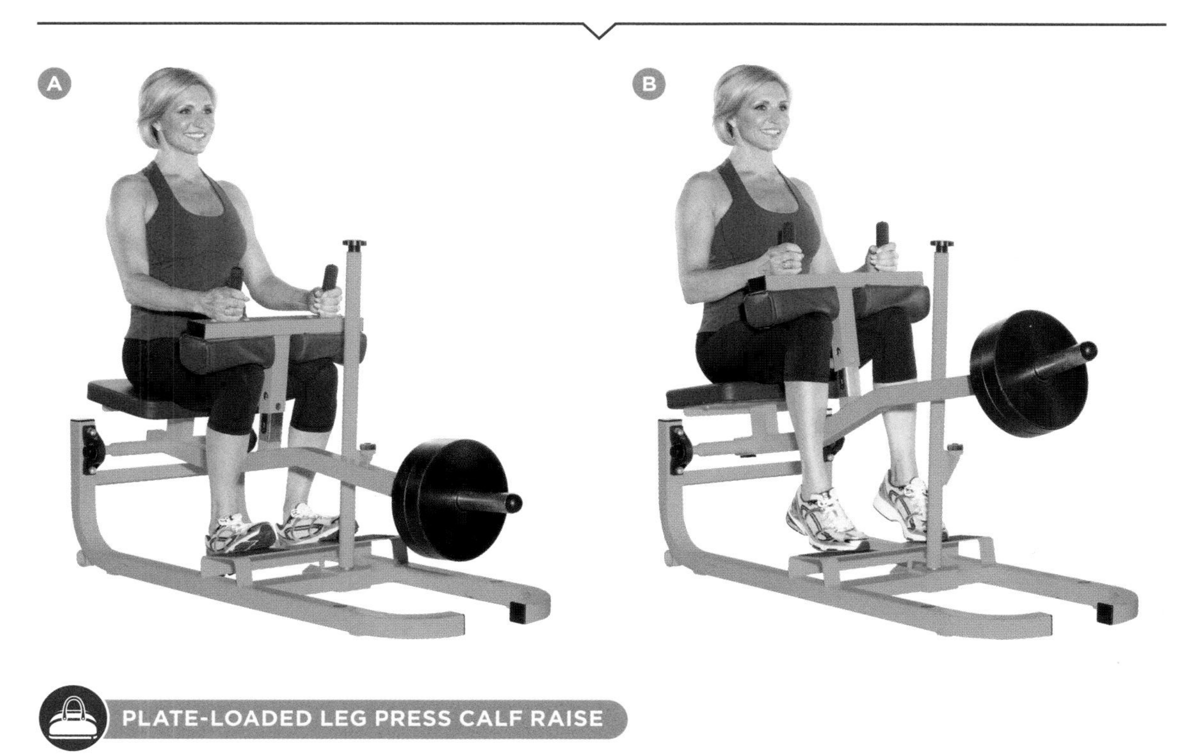

PLATE-LOADED LEG PRESS CALF RAISE

Sit in a leg press machine, tucking your butt firmly in the seat and placing your feet shoulder-width apart, toes and balls of feet only on the footplate. Release the rests and let the weight rest on the balls of your feet and your toes. Extend your feet, pressing the weight up with your toes and balls of feet. Lower the weight down and repeat.

SINGLE LEG SQUAT

Ⓐ Stand alongside a sturdy table or chair with one hand on top to balance. Ⓑ Extend your right leg out to the front while squatting down with your left leg. Return to standing position and repeat. Work both legs.

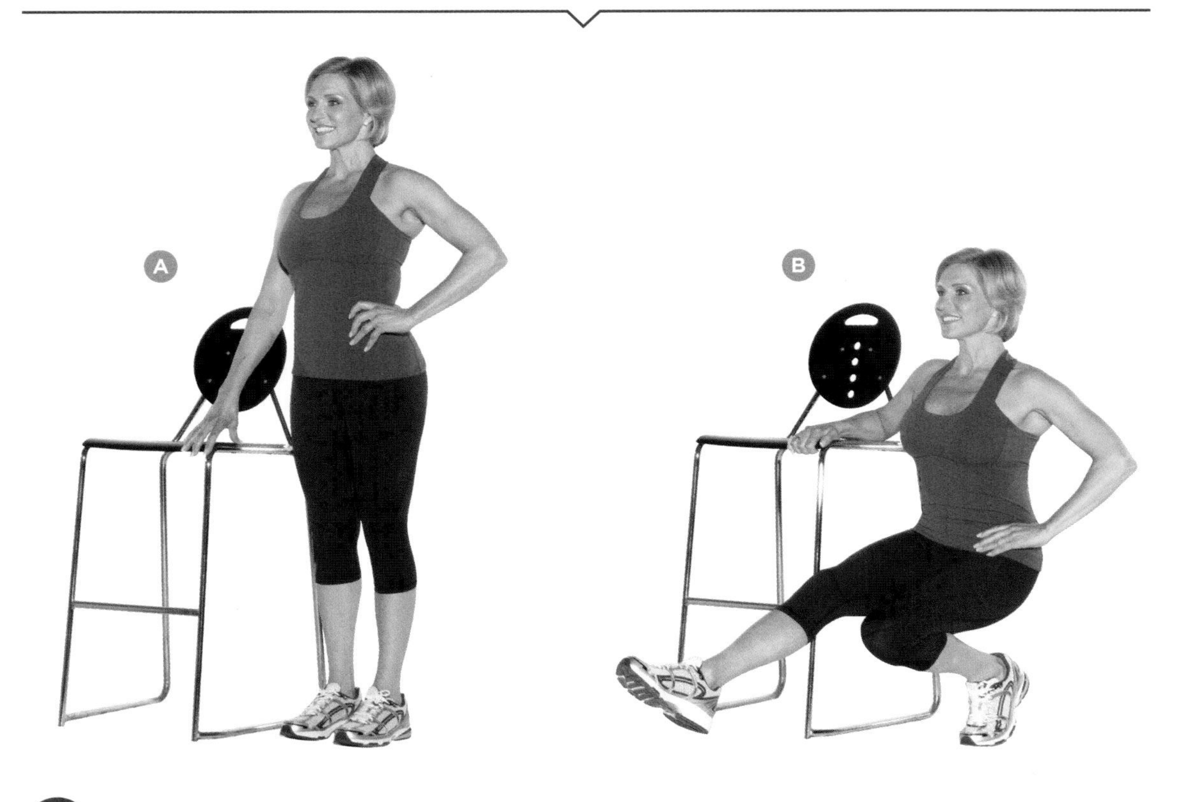

SQUAT WITHOUT WEIGHT

Place a 2" x 15" x 4" (approximately) board under your heels. Stand on the board, heels only, keeping the feet roughly shoulder-width apart while standing erect. Arms are placed behind your head. Keeping your head up and back flat, bend at the knees, lowering your butt down and out behind you until your upper thighs are parallel with the floor. Return to standing position and repeat.

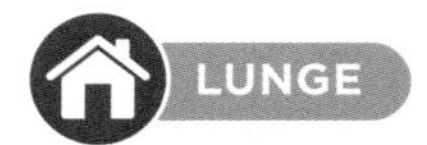

LUNGE

(Great for glutes, too.) Stand erect with feet together. Step forward with your left foot and sink to the floor so that your right knee is almost touching the floor. Return to upright start position and continue to work each leg, alternating the lunging action. Increase intensity by adding dumbbells.

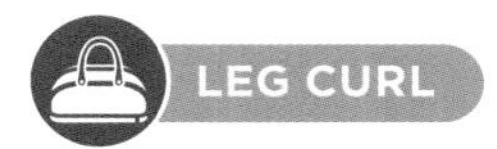

LEG CURL

Ⓐ Position yourself in the leg curl machine. If there are handles, you can grasp them. Place your calves under the calf pad. Ⓑ Slowly curl the legs/weight upward from a straight leg position until the leg bar touches the back of your hamstrings. Lower slowly and repeat.

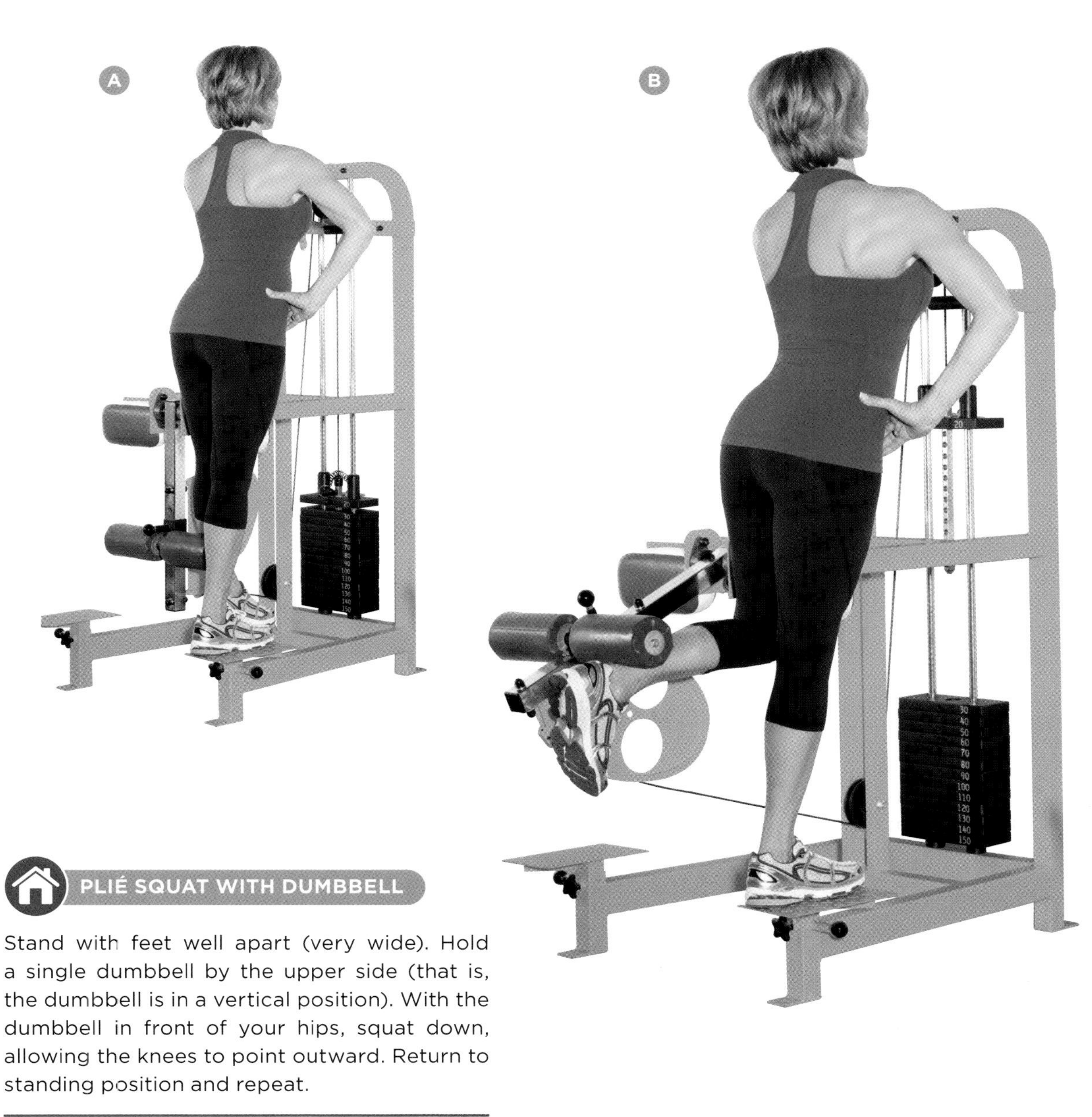

PLIÉ SQUAT WITH DUMBBELL

Stand with feet well apart (very wide). Hold a single dumbbell by the upper side (that is, the dumbbell is in a vertical position). With the dumbbell in front of your hips, squat down, allowing the knees to point outward. Return to standing position and repeat.

FRONT SQUAT ON SMITH MACHINE

Ⓐ Position a loaded Smith machine bar across your chest and shoulders in front of your neck. Cross your arms in front of your chest and rest your hands on the bar. Ⓑ With your back slightly arched and your head up, bend at the knees and hips to squat down until the upper legs are parallel to the floor. Return to upright position and repeat.

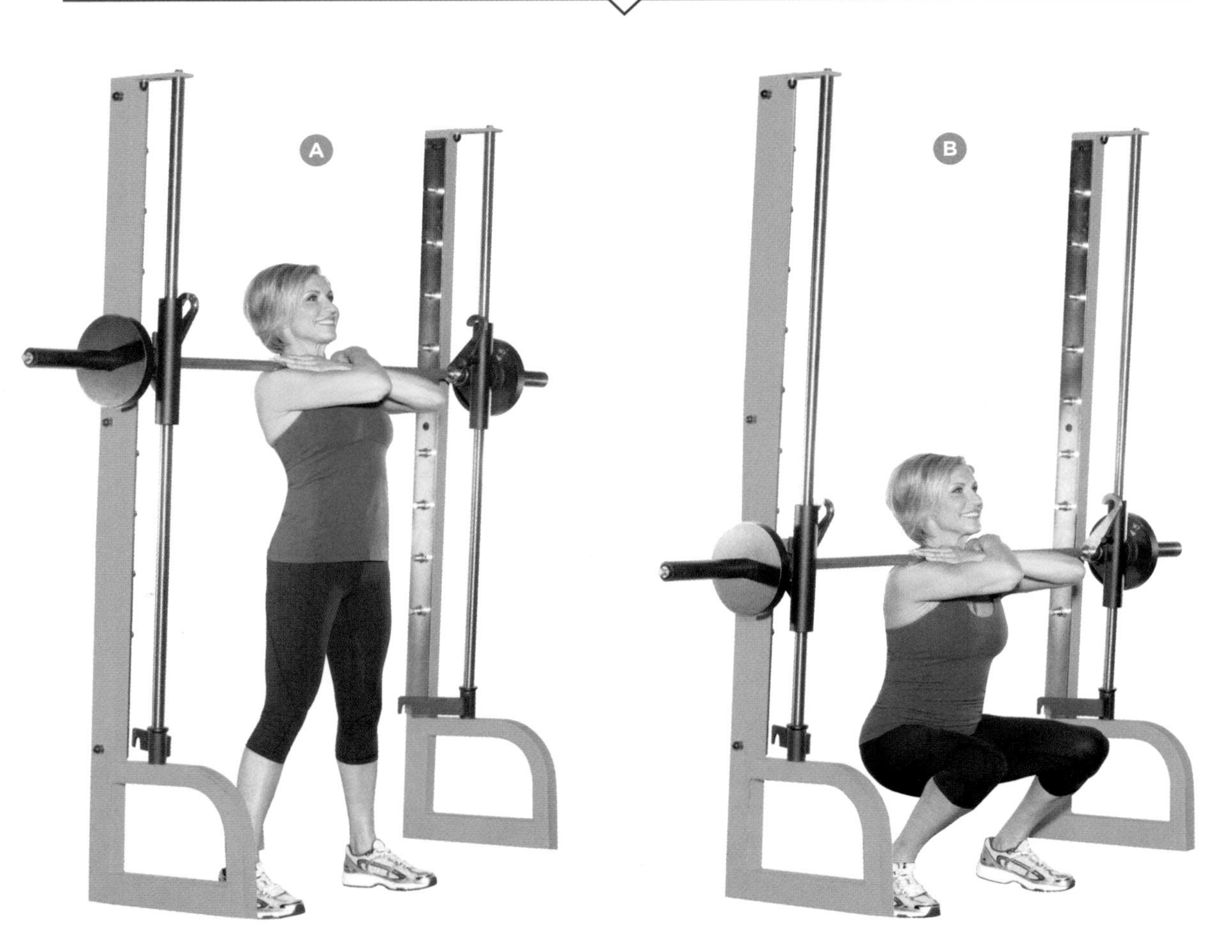

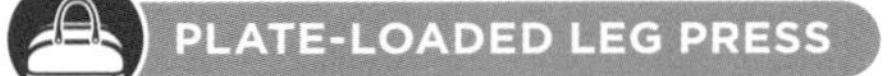

PLATE-LOADED LEG PRESS

Sit back in a 45-degree leg press machine. Make sure your back is tight against the backrest. Place your feet about shoulder-width apart on the footplate. Release the release handle. Lower the weight resistance until your knees are pulled tight into your chest. Press out and repeat.

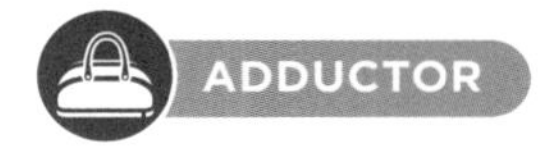

ADDUCTOR

Ⓐ Sit down in an adductor machine. Place legs on the pedals on either side of the seat. If the machine has handles, lightly grasp them. Ⓑ Slowly draw the legs close together against the resistance. Open and repeat.

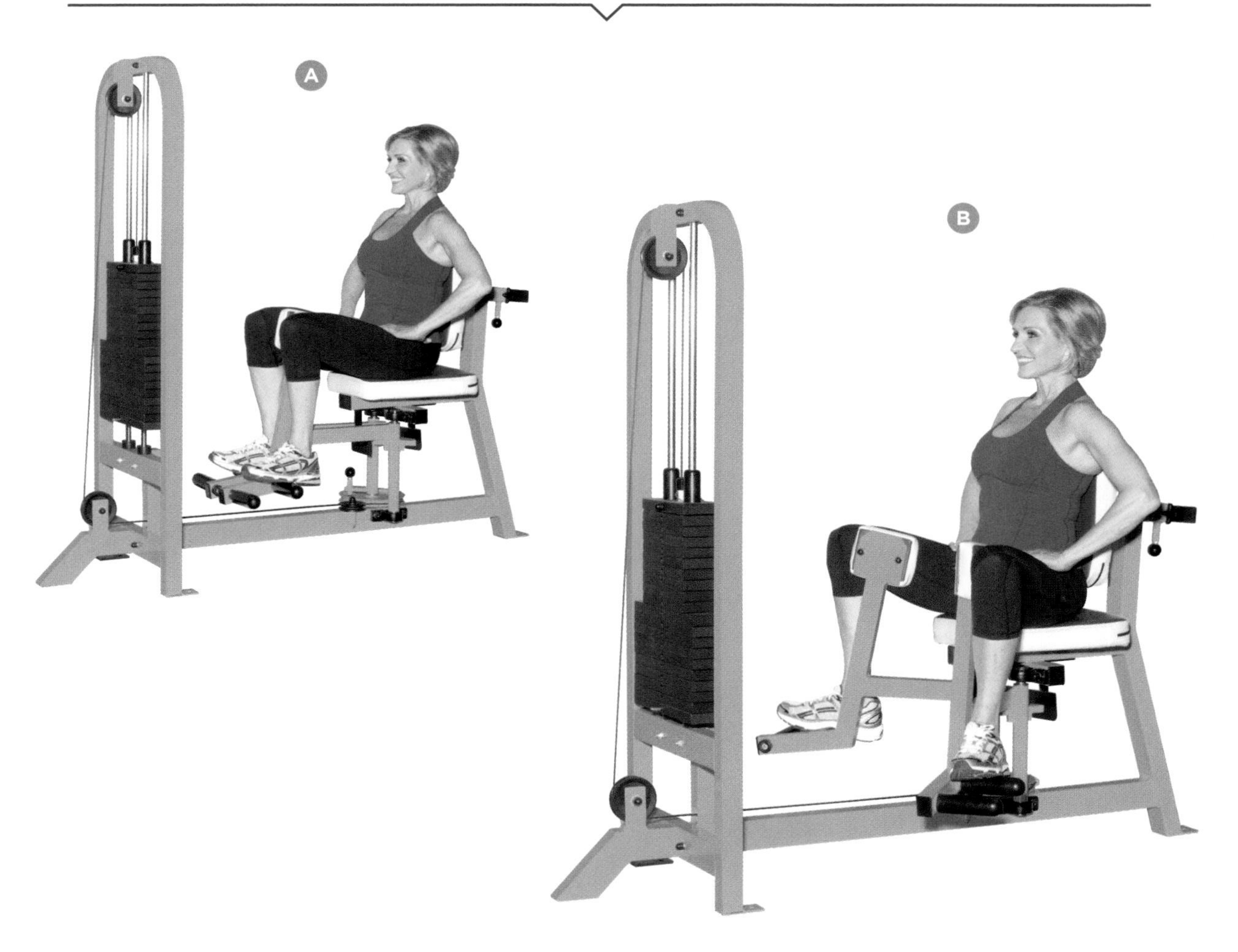

BARBELL BACK SQUAT

Take a loaded barbell from the squat stands and place it on shoulders behind neck. Palms are facing forward. Step back from the apparatus and, with back slightly arched and the weight over your feet, bend at the knees and hips to squat down, slowly and under control, until the upper thighs are parallel to the floor. Return to standing position and repeat. For beginners, a spotter is recommended.

MACHINE LEG EXTENSION

Ⓐ On a leg extension machine, adjust the backrest so your back is firm against it. Knees should hang over the seat. Adjust the shin pad so it sits tight against your ankles. Grip the handles on either side of you. Select a weight. Ⓑ Flex your feet and inhale as you lift the weight until your legs are fully extended in front of you. Exhale and lower the weight. Repeat.

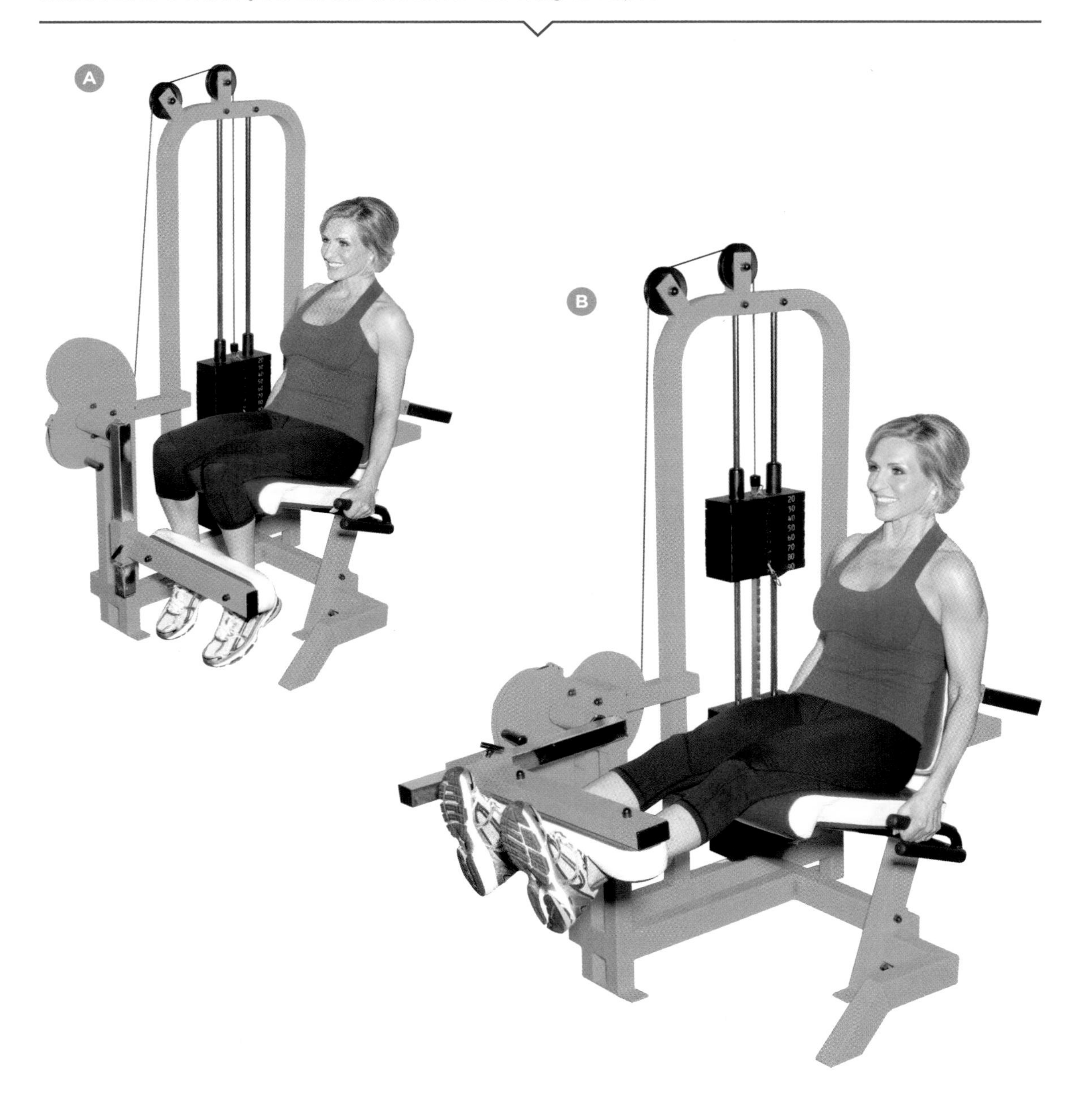

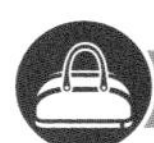

SMITH MACHINE WIDE-GRIP BENCH PRESS

Ⓐ Place a flat bench under the Smith machine bar. Load weights and lie on the bench faceup with your feet flat on the ground and the bar over you at about chest level. Hold the horizontal Smith machine bar with a wide overhand grip, hands shoulder-width apart. Lift the bar off the rests and lower it slowly to your chest. Ⓑ Keeping the arms in, close to the torso, press the bar upward from the chest to the arms-straight position. Lower and repeat. For beginners, a spotter is recommended.

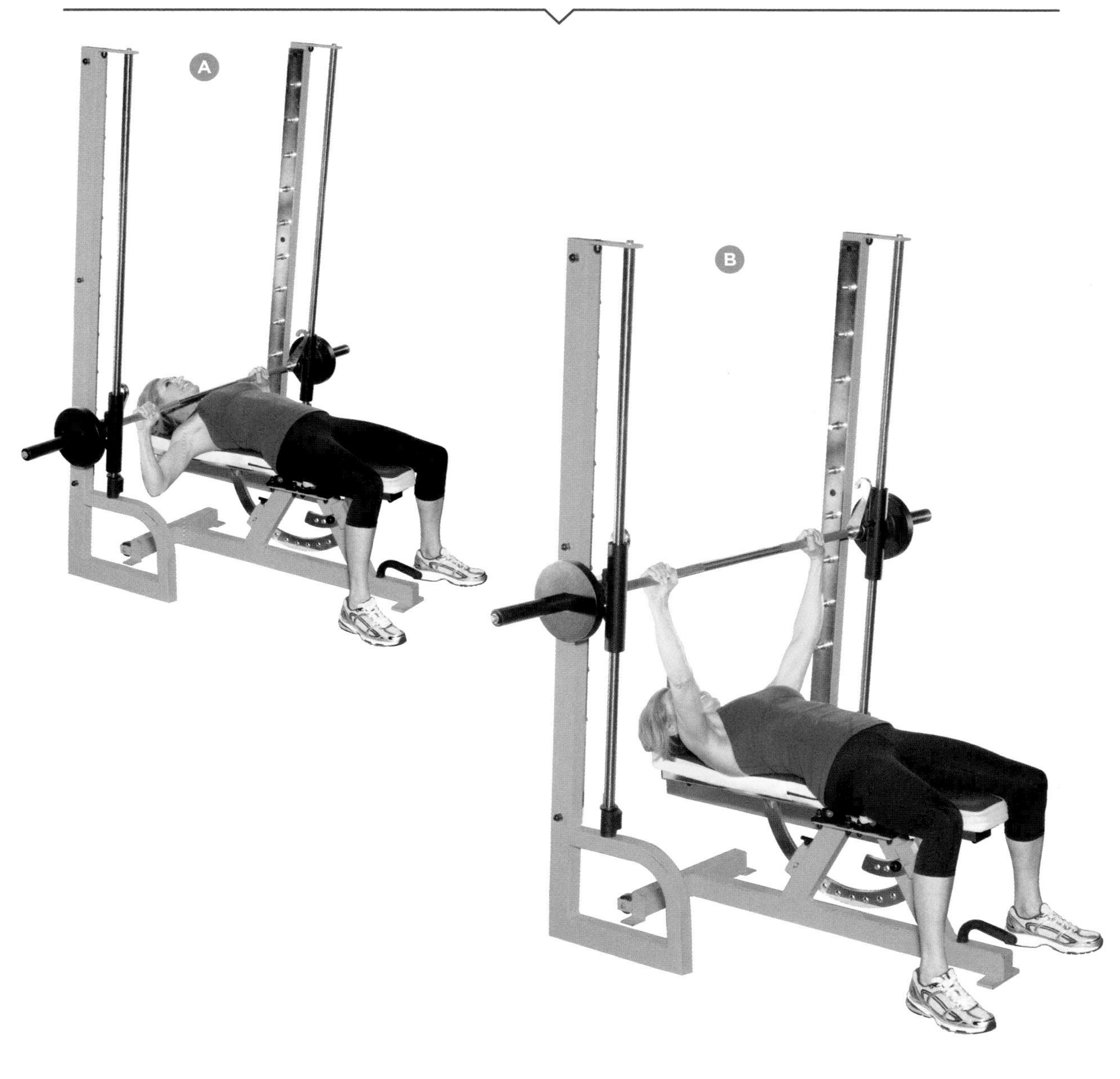

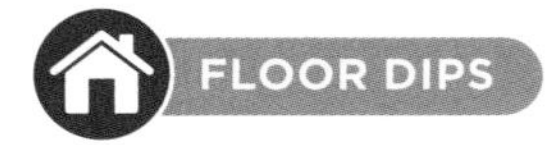

FLOOR DIPS

Support yourself facedown on the floor with both arms straight and set a little wider than shoulder-width apart. Feet are out behind you and your weight is resting on your toes. Keeping the butt up and the body stiff, lower into a dip until the face almost touches the floor. Press up to start position. Do not hinge at the waist. Repeat.

SUPINE DUMBBELL BENCH PRESS

Lie faceup on a flat bench, feet firmly planted on the floor. Hold a dumbbell in either hand, keeping arms bent and resting the weights lightly on your chest. Press both weights simultaneously straight up to arm's length above shoulders using control. Lower and repeat.

STRAIGHT-ARM PULLOVER

Lie on your back on a flat bench. Grasp a barbell with hands shoulder-width apart and at arm's length above your chest. Keeping the arms straight, lower the bar behind your head as far as possible. Return to start position and repeat.

ROUND THE WORLD

Lie on your back on a flat bench holding a dumbbell in each hand. With your legs bent and feet flat on the ground, take the dumbbells from the upper legs to behind the head. Return to upper legs and repeat.

SUPINE DUMBBELL FLY

Sit on the end of a flat bench with feet planted firmly on the floor, holding a dumbbell in each hand resting on your upper thighs. Lie down on the bench, letting the dumbbells lift off your thighs. Press the dumbbells to arm's length above the chest. Unlock the elbows slightly and maintain this arm position while lowering the arms out to the side so that the chest muscles are fully stretched. Return to start position and repeat.

INCLINE DUMBBELL BENCH PRESS

Ⓐ Lie faceup on an incline bench set at approximately 40 degrees. With elbows bent, hold a dumbbell in each hand, palms facing forward, at shoulder level. Ⓑ Press the dumbbells upward, keeping the palms facing out, until the arms are straight and fully extended. Lower and repeat.

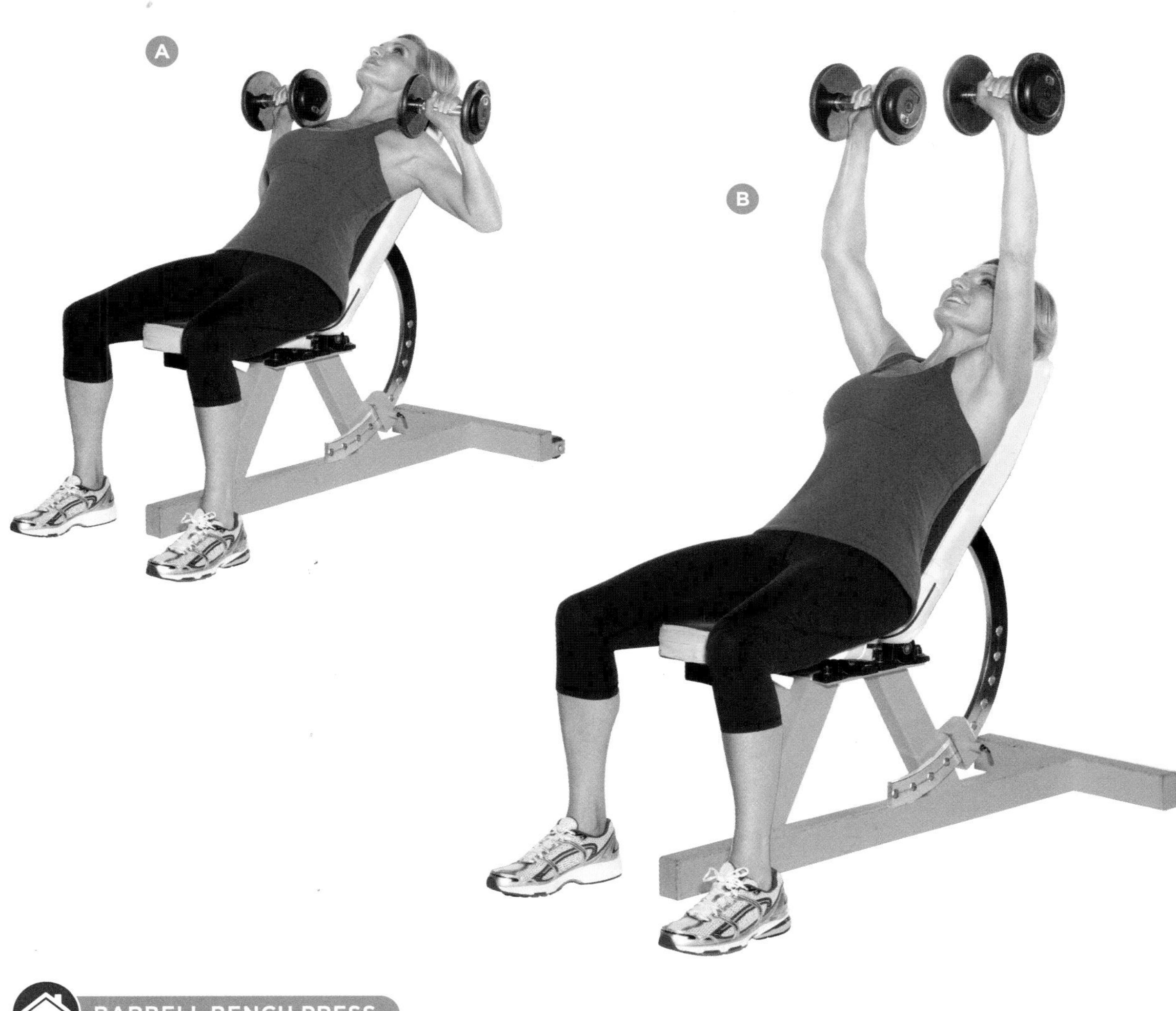

BARBELL BENCH PRESS

Lie faceup on a flat bench. Grip a loaded barbell with hands shoulder-width apart. Breathe in and lift the bar to the start position, resting lightly on your chest. Exhale as you press the bar up until arms are fully extended directly over your chest. Inhale and let the bar come down slowly. Repeat.

CROSSOVER PULLEY

Ⓐ Attach handles to either side of a twin cable pulley machine and set the cables to their highest height. Stand halfway in between the uprights with a handle attached to a cable in either hand. Lean slightly forward from the waist. Ⓑ With elbows bent and arms extended away from your sides as your start position, begin to pull the cables across your chest until the handles meet in front of you. Maintain the contraction for a few seconds. Slowly bring the arms back to the start position. Repeat.

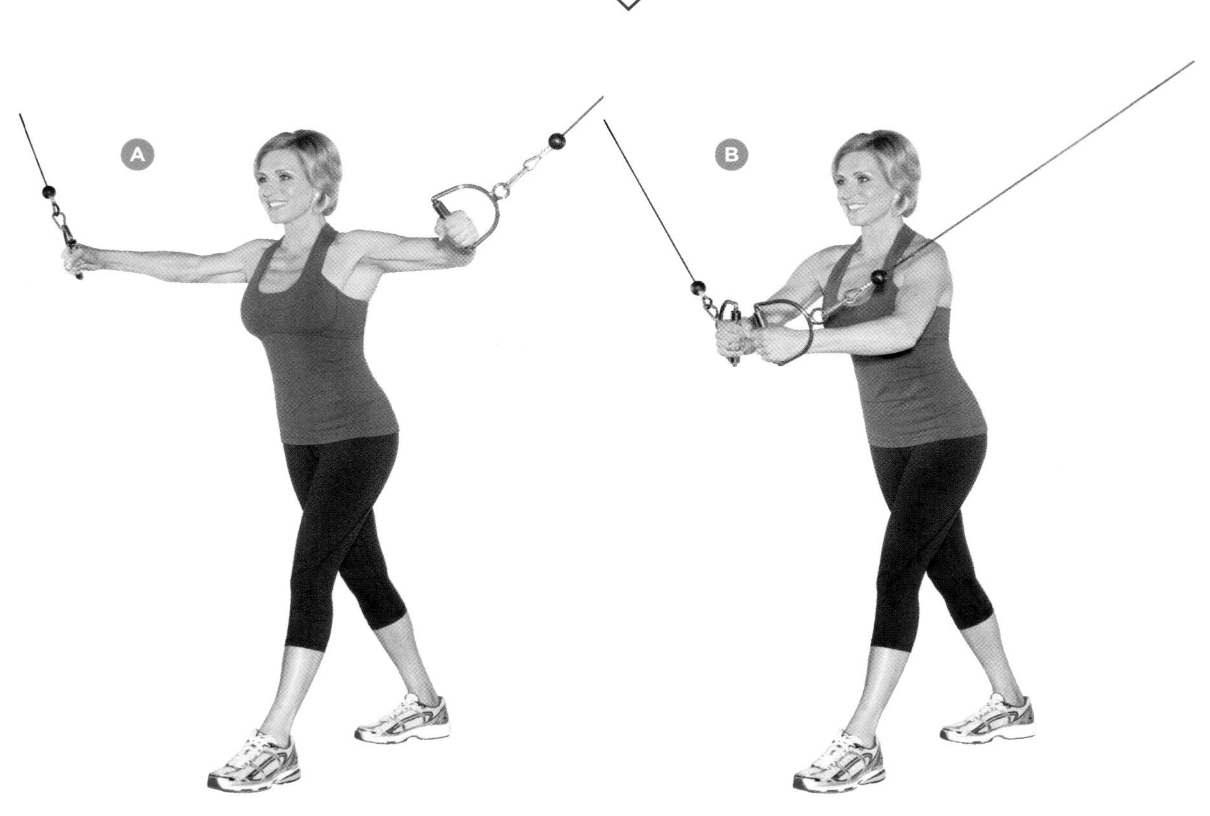

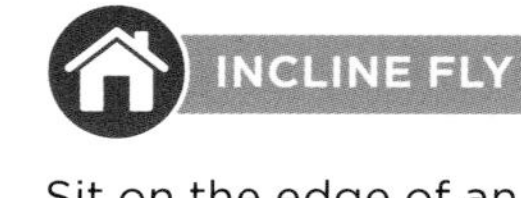

INCLINE FLY

Sit on the edge of an incline bench holding a dumbbell in each hand, feet flat on the floor and body facing out. Lie back on the bench as you raise the dumbbells off your upper thighs, palms facing each other. Press the dumbbell up straight above the chest and let the elbows bend slightly. Lower the dumbbells out to the side, maintaining a slight bend in the arms. Bring the dumbbells up to the start position and repeat.

FACEDOWN LEG RAISE

Lie on the floor facedown, arms by your sides. Raise your right leg, keeping it reasonably straight as you lift it to its highest point. Lower and repeat. Work the left leg in the same manner.

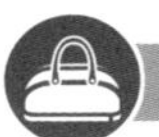

PRONE HYPEREXTENSION WITH OR WITHOUT WEIGHT

(A) Position yourself in a Roman chair so that your thighs are flat against the pads and your feet are shoulder-width apart on the footplate. You should be facing forward in the machine. Place your hands behind your head whether you are holding weight or not. Lean forward. (B) Bend at the hips until your head is pointing down to the floor. You will be at about a 60-degree angle. Slowly return to the start position. Repeat.

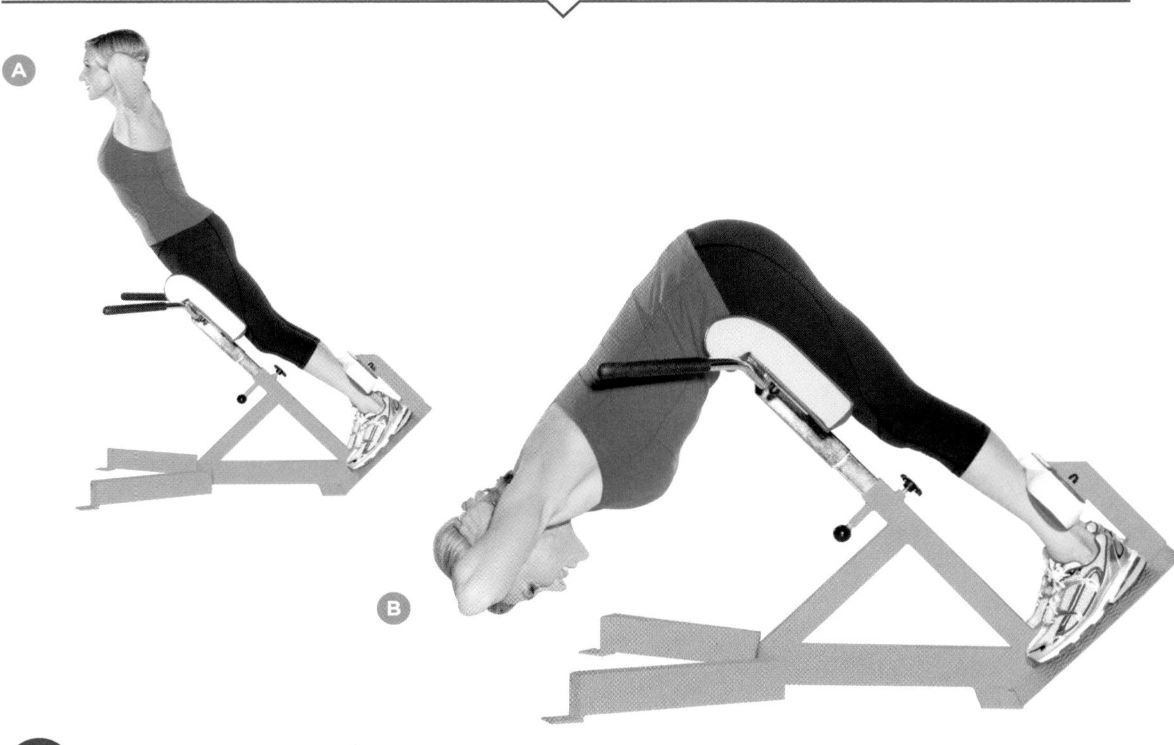

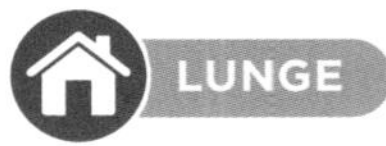

LUNGE

Stand erect with feet together. Step forward with your left foot and sink to the floor so that your right knee is almost touching the floor. Return to upright start position and continue to work each leg alternating the lunging action. Increase intensity by adding dumbbells.

GLUTES

STIFF-LEG DEADLIFT

Stand erect holding a loaded barbell in front of your upper legs at arm's length. Grip is overhand, palms facing down, and hands are shoulder-width apart. Lower the weight to the floor by bending forward at the waist, keeping the legs and back straight. The barbell should now be hanging down at arm's length directly below your shoulders. Keeping your knees tight, slowly return to the start position. The barbell is now hanging in front of your upper thighs. Repeat.

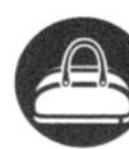

KNEELING CABLE KICKBACK

Ⓐ Position a flat bench lengthwise in front of a pulley machine. Set the pulley at its lowest position. Attach an ankle cuff to the pulley. Attach the ankle cuff to your left leg. Kneel on the bench with your right leg and plant your right arm firmly in front of you or grasp the upright for support. Ⓑ Keeping the left leg straight and free of the bench, kick slowly backward, taking the leg to its fullest range of movement. Lower and repeat. Work the right leg in a similar manner.

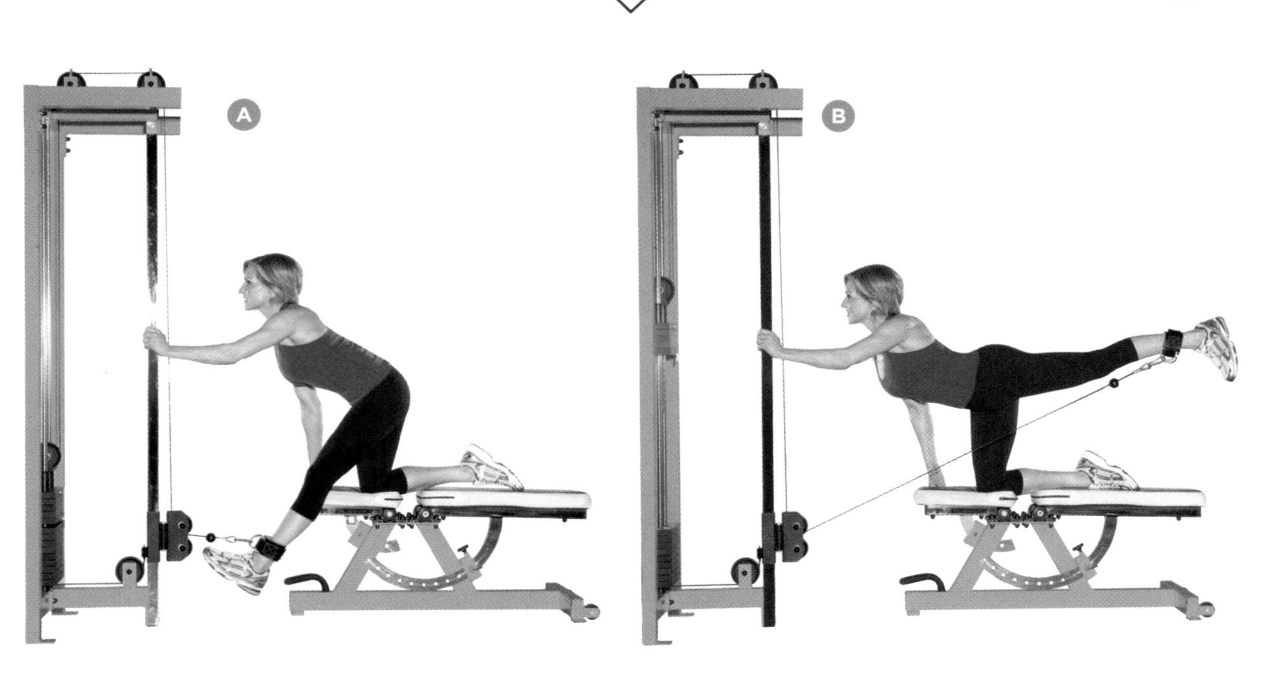

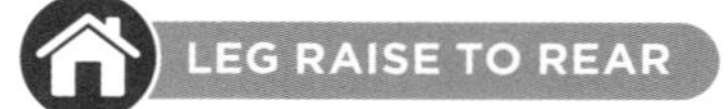

LEG RAISE TO REAR

Stand upright, holding on to a support for balance. Using the strength of your glutes only, raise your right leg backward, keeping it straight, and lift your leg as far as it will go. Lower to start position and repeat. Work the left leg in the same manner.

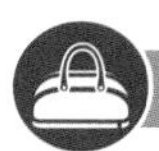

STANDING CABLE KICKBACK

Ⓐ Position yourself in front of a pulley machine. Set the pulley at its lowest position. Attach an ankle cuff to the pulley and then attach the cuff to your left ankle. Stand facing the cable machine. You may lean forward to grasp an upright to help maintain your balance. Ⓑ Kick the left foot backward through its entire range of movement. Lower and repeat. Work right leg in a similar manner.

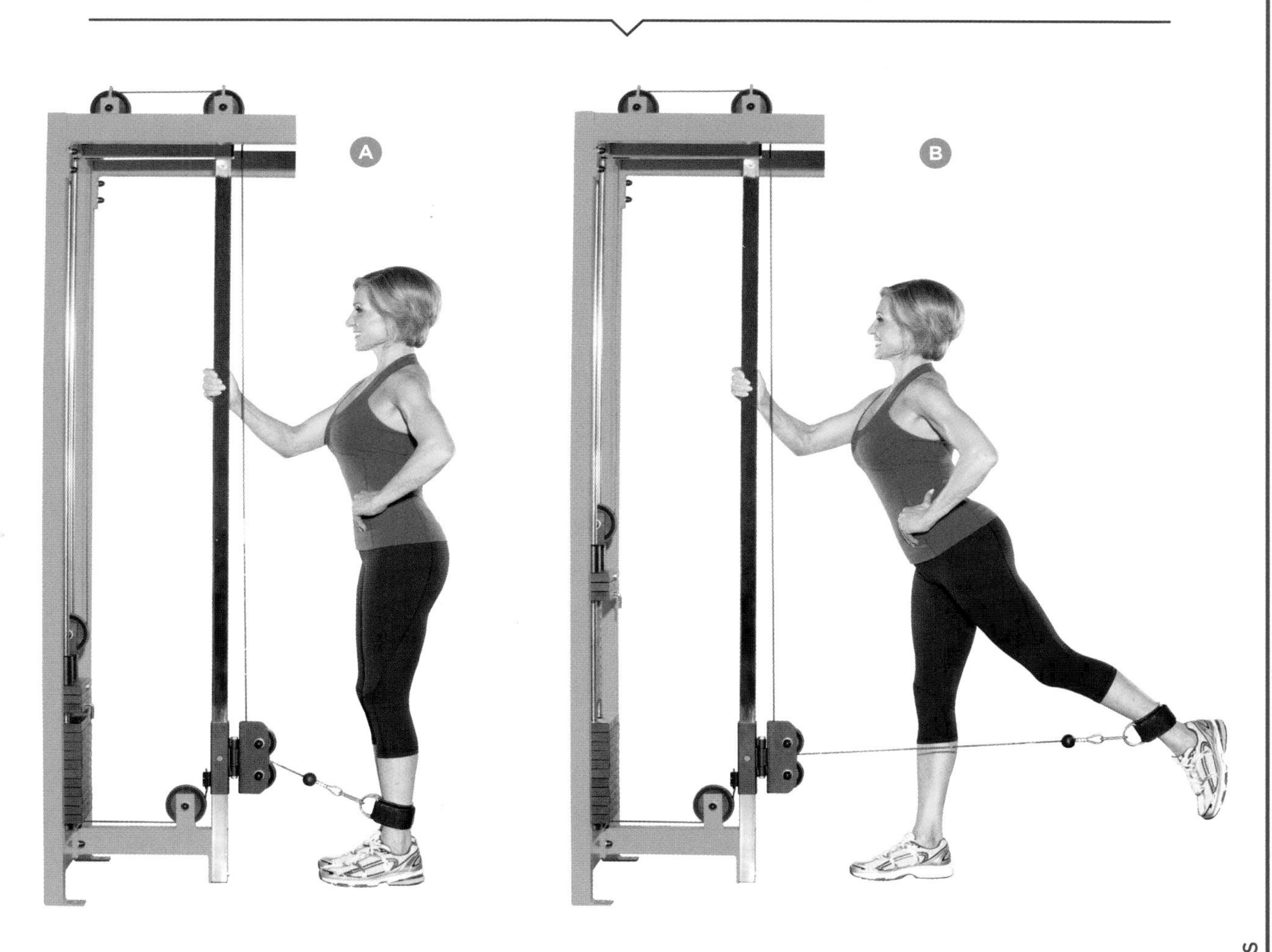

BUTT MACHINE KICKBACK

Adopt the position as shown in the butt machine directions. Press or curl the weight stack resistance according to the individual mechanics of the machine.

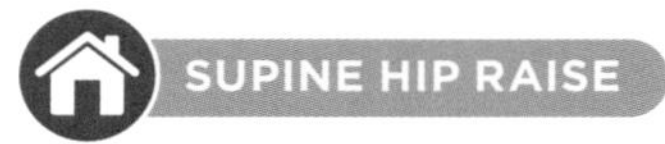

SUPINE HIP RAISE

Ⓐ Lie on the floor with your legs apart and knees drawn toward your body. Ⓑ Using the strength of your glutes only, raise your hips as high as possible. Hold the contraction and then slowly lower and repeat.

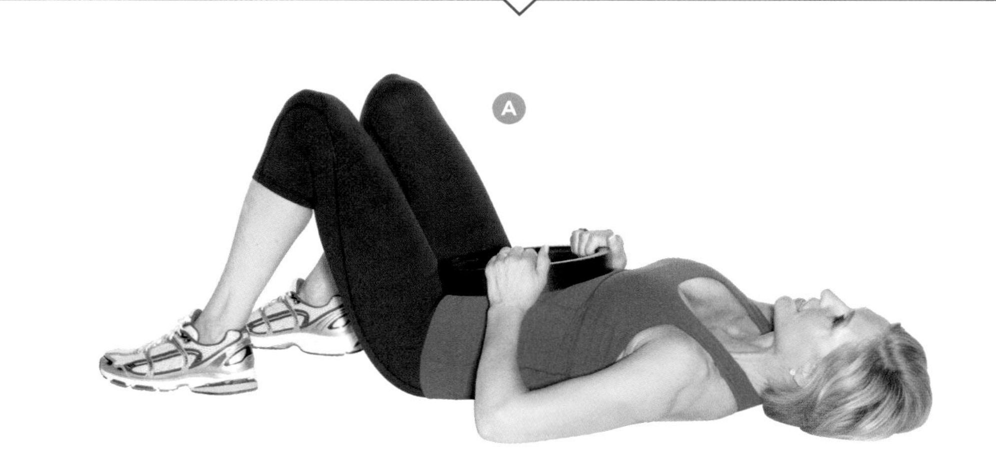

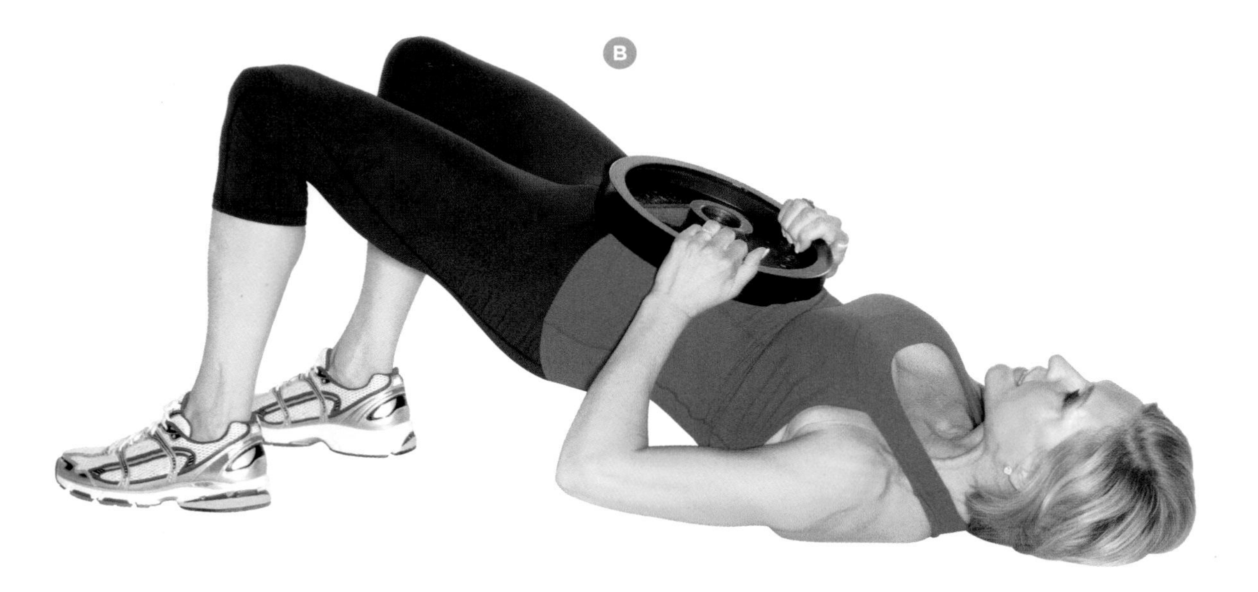

BEST BODY NOW Fitness Benefits

What are some of the lean body benefits you'll experience from this strength-training plan?

A revved-up metabolism
Lean, sculpted muscles and an overall tighter physique
Greater flexibility
Unlimited energy
Better posture
Sounder sleep
Rock-solid self-esteem
A boost in the libido with a body to match
Increased stamina and endurance
A greater desire to be active
Greater concentration
Improved health and immunity

While your muscles respond to the Best Body Now eating and training program, your self-esteem simultaneously experiences a significant boost as well. There is something satisfying about spending time in the gym with just you and the weights if you can see past the notion that gym time is punishment. Your diligence and commitment will help you get the job done, which can't help but produce an empowering sense of accomplishment. I haven't seen anyone come out of a gym with less confidence.

I haven't seen anyone come out of a gym with less confidence.

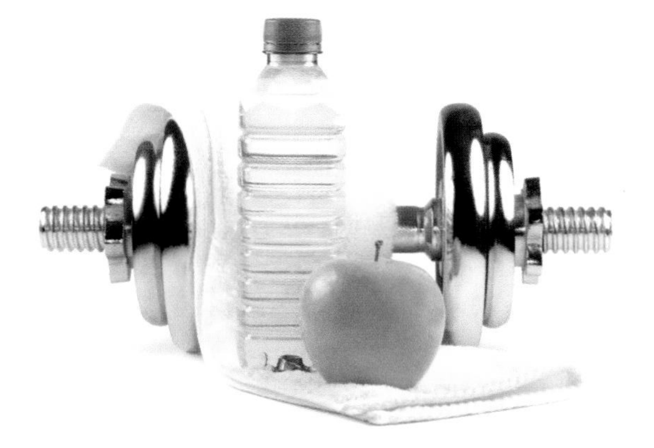

TAILORED FITNESS GUIDELINES FOR EVERY AGE

THE BASICS OF THE BEST BODY NOW FITNESS PLAN REMAIN THE SAME for every age, and the more you practice them, the more they become healthy habits that will stay with you for the rest of your life. However, the body is supremely adaptive, and you will have to make a concerted effort to stay ahead of this adaptive response by tweaking the regimen as your body evolves and your muscles adapt to the program. Next, we'll look at how your fitness needs evolve in your thirties, forties, fifties and beyond and how to leverage savvy workout strategies to create your Best Body Now at any age.

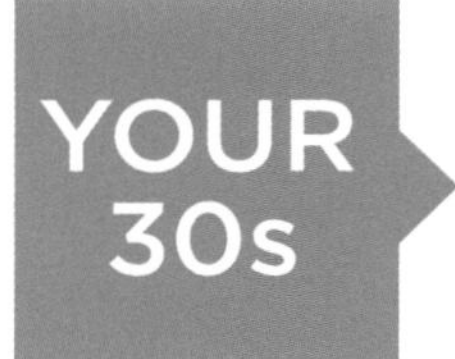

Start Strength-Building, Life-Enhancing Healthy Habits

In my thirties, I was completely out of touch with my body and didn't realize how my body was changing as I got older or that I had the power to prevent or lessen the aging process through improved nutrition and fitness. Although I went to the gym, it was by no means with regularity. My fitness routine lacked both *fitness* and *routine*—forget commitment, forget focus and forget consistency. The result was bouts of weight loss and gain, with no real physique or tone. Everything about me suffered, from my self-esteem to my appearance to my zest for life, and ultimately my health as well. I felt tired, weak and depressed. And, frankly, spending time in the gym rather than with my family wasn't an option. When I finally learned to make myself a priority, I began working out and making better decisions about what's right for my body and health. The result? I set myself up for robust health, an incredible physique and energy that you'll have to experience yourself to believe. Stay tuned, because with the Best Body Now program you are about to experience the same for yourself.

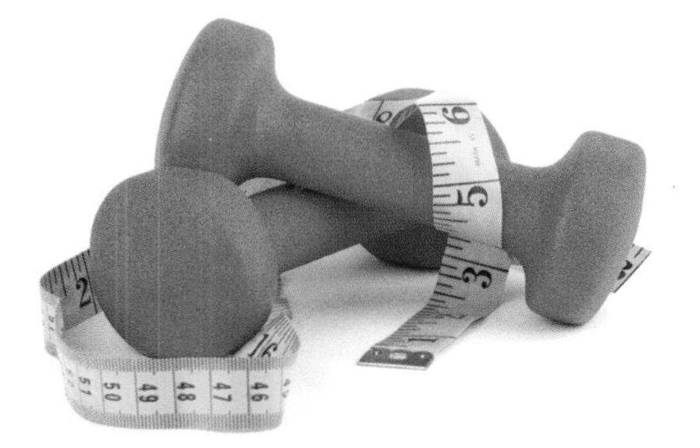

YOUR 30s What's Happening in Your 30s That Impacts Your Fitness Needs

Significant life changes can increase your anxiety level, including such milestones as marriage or divorce, pregnancy, young children, job relocations, career advancement and much more, which can cause you to skip workouts. An on-the-go life often means that family comes first and gym time last, if at all.

Busy work schedules, multitasking and fast-paced lifestyles can cause stress and anxiety, which triggers a fight-or-flight response in your body that in turn increases levels of cortisol, a hormone produced by the adrenal glands in response to stressful situations. A study in *Psychosomatic Medicine* has shown this hormone can cause weight gain, particularly in your abdominal area, over time.

Naturally occurring bone loss, which can weaken bones and lead to osteoporosis and fractures, begins in your thirties and can increase more rapidly through lack of exercise or a sedentary lifestyle. Strength training, however, builds muscles, which in turn improves bone density and prevents breaks. That's because when muscles contract, they pull on bone, which increases circulation and triggers bone cell growth that eventually increases mass.

More items on the to-do list can result in fewer hours of sleep each night, which means you're more likely to cancel a sweat session if you feel tired. Less sleep also contributes to weight gain.

THE FIX? New Fitness Strategies for Your 30s:

1 PLAN WORKOUTS EACH WEEK. Know before the week starts when you'll work out, and carve that time into your calendar so that exercise doesn't become the first item you skip when multitasking gets out of control. I always have a plan B in case life gets in the way of my schedule. This ensures that momentum isn't lost and that focus isn't lessened, especially in the beginning, when new habits must be carefully nurtured.

2 ADD CARDIO SESSIONS ONE OR TWO TIMES A WEEK. In addition to pumping iron, add a couple of thirty-minute bursts of cardio activity each week. Studies, including one published in *Journal of Family* *and Reproductive Health*, suggest that regular aerobic activity can reduce the effects of premenstrual syndrome (PMS), such as bloating, pain, irritability, fatigue and more. Heart-pumping workouts at any age also contribute to a reduced risk for cancer and cardiovascular disease by lowering your weight, blood pressure, cholesterol and more. Even if you only look at cardiovascular exercise from an emotional perspective, engaging in it in some form regularly makes you feel vital and more content with your life. This is a good thing!

3 INCORPORATE INTERVAL TRAINING. To maximize fat burning, especially if you're only doing a quick thirty-minute lifting session, add intervals, which are short bursts of cardiovascular activity, between strength-training sets to get your heart rate up. I like to alternate between jumping rope, doing lunges or squats with hops, jumping jacks and more. Start with thirty-second breaks between weight sets and mix it up. Don't be afraid to employ interval training while lifting, too. Do three regular-paced repetitions of an exercise followed by three faster-paced ones, three more regular-paced, and finally three more faster ones. You'll notice a difference in intensity by training this way.

4 TONE TROUBLE SPOTS EACH WEEK. Even if you don't have many stubborn areas yet, this is the time to start focusing on those notorious trouble spots, like the abs, glutes and triceps. Start focusing on those difficult areas by training them at least one more time each week in addition to the basic plan outlined in the beginning, to prevent sagging before it starts. For example, if glutes are your trouble spot, instead of training them only on day 5, add three more sets on another training day so you're working them twice in one week.

5 RETHINK FITNESS AS A LIFESTYLE, NOT JUST A WORKOUT. In weeks when I'm unusually busy, I'll just squeeze in heart-pumping exercise where I can. The American College of Sports Medicine and the American Heart Association agree that this strategy is effective. They've updated their physical activity guidelines to include that cardiovascular activity can actually accumulate during the day, rather than having to be done all at once.

TOSCA TIDBIT

Training time is Tosca time. This means all distracting gadgets—phones, PDAs, pagers—are off. Make your workouts "me time," too, for the best results.

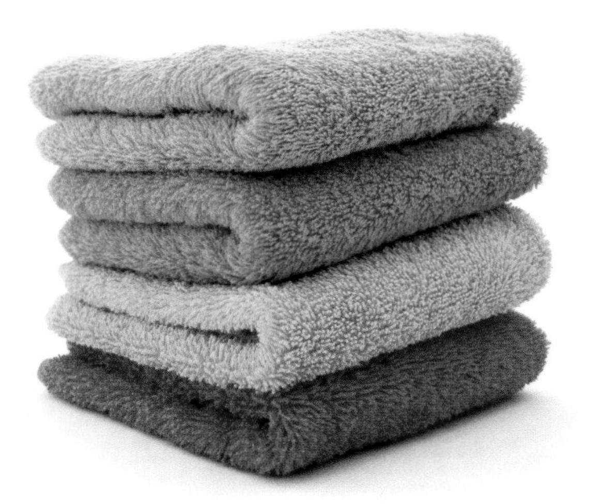

This means you can take a ten-minute walk to work, a ten-minute walk break at lunch and another ten-minute bike ride with the family after dinner for a total of thirty minutes daily. Start to identify areas where you can add more calorie-burning sessions, even if just short bouts, including climbing stairs, walking to the grocery store or doing laps around the school football field while you wait to pick up your kids. Because cardio minutes add up and because the benefits of just living a healthy life are cumulative, try to replace sedentary minutes with fun activities, such as dancing, kicking around a soccer ball, playing the Wii or chasing your toddler around the park—this is a smart way to get your family moving, too.

6 KEEP A GYM BAG HANDY. If you're always running errands and juggling a million agenda items, keep a gym bag in various places—your office, the house, the car—so that when you get some time to spare, you can be prepared for a workout anytime. Even if you've just got an extra fifteen minutes, lace up your sneakers and go for a quick walk. Every little bit counts, and at the end of the day, if you've logged additional walking minutes, you're that much closer to your Best Body Now goals.

> Take classes that challenge you to learn new exercises or move muscles in a different way.

7 EXERCISE WHEN YOUR BODY HAS THE MOST ENERGY. If you wake up with boundless energy, work with your natural biorhythms and try to get your workouts in early. On the other hand, if you tend to have more energy midway through the day, move your routine to lunch or after work. If you work with your normal energy levels, you'll be more likely to get motivated to exercise and to remain that way.

8 ADD YOGA FOR STRESS RELIEF. A smart way to reduce anxiety while still toning muscles is practicing yoga. The practice has been shown in studies, such as the one published in *Complementary Therapies in Clinical Practice*, to have a calming effect on the body, in addition to creating lean, gorgeous muscle tone. Putting at least one class a week on your schedule can help you create a calm, stress-free week, while improving your balance and flexibility at the same time. Legions of celebs including Madonna, Jennifer Aniston and Christy Turlington rely on yoga to help create noteworthy physiques.

9 TRY NEW ACTIVITIES TO STAY MOTIVATED AND ENGAGED.

Take classes that challenge you to learn new exercises or move muscles in a different way. You'll get more comfortable with the gym and socialize with a community of like-minded people when you stretch yourself into new adventures. You may find that you fall in love with a new sport or discover a skill you didn't know you had.

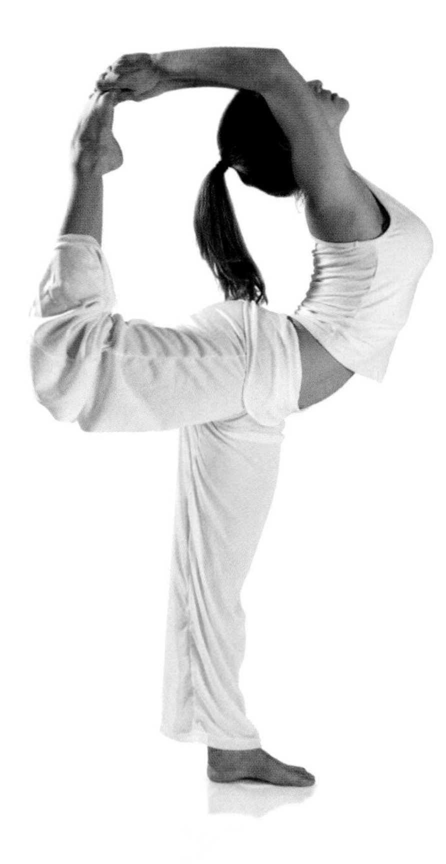

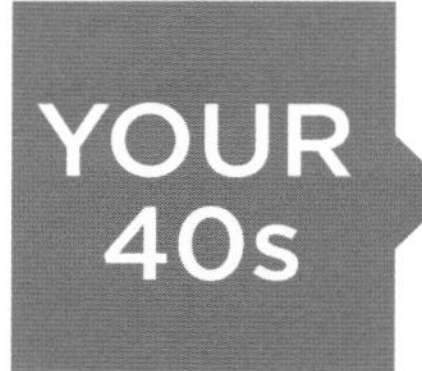

Protect Against Aging-Related Health Risks and Diseases

Although when I began working out in my late thirties my focus was cardio, by the time I reached my forties, I began to incorporate more strength training and saw incredible results. My new plan allowed me to combat much of what people think is the natural physiological decline of the body, strength and endurance that happens when we age. Natural decline? This couldn't be further from the truth. I'm actually doing more physically now than I was in my twenties. Over the past decade, I've watched my body continue to respond to my challenging it with new moves and more weight training. I remain intensely focused on each exercise and committed to a healthy, active lifestyle. Even though I'm ten years older now, I'm using the same principles, but with a few tweaks to respond to my body's changing needs, and the results are better than ever.

YOUR 40s

What's Happening in Your 40s That Impacts Your Fitness Needs

- Hormone changes related to perimenopause, the time when the body begins to transition into menopause, include irritability, depression, fatigue, weight gain and more, all of which can be successfully combated through exercise.

Exercise can help reduce cancer risk.

Heart disease risk and stroke risk in women increase with age. Major contributing risk factors include being overweight, high cholesterol and high blood pressure, which can be prevented or lessened by working out.

Cancer risk increases with age. The most prevalent types of cancer in women, including breast, lung, colorectal, uterine and ovarian, tend to appear in the forties on average. These cancers are all linked to obesity, among other unhealthy lifestyle factors, including being sedentary. Some studies, such as one from the University of Wisconsin, have shown that exercise can help reduce cancer risk.

Changes in our brain happen earlier than we think. Remember, in a study published in *Nature*, researchers from Harvard and the Children's Hospital Boston have shown aging can begin impacting brain function as early as forty, including slowing or affecting changes in memory, learning ability and attention span. Research has found that exercise can improve concentration levels, memory and information retention.

Because the metabolism begins to slow down in the thirties at a rate of about 2 to 5 percent every ten years, you burn between 50 and 100 fewer calories a day. By the time you reach your forties, you're losing as much as 8 percent of your muscle mass every decade, contributing to the gradual decline in the body's natural fat-burning capacity. This is another significant reason to lift weights, since increased muscle mass in turn accelerates the metabolism.

While bone loss begins in the thirties, the rate at which you lose it increases in your forties. Now more than ever, it is essential to increase muscle strength, which in turn improves bone density and can help prevent osteoporosis. The answer always seems to be pointing in the direction of weight training in every way.

Increased muscle mass accelerates the metabolism.

Muscle may have memory, but it might not completely remember how tight it once was! You'll need to be even more diligent about your workout routine this decade to stay in top shape.

THE FIX? New Fitness Strategies for Your 40s:

1 **TRAIN TROUBLE SPOTS MORE OFTEN.** In my forties, I added an extra training segment to my workouts to tone stubborn areas, including abs, glutes and underarms, at least two to three times a week. While I don't advocate "spot training," focusing a little extra on certain body

parts as a component of a head-to-toe regimen can keep flab at bay, especially if you've got a solid lifting and cardio plan in place. I also incorporate new exercises every two to three weeks to surprise my muscles and keep them challenged, especially in my trouble spots. It is also a good strategy to increase the number of repetitions performed from beyond twelve to as many as fifteen to twenty to remain lean and toned. According to a UCLA report, strength training three times a week for two months can help you recover from a decade of muscle loss.

2 SUPPLEMENT STRENGTH TRAINING WITH ADDITIONAL CARDIO. If you've got a solid lifting routine in place, adding a few cardio sessions each week to your training habit in your forties helps increase weight loss and promotes fat burning, as well as reducing cancer risk. One study showed that women who did up to three hours of strenuous exercise each week dropped their risk of breast cancer by 23 percent. I usually do my cardio in the morning, and if I'm really trying to increase my metabolism, I'll break up doing cardio and weight training by doing cardio in the morning and weights at night to burn fat twice in one day. This is especially helpful when you may have just enough time to run your three miles in the morning and know that you can attack resistance training of three body parts later in the day.

Strength training three times a week for two months can help you recover from a decade of muscle loss.

3 INCREASE CIRCUIT TRAINING TO BURN MORE FAT. If you're already doing thirty-second cardio intervals between lifting sets, as suggested in your thirties, increase your time by fifteen to thirty seconds, particularly on days when you're not doing any other cardio or flexibility work. You'll increase your heart rate for a longer period and rev up your metabolism, as well as engage different muscle fibers than those normally in action when you're just lifting.

4 TRACK MILEAGE TO BOOST HEART AND BRAIN HEALTH. Walking is one of the easiest activities I can think of, and it's often my workout of choice on the road. Just twelve miles of walking per week can improve heart health and help ward off cardiovascular disease before you reach your fifties. It's also my favorite way to reduce stress and shed the to-dos of the day, which ultimately lowers blood pressure. Turns out walking is also great for your memory. Studies from the University of Illinois–Urbana show that just thirty minutes of brisk walking a few times a week can be enough to improve blood sugar levels, which in turns heightens brain function and memory. Nothing could be easier

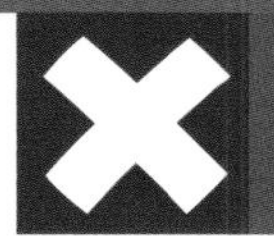

THE WORST FITNESS HABITS

Some workout habits arise out of laziness, and some are downright dangerous. Check out the worst fitness mistakes you can make and the simple corrections that can help you stay focused.

1 FORM. I can't say this enough...form is your safety net. Once you compromise the way you do the move, you're no longer getting the greatest benefits from the exercise and you're seriously increasing your risk of getting hurt. Even if it means lowering the amount of weight you are lifting, follow the correct form for the most outstanding results.

2 OVERTRAINING. I believe in staying motivated, but don't expect that you're going to dive right in and pound your body into its best shape ever overnight. Not only will this all-or-nothing attitude cause burnout, but you also risk injury and you will definitely give up on yourself because this is an unreasonable expectation. Instead, you're going to gradually build up your muscles so they get the most effective, efficient workout possible. If you follow the Best Body Now program, more doesn't always mean better, faster results. And remember, rest is good for your body. Take days off between training to repair and rebuild, or if you're training daily, don't work the same muscle groups back to back.

3 UNDERTRAINING. Once you're dressed and ready to sweat, commit to giving it your all for the next thirty to sixty minutes. Just going through the motions doesn't do anything for your body and makes it easy to let boredom creep in. You owe this time to yourself—you deserve it—so make sure you give it your all. As *So You Think You Can Dance* choreographer Debbie Allen says, "Put on your short stuff and sweat!" I like it!

4 DAYDREAMING. It's so easy to let your mind wander while you're lifting weights, but studies, such as those published in *Athletic Insight* and the *Journal of Motor Behavior*, have shown that when you're completely focused on each rep, more muscle fibers are used. You can develop a laser-sharp focus by actively involving your mind in every set and rep, thinking about how your body moves, how the muscle engages, which muscle or muscles you're using and correct form. This adds up to a better workout and faster results. So forget about the laundry, your kids' schedules and your afternoon conference call, and stay 100 percent in the moment.

5 STAYING WITH A FEW EXERCISES YOU KNOW. Your muscles love being challenged, so if you just stick to the same routine, they'll eventually adapt and won't have to work as hard to do the same moves. But if you change the exercises and even the order you do them in, you ensure that muscles don't get too efficient at any single routine. Not only is this better for toning, but it also helps your mind stay focused and engaged.

6 HOLDING YOUR BREATH. Regular steady breathing has many benefits, including keeping you from passing out. The upsides are that proper inhalations and exhalations can help you power through moves, keep lactic acid (a by-product that builds up in the muscles during exertion) at bay and help maintain a steady heart rate. A full breath delivers the maximum amount of oxygen to the blood, which in turn delivers more energy to the working muscles.

than using the simple activity of walking as your default exercise plan from here on in.

5 ADD ONE MORE YOGA SESSION TO YOUR CURRENT ROUTINE.

To keep my muscles strong and limber, I increased my yoga sessions to two or three a week in my forties, which helped combat the bone loss that occurs in this decade. I found it improved my mood by lessening anxiety and creating a long, lean physique. I love doing it right after I lift weights—yoga positions lengthen the muscle you just finished training and help you maintain flexibility, which prevents injury. Yoga also requires that you work on practicing your balance, and this also is an effective way to avoiding injuring yourself. Studies, including those cited in the Harvard Health Publications report titled "Yoga for Anxiety and Depression," have also shown that yoga's positive effects on mood and anxiety level can also help you sleep better, as well as lower your blood pressure.

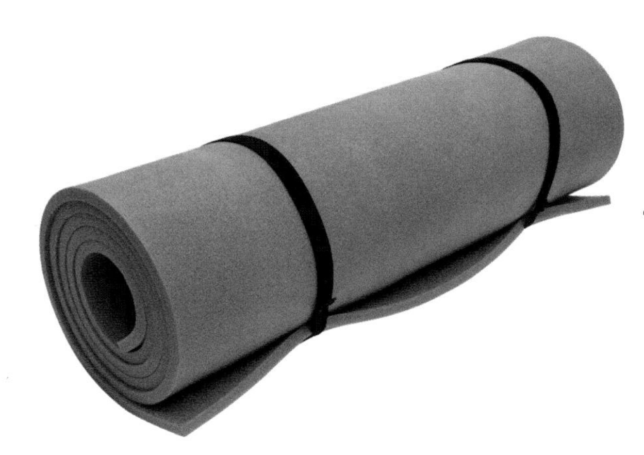

> Even low-impact exercise, the type that doesn't strain your joints or put stress on your body, boosts energy and reduces depression and fatigue.

6 PUSH THROUGH THE BLAHS.

Even I get them sometimes—it's normal. But studies show that even low-impact exercise, the type that doesn't strain your joints or put stress on your body, boosts energy and reduces depression and fatigue. One such study, published in *Psychotherapy and Psychosomatics*, showed that low-intensity workouts were just as effective as moderate-intensity workouts in increasing energy levels and countering fatigue. This effect lasts throughout the day because your metabolism increases, plus you strengthen the immune system in the long run. Fatigue from training is one thing—yes, you deserve a rest day—but if you're lacking enthusiasm or motivation, a common side effect of perimenopause and stress, just *start* working out. You'll see that once you get moving, you'll love the feel-good endorphins (the pain-reducing brain chemicals that create "runner's high") and energy rush so much that you'll be unlikely to stop. When you're finished, you'll feel the success of a job well done. You probably won't even remember how tired you were before you started.

7 SLOW DOWN YOUR MOVEMENTS TO GET THE MOST OUT OF EXERCISE.

Focusing on form and technique is a fundamental part of the Best Body Now fitness plan, and for good reason. A study from the University of Salzburg compared women in their forties and fifties using traditional resistance training with those trying a new method called SuperSlow, which simply means the moves are done much slower with fewer reps. Researchers found that the SuperSlow group built more muscle mass than the non-SuperSlow group even though they were using the same size weights—likely because they were concentrating more and focusing on the right technique, form and challenge. Even if you don't go SuperSlow, just decreasing your speed enough to ensure you're doing the moves correctly, concentrating on the muscle contractions and not using momentum to do the moves will help you work out more efficiently. Bear in mind the SuperSlow method is just one variation—use it to add variety when needed. In my case I find myself performing quicker reps most of the time and using slow reps for certain exercises that demand it, particularly curls and leg work.

> Once you get moving, you'll love the feel-good endorphins and energy rush.

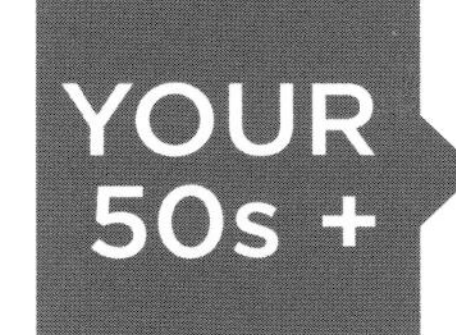

Strengthen Your Physique

My fitness approach for fifty is fundamentally similar to what I did in my forties but with a few tweaks to deal with age-related changes. The key is listening to my physiological signals about what needs to be different. For example, am I sufficiently challenging my mind and body, following my natural curiosity to explore new moves and responding to issues such as age-related loss of muscle and flexibility? By following the Best Body Now fitness plan, I'm doing all of this and more. Today my challenge is training for a sprint-distance triathlon, which will challenge my swimming, running and cycling abilities. I can't wait!!

YOUR 50s +

What's Happening in Your 50s + That Impacts Your Fitness Needs

- Loss of muscle, bone density and flexibility continues into the fifties and beyond, but can be countered or managed by lifting weights. As I mentioned before, when you lift weights, the muscle contraction pulls on the bone, increasing blood flow and spurring the growth of new bone cells that build density and prevent the onset of osteoporosis.

- The metabolism naturally slows down as you become less active, making it more challenging than ever to keep weight off, even if your nutrition is in tip-top shape. By the time you reach sixty-five you may have lost up to one-third of your muscle mass thanks to gradual losses of 3 to 6 percent in metabolic efficiency each decade.

- You become more prone to dehydration as you age for a variety of reasons. One is that your ability to recognize thirst is diminished and drops in intensity. This means you need to be even more diligent about drinking water before, during and after workouts. Every three hours you should be drinking at least 16 ounces of water.

- The body experiences a steady increase in blood pressure with each decade; however, after fifty or postmenopause, blood pressure tends to rise more steeply. Although changing hormones, genetic predisposition and poor diet are believed to be the main contributing causes, hypertension, or high blood pressure, can be controlled and possibly prevented through exercise and diet.

- A Northwestern University study shows that the risk of cardiovascular disease increases fifty percent by the time we reach fifty if we have two or more contributing risk factors. These may include high cholesterol, high blood pressure and obesity, most of which can be controlled or lessened through strength training and improved nutrition.

- Loss of brain function, and even the early signs of dementia, can start by the fifth decade, where significant changes can happen in memory, learning and attention span. But research published in the *Annals of Internal Medicine* has shown that just fifteen minutes of exercise three days a week can reduce your risk of developing dementia and Alzheimer's by 30 to 40 percent.

- Bone loss continues, which increases your risk for osteoporosis. The National Osteoporosis Foundation reports that one in two women over fifty will have at least one fracture from the disease. Dropping weight in your fifties can reduce your risk of developing osteoporosis, according to UCLA experts.

- Hormonal changes caused by menopause can lead to depression, irritability, fatigue, lack of sex drive, insomnia, a compromised immune system and more. Studies, like one published in the *Journal of Advanced Nursing*, show many of these symptoms can be improved through exercise.

> Fifteen minutes of exercise three days a week can reduce your risk of developing dementia and Alzheimer's.

THE FIX? New Fitness Strategies for Your 50s +:

> I dedicate a portion of all my workouts to toning stubborn areas such as abs, glutes and underarms.

1 INCREASE CARDIO FREQUENCY AND INTENSITY FOR HEART HEALTH. The risk for heart disease rises when you reach fifty, but you can lower your odds by increasing the number of cardiovascular workouts you do in a week. When I turned fifty, I started to do five per week. Make sure these sessions are significantly strenuous. For example, I like to run during warm-weather months and snowshoe during winter. If you're just beginning, start slowly with three cardio sessions, adding one session every four to six weeks to stay challenged. Also, I make sure to do cardio first thing in the morning, before eating, to maximize fat burning. A study of women fifty-five and older from the University of Illinois–Urbana shows that those who are most physically fit had the healthiest brain function and the strongest memories.

2 FOCUS EVEN MORE ON TROUBLE SPOTS. Now that I've reached my fifties, I dedicate a portion of all my workouts to toning stubborn areas such as abs, glutes and underarms. My personal weakness is my lower legs, so I put in extra calf training when time permits. Not only do I dedicate time in each sweat session, I also make sure to change exercises each time to surprise muscles and keep them working at their peak. If you're still getting comfortable with the exercises, simply vary the moves every week rather than every workout so you can perfect your technique and improve your form at the same time. I'm also constantly monitoring my reps—when a move gets simple, I increase the number of times I perform it. You'll help eliminate the sag in places such as right under your butt if you do this. It works for me.

3 STAY CHALLENGED BY ADDING INTERVAL TRAINING. If you're already doing cardio bursts between your weight-training sets to elevate your heart rate, increase the time by fifteen to thirty seconds per burst for even more calorie burning—it's an incredible challenge. Studies show that interval training, which is increasing your heart rate for a short period of time, then letting it return to normal during exercise, can ultimately cause you to burn more fat during and after workouts. It's also good for your heart and keeps energy levels high.

4 ADD A STRETCH MORNING AND NIGHT TO STAY FLEXIBLE. I love my morning stretches to get my muscles flexed and warmed up. Because our flexibility naturally decreases with age, I make sure that in addition to pre- and postworkout stretches, I add some light flexibility moves for two to three minutes when I wake and before bed. Often I perform my morning stretches in the shower under hot water to save time and still squeeze this important habit into my Best Body Now day. This helps joints and muscles stay limber as well as improving stability, range of motion and functionality, which can prevent falls as you get older.

5 INCORPORATE MORE YOGA TO ALLEVIATE MENOPAUSE SYMPTOMS. Nothing makes me feel as relaxed as a yoga session, but that's not the only reason I practice. Yoga can help reverse the aging process by minimizing or countering the effects of a sedentary lifestyle, including poor flexibility, arthritis, high blood pressure and more. A study published in the *Archives of General Psychiatry* showed that menopausal women who did ninety-minute yoga sessions twice a week experienced fewer hot flashes and night sweats, and their overall mood improved. Adding more sessions also keeps muscles strong and limber while increasing your energy, keeping stress at bay, improving tone and definition, building endurance and reducing fat stored around your middle that's caused by changing hormones and stress levels. I take a yoga class whenever I can—and if there's no time for a full hour, I'll do a set or two of my favorite positions just to move and calm my body.

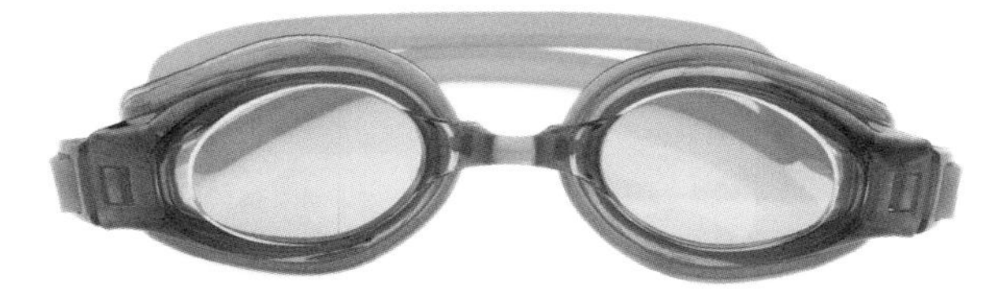

6 CONSIDER ADDING A SWIMMING WORKOUT THAT'S GENTLE ON THE JOINTS. I love swimming because it's low-impact but a superb fat-burning and muscle-toning activity. It's gentle on the joints thanks to the buoyancy of water, so it allows you to push yourself without the feeling of exertion you get from supporting your body

TOSCA TIDBIT

Secretly sculpt when not at the gym by keeping your abs contracted when you walk, and clench your booty with each step for extra toning. I do this all the time—and, trust me, no one can tell. Only the results are noticeable.

weight. Many gyms offer water classes, in addition to free swims, if you don't have access to a pool.

7 **INCORPORATE STEP CLASSES OR JUMP ROPE AS CARDIO.** It turns out these weight-bearing exercises are great not just for cardiovascular exercise but also for bone health. Studies from the University of Oregon showed that postmenopausal women increased bone density from doing weight-bearing exercises that included jumping and resistance exercises with weights. The five-year study incorporated weights up to just 10 pounds with everyday exercises including squats, lunges and jumps. Try substituting one or two classes a week using these types of moves for your cardio sessions. As an alternative, work in thirty seconds of rope jumping or skipping in place between weight-lifting sets—you'll increase your heart rate and burn more calories while adding extra weight-bearing moves. And remember, if you're in a conditioning class that uses weights, this also counts as a strength-training session.

> Short bursts of activity, even just ten to fifteen minutes at a time, can improve your energy and mood.

8 **USE EXERCISE TO BOOST YOUR MOOD.** When I'm feeling sluggish or unmotivated, I do a set of jumping jacks or jog in place for a minute or two. That might sound silly, but it's not. Research from the Mayo Clinic shows that not only does thirty minutes of daily exercise five days a week improve depression symptoms greatly, but short bursts of activity, even just ten to fifteen minutes at a time, can improve your energy and mood in the short term. Fatigue, sadness, stress, self-doubt and irritability, common in postmenopausal women, can be lessened temporarily with a brisk walk, jumping rope or dancing around the living room. And remember, cardio activity accumulates during the day, so doing a ten-minute energy booster three times a day gets you to your thirty-minute daily goal.

9 **STAY HYDRATED.** Sweat sessions leave your body with the need to refuel. The few times I've forgotten my water bottle or just whipped through a workout without drinking, I've noticed the results—my workout just isn't as strong and I'm sluggish later. Now I always drink 8-ounce glasses of water before, during and after exercise to keep hydrated. You'll see that water intake is programmed into the Best Body Now eating plan for all ages, but this is particularly important as you age, especially when you're working out. Water keeps energy high, helps

muscles rebuild, flushes out toxins and ensures that you stay healthy.

10 WALK WHENEVER YOU CAN FOR EVEN MORE EXERCISE.

At least once a week I schedule walks with my family—it's the perfect way to spend quality time catching up on our lives while we log some steps. As it turns out, this also helps reduce some of those annoying symptoms associated with menopause. In a study published in the *Archives of General Psychology*, a group of menopausal women who walked just three times a week for an hour reported fewer night sweats and hot flashes, as well as happier moods. Our dogs love it, too.

Menopausal women who walked just three times a week for an hour reported fewer night sweats and hot flashes, as well as happier moods.

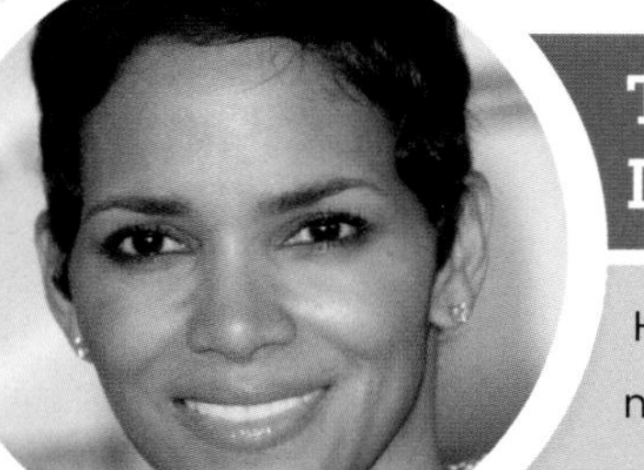

The "H" Factor: A-List Proof That Life Gets Better at 40

Halle Berry, forty-two, takes the term "hot mom" to a whole new level. My guess is she's one of the few fortysomething new mothers with a dozen or so appearances on *People* magazine's 100 Most Beautiful list and the only one to land on the November 2008 cover of *Esquire* with the headline "Halle Is the Sexiest Woman Alive." Part of what I love most about her is that unstoppable confidence and joyful radiance that seem to bubble up from within. Her Academy Award–winning performance in *Monster's Ball* seems to only have fueled her fire. She's done another dozen movies since then, playing the sexy leading lady, and has more in development. I believe she's going to sweep *People*'s lists for decades to come.

MY BEST BODY NOW

Triumph of the Not-So-Average Jane
Christine Cmolik's Journey

THEN
5', AGE 59
170 POUNDS

NOW
AGE 61
110 POUNDS

At my worst point, I hid behind shapeless clothes and low self-esteem. I didn't like myself. I hated going into dressing rooms in clothing stores because nothing looked flattering and I didn't want to see the blubber. I was ashamed.

My push to change came when I began a new job and was the oldest and least fit in the group. At the time, my weight had climbed to 170 pounds and my health had dropped to rock bottom, including periods of depression, aches and pains, irritable bowel syndrome, high blood pressure, high blood sugar, asthma and lack of energy. I ate just two to three times a day, living on junk food, gourmet meals and desserts, whether I was hungry or not.

I began working out on the treadmill and lost some weight, but I really got my body into shape with Eating Clean and strength training with the help of a home gym and a trainer to teach me techniques and moves. In fact, I got so into it, I set a goal to compete in bodybuilding, am working on getting a fitness certification to help older women learn to train, and even feel confident enough now to call myself an athlete. The results have been incredible: my resting heart rate dropped from 90 to 100 beats per minute to 68. I went from taking multiple medications to *none*. My hair and skin are healthier than ever, my energy is off the charts and conditions such as depression and IBS vanished. It took just four to six months to see these life-changing results.

Now I eat several times a day, Eating Clean 90 percent of the time and never feeling hungry. I have a flat stomach for the first time in years. To help, I carry a cooler so I'm never without healthy options.

I have a more positive outlook and high self-esteem, and I spend time and effort on my appearance—I even love trying on clothes because everything looks good. I now believe the body should be nurtured and respected, and being my best physically helps me emotionally and socially. Caring for my aging parents, working, and financial and home responsibilities are easier because I have the energy, health and emotional strength to do it. I feel more valuable.

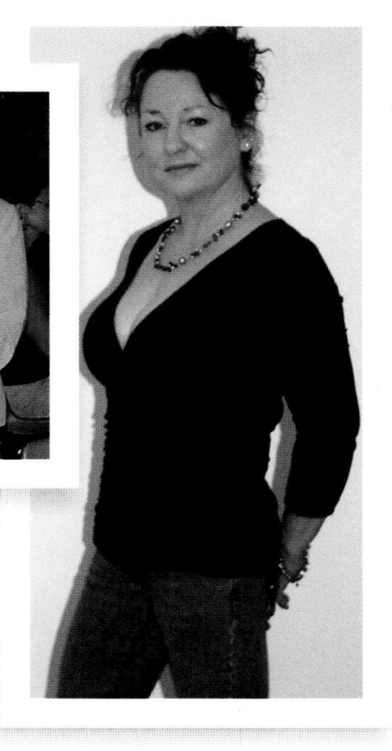

To stay motivated, I read women's fitness magazines cover to cover, looking for new moves for inspiration and challenge. I hang up pictures of women with bodies I aspire to, and reward myself with spa appointments and manicures. Best of all, this lifestyle gives me the attention and time I need for myself in times of overload from every aspect of my life. It's not a diet or a weight-loss plan—it's a way of life, and one that is much easier to live than the one you are currently living. It is a very small investment with huge rewards.

Today, my only problem is remembering to dress my age!

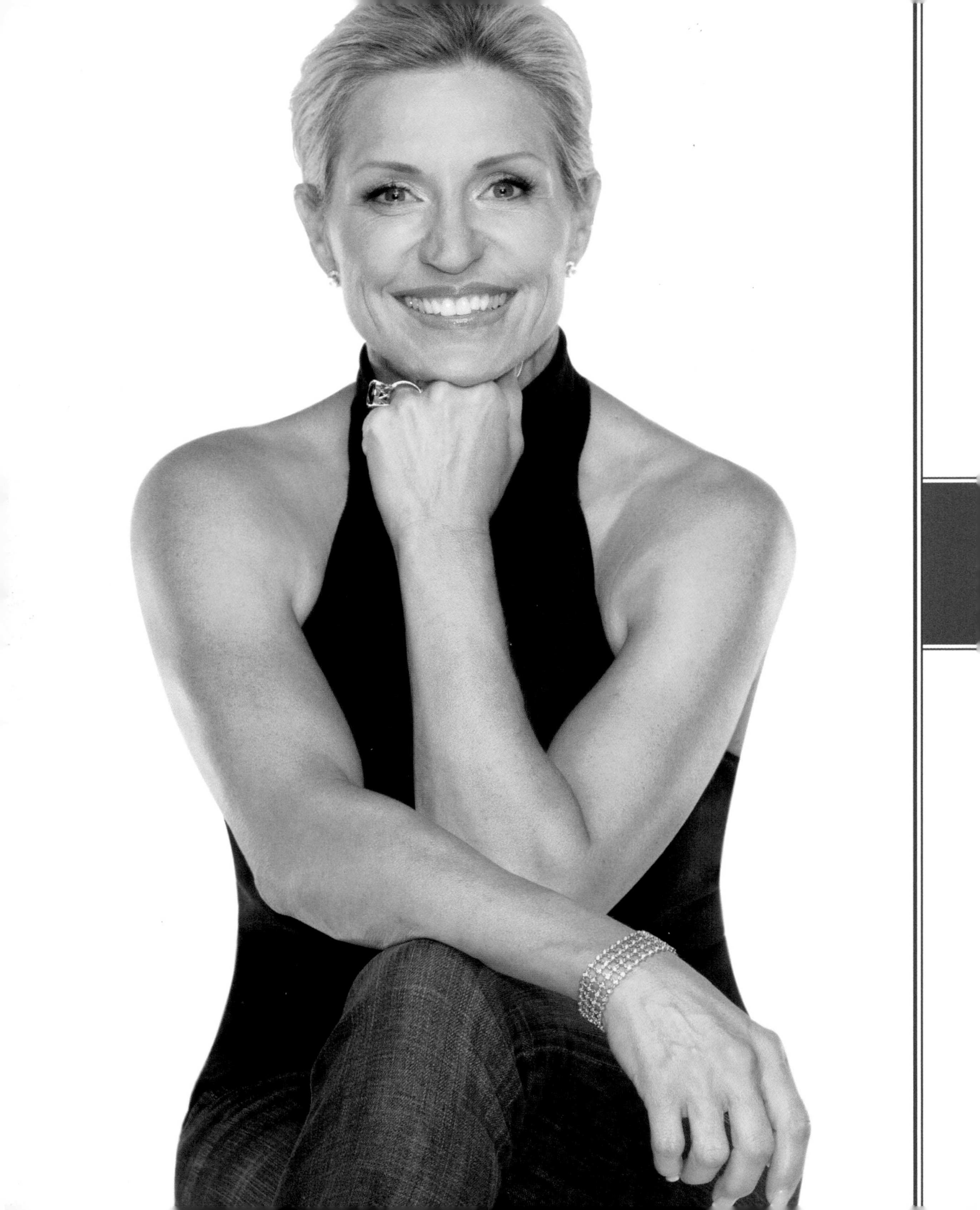

Best Body Now Health 6

AGING IS INEVITABLE, AS ARE THE DIFFERENCES WE SEE in our hormones, those powerful substances in our bodies that regulate certain cells, organs and sexual functions, including menstruation, pregnancy, menopause and even appetite. But the symptoms and side effects commonly associated with these body changes don't have to be *your* experience. I know, because I saw a radical reversal in how I looked and felt, head to toe, after incorporating very simple smart-health strategies into my life—the same ones hormone specialist Dr. Uzzi Reiss recommends in his practice. Not only did my appearance improve, from body shape to skin to hair, but also the conditions

Hot flashes? Gone. Irritability? Also gone. Fat around my stomach? Nowhere to be seen!

I've lived with nearly my entire adult life—from stress to fatigue to hypoglycemia—vanished. Hot flashes? Gone. Irritability? Also gone. Fat around my stomach? Nowhere to be seen!

I'm also happier, more sexual and more energetic than ever before. That makes sense: the building blocks of this program—supplementing your body with nutrients, natural hormones, natural antivirals that kill or stop the growth of viruses and antioxidants that stop cell-damaging free radicals—successfully work because they use the same effective alternatives found in plants, our environment and even your

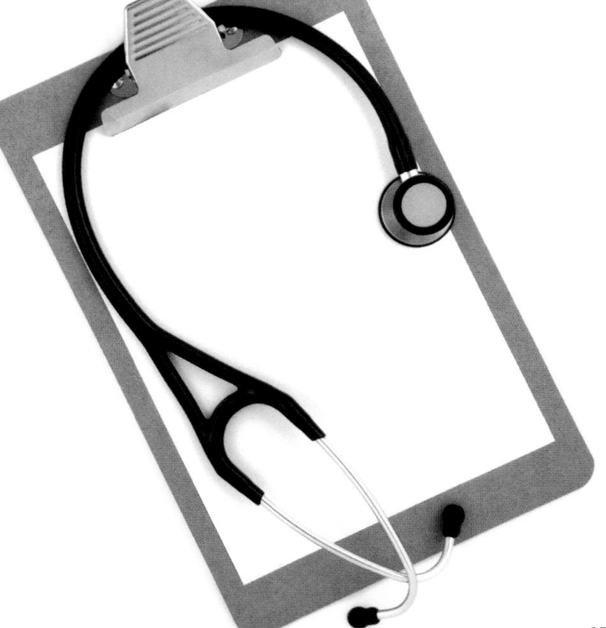

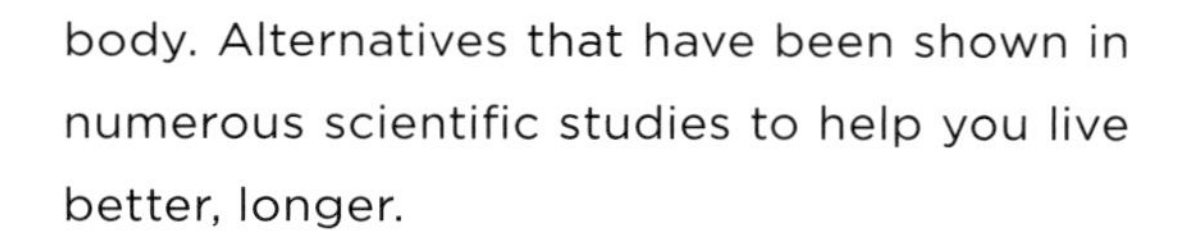

body. Alternatives that have been shown in numerous scientific studies to help you live better, longer.

The Best Body Now health plan described in this chapter is based on the recommendations, advice and guidance of Dr. Reiss, an ob-gyn, founder of the Beverly Hills Antiaging Center and bestselling author of *The Natural Superwoman* and *How to Make a Pregnant Woman Happy*, as well as on the latest research, strategies and findings from the medical community. I turned to Dr. Reiss for advice because of his unique specialty in natural hormones, a scientific approach that differs from that of traditional gynecologists, who use synthetic options. His treatments and philosophies, which resonate with my own, come from his successful work with more than fifty thousand women over the past twenty-five years, helping them feel healthier and more vibrant in their thirties, forties, fifties and beyond, than ever before. Following his counsel, I've boosted my energy levels and physical health more than ever, as well as countered many of the effects of aging.

I'm also happier, more sexual and more energetic than ever before.

A Customized Rx for Your Best Body Now

AS DR. REISS EXPLAINS, IF YOU ATE perfectly, you wouldn't have to adjust your health plan by using supplements or other treatments—you would be getting the right amount of nutrients and fuel from food. Unfortunately, women are so busy being the ultimate caregivers or career women, they sacrifice their health by making poor food and lifestyle choices, including sleeping less, giving in to stress and undernourishing their bodies and minds. Not only that, but thanks to pollution, chemicals, processing methods and growing/raising conditions, food choices are often stripped of nutrients and vitamins, injected with hormones or antibiotics, or subjected to toxins.

> Your body responds to smart health choices the second you make them.

The upside is it's never too late to make a change. Dr. Reiss sees amazing Best Body Now transformations at every age in his practice, just as I've seen in my own body. We've customized this plan for you, because your body responds to smart health choices the second you make them.

While you may want to believe supplements are like a magic pill or cure-all promising life-changing weight loss, health or beauty, the truth is that no such pill exists. The best way to supercharge your body is through nutrition first. My challenge to you is to consider the Best Body Now superfoods listed in Chapter 4—nutrient-dense fruits and vegetables, whole grains and lean protein—as your primary "supplements." Nourishing your body with wholesome natural foods is your first step toward a lifelong health transformation. Look to vitamin and mineral supplements as necessary to round out your eating plan and achieve complete health benefits. That's what I do and what Dr. Reiss recommends to clients.

> Consider the Best Body Now superfoods listed in Chapter 4—nutrient-dense fruits and vegetables, whole grains and lean protein—as your primary "supplements."

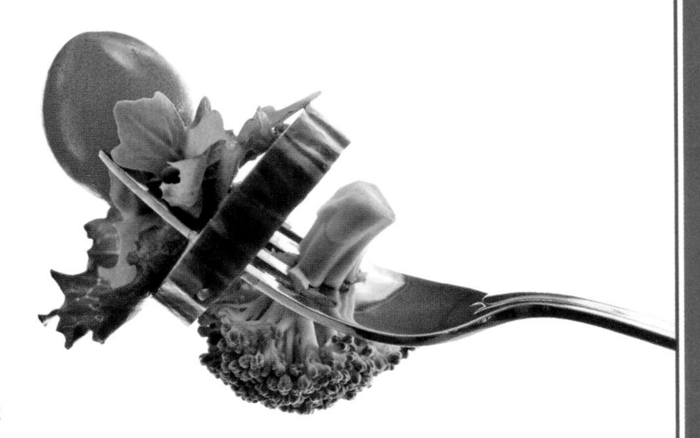

BEST BODY NOW Health Basics

NEARLY EVERYTHING YOU NEED TO ARM YOUR BODY AGAINST AGING ALREADY EXISTS IN NATURE. We know that vitamin C, found in oranges and other citrus fruits, boosts our immune system when we get a cold, and that B vitamins, available in foods such as tuna, soybeans and garlic, relieve stress and fight depression. But these vitamins are only the beginning: there exists an entire host of disease-fighting vitamins, minerals and antioxidants found in fruits, vegetables, plants, spices and herbs. When you consume them, they fuel the body with nutrients that strengthen the immune system, fight cardiovascular disease, build bones, regulate hormones, help cells function better, and more. They're the substances that help you fight aging and age-related conditions, and they're all available in the foods you eat. Once you begin to eat mindfully, such micronutrients become available to the body in greater quantity and supplementation becomes a matter of choice.

GET YOUR NUTRIENTS FROM FOOD FIRST, IF POSSIBLE. In nearly all cases, it's better to get your nutrients, vitamins and minerals from natural food sources, rather than supplements. For example, you'll get heart-healthy omega-3 fatty acids from eating fish and disease-fighting curcumin from foods seasoned with turmeric. In some cases, where supplement forms are advised, it's because research has shown no quantifiable difference in supplement versus nature or because you'll likely get only very small amounts from food, which is especially important if you're treating a condition you currently have versus preventing disease in the future.

EVERY HUMAN BODY IS DIFFERENT. The only way to know exactly how much you really need of any supplement, vitamin or natural hormone is to get tested. Your doctor can do this for you, as well as tailor your dosage to your specific needs. It doesn't make sense to add substances you don't need, even if they're good for you. Supplements are most efficient when used properly.

YOUR BODY CHANGES EVERY DAY. Hormone levels constantly change. For instance, estrogen, the main female hormone, ebbs and flows each day throughout a woman's normal cycle—estrogen levels are low just before your period and rise again the week after it's finished as your body prepares for pregnancy. Not just estrogen, but other hormones constantly fluctuate based on how stressed you are, how much exercise you're doing, what you eat and more. The hormones produced by the thyroid gland

> With every bite you take you have two choices: protect and enhance cells or work against them.

regulate your body's temperature, weight and heart rate, and the adrenals secrete cortisol when you're anxious or worried. This is why a "one pill fits all" solution doesn't work for everyone, nor does everyone's body stay the same every day.

EVERY FOOD OR SUPPLEMENT WORKS IN ONE OF TWO WAYS. There are no such things as foods or supplements that have neutral or zero effects on your body. Absolutely everything you ingest either works for you, by promoting what's good or suppressing what's bad in your body, or does the opposite, enhancing negative activity or suppressing the positive. With every bite you take you have two choices: protect and enhance cells or work against them. I keep this in mind whenever I'm tempted by a handful of M&Ms or (seemingly healthy) low-calorie, chemical-filled frozen yogurt—saying "no thank you" is easy.

LOW ESTROGEN LEVELS OFTEN GO UNTREATED. Many women stopped taking synthetic hormones, chemical substances designed to do what your body's natural hormones are supposed to, during the menopause transition because of negative press. Unfortunately, that can cause your estrogen levels to drop and symptoms including depression, disinterest in sex, anxiety, forgetfulness and more to rise in response. Bioidentical hormones—those identical to ones already in our bodies—however, are a safe, natural alternative for alleviating common symptoms in our thirties, forties and fifties because our bodies recognize and respond to their molecules.

> Bioidentical hormones are a safe, natural alternative for alleviating common symptoms.

LOSE THE "I HAVE TO TAKE EVERYTHING" MIND-SET. I use this health program in combination with what my doctor has shown through tests or family history to do what's right for me. Rather than take every supplement on the menu, I pick and choose what I know is right for me. Taking what your body isn't lacking or doesn't require doesn't help, Dr. Reiss explains. Understanding your family's health issues, as well as your lifestyle today and in the past, is critical to helping you determine how to supplement your health plan. Following the Best Body Now eating plan is the first step. Next, collect information about your family's medical history and your lifestyle and share it with your physician, along with advice from this chapter. He or she can help you arm yourself against illness and disease, as well as monitor your body's health transformation as you begin to make changes in how you eat and supplement your nutritional plan.

ANTIVIRALS ARE THE NEW ANTI-OXIDANTS. Antivirals are the newest substances to be found in nature, possessing even more disease-fighting power than antioxidants. Specifically, antivirals are substances found in nature or manufactured by humans that stop the spread of viruses in your body, explains Dr. Reiss. They're considered the new immune system strengtheners, similar to antioxidants but more powerful. They can be used daily when you're trying to treat a problem, and Dr. Reiss recommends using some types before you travel, after you've been in contact with someone who has the flu, or you're in very crowded spaces, such as a concert, airport or plane, just to keep yourself protected from illness.

You can't get enough of these incredible antivirals. The following types, combined with cell-strengthening antioxidants, should be on the top of your radar every day, at any age, because of their strong disease-fighting, age-proofing and immune-system-boosting properties. They're all available as nutritional supplements from qualified physicians, pharmacies or health food stores.

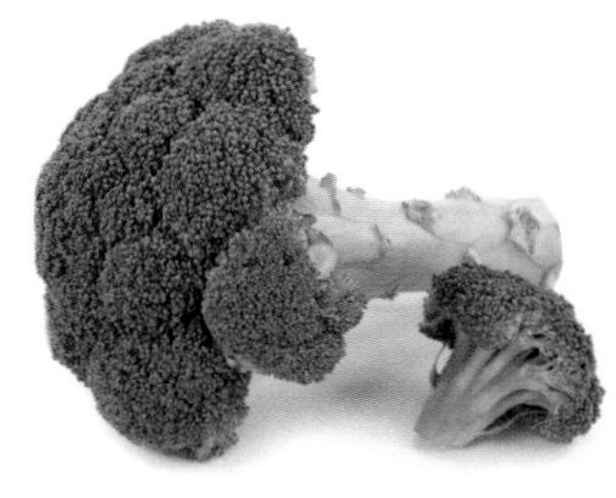

SULFORANAC. Just as walking boosts heart health, so does eating fresh broccoli. It contains sulforanac, an antiviral that helps to prevent cardiovascular disease and cancer.

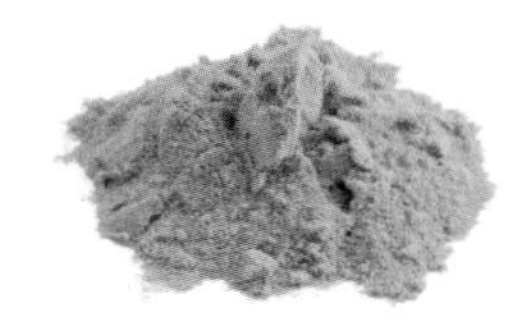

TURMERIC. You've probably seen this popular Indian curry spice as an ingredient in recipes. It turns out the turmeric plant contains the antiviral curcumin, which reduces inflammation in the body and helps prevent diseases such as cancer, arthritis and Parkinson's.

ROSEMARY. Experts tell us to work on crossword puzzles in order to keep our memory sharp and lift weights to increase blood circulation. You can also eat more rosemary. This flavorful herb does more than enhance the taste of roasted vegetables. It's a powerful antiviral shown to improve brain function and circulation, as well as help to prevent cancer.

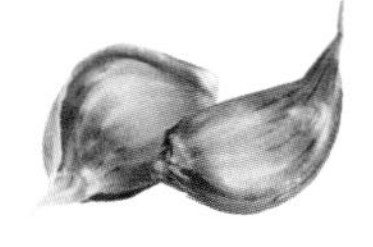

GARLIC. One way to protect yourself against a variety of cancers is to reduce your level of stress, which is linked to this disease. Another way is to fill your diet with garlic, which has been shown to guard against breast, colon and prostate cancers.

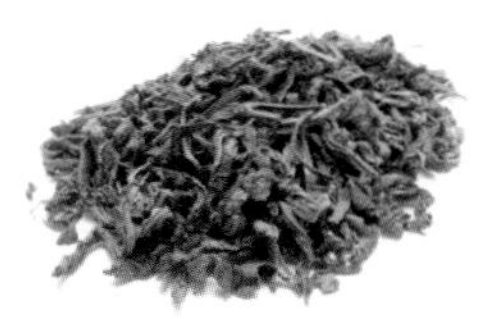

GREEN TEA. Teas are made up of herbs containing extremely healthy ingredients, including antivirals and antioxidants. Green tea contains incredible disease-fighters known as catechins that lower cholesterol and help stop cancer cells from forming and spreading.

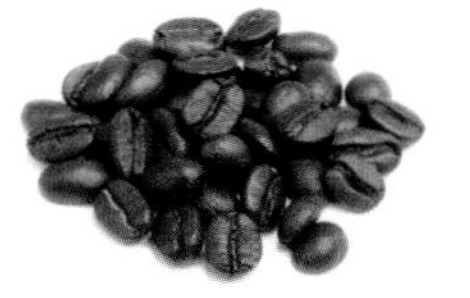

COFFEE. Most of us drink coffee because the caffeine gives us energy in the morning or a pick-me-up in the afternoon, but scientists are discovering that it also contains powerful antivirals capable of lowering our risk for diabetes, Parkinson's and cancer.

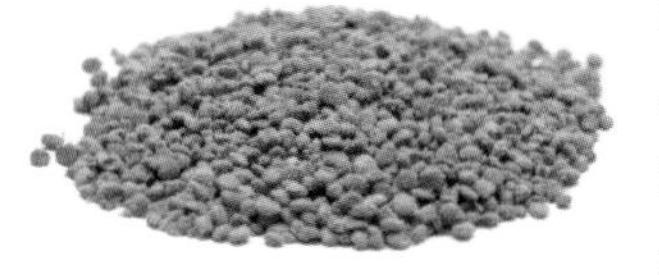

BEE POLLEN. Fresh fruits and vegetables contain large amounts of B vitamins and vitamins A C, D and E, which enhance the immune system and heighten energy levels. It turns out bee pollen also contains very high concentrations of these same nutrients, making it a powerful disease fighter.

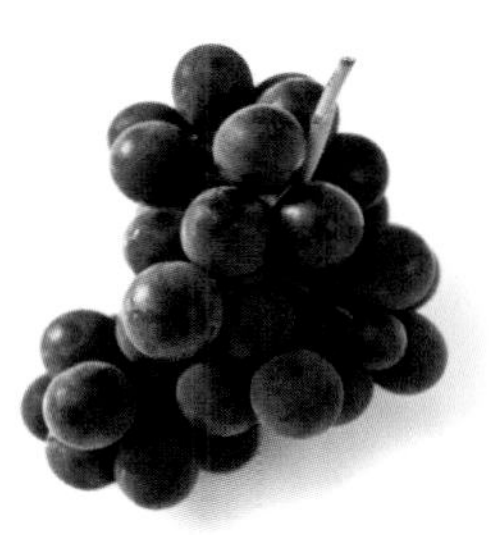

RESVERATROL. Scientists have long observed the "French paradox," wherein French people eat a relatively high-fat diet and drink large amounts of red wine, yet have low incidences of disease, including heart problems and cancer. They now believe a natural component of the grapes used to make red wine, called resveratrol, protects against cancer, heart disease and inflammation. You would have to drink thousands of glasses of wine to get the full benefits (which wouldn't help create your Best Body Now), or you can take supplements that contain the extracts.

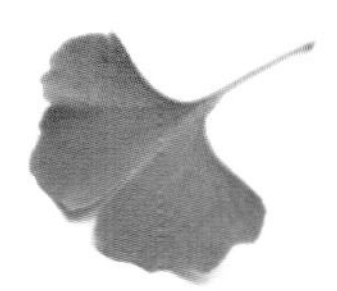

GINGKO. There are plenty of natural mood boosters, including exercise, laughter and time spent with people we love, all of which increase circulation and trigger brain chemicals that make us happy. Scientists have discovered that gingko acts similarly and can reduce depression and enhance memory and brain function by increasing circulation in the brain.

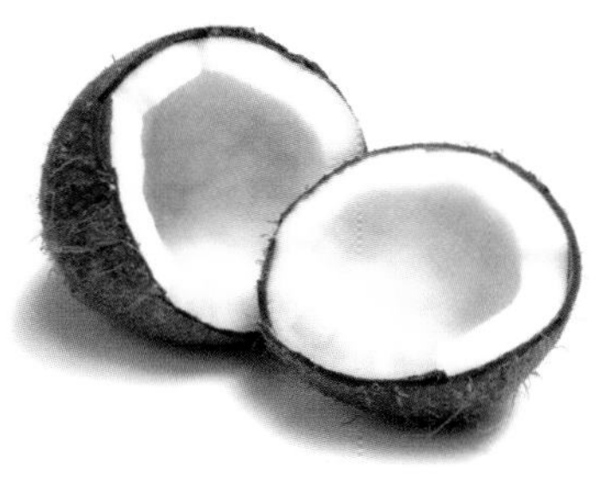

COCONUT OIL. Researchers have often wondered why people living in tropical climates have lower rates of high cholesterol, heart disease and cancer. One conclusion is the use of coconut oil in cooking. Scientists have also found a correlation between the oil and weight loss due to its natural ability to stimulate the thyroid.

START YOUR BEST BODY NOW

CHANGING HEALTH HABITS CAN BE daunting, but you'll begin noticing benefits immediately once you start, and that is encouraging news. Try the tips below to hit the ground running on the road to your Best Body Now.

1 DO SOME RESEARCH. Arming myself with information helps me stay engaged and involved, and helps me make the best choices for my health. Investigate the supplements listed in this chapter to really immerse yourself in all their benefits, so you fully understand how and why nutrients are working for you. Look for reputable sources such as the Mayo Clinic and UCLA for published studies, additional information and brand recommendations.

2 MAKE AN APPOINTMENT WITH YOUR DOCTOR. You get the best results when you treat your body's exact requirements. Through testing, your doctor can identify where you may need additional supplementation, as well as determine specific doses that will maximize your results.

3 CHART WHAT YOU NEED. Once you talk to your doctor and purchase the vitamins, nutrients and supplements you need, write down your daily plan of what you need to take, when, with food, etc. It will save time during rushed mornings and help you stick to the program.

4 RE-EXAMINE YOUR MEDICINE CABINET. Toss out old or expired meds, vitamins, supplements, etc., as well as those your doctor determines you no longer need.

5 RE-EVALUATE YOUR SHOPPING LIST. Even if you supplement with nutrients, make sure the following high-power fruits, vegetables and plants are available in your kitchen every week: green tea, rosemary, garlic, turmeric, pomegranate, kale and coffee.

STAY ON TRACK

ROBUST HEALTH DOESN'T HAVE TO BE COMPLICATED OR DIFFICULT. Give yourself some time to adjust to the changes, and move through this checklist to help stay the course. Your efforts and investment in yourself *will* pay off sooner than you imagine.

1 EVALUATE YOURSELF HONESTLY. If you know, for instance, that you hate fish and the odds of you consuming more of this food are similar to winning the lottery no matter how nutritious it is for you, then commit to taking omega-3 supplements. Being realistic about your lifestyle and habits makes it easier to succeed.

2 CONSIDER YOUR LIFESTYLE. Have you lived on junk food, or are you an organic food junkie? Is your life high-stress or pretty calm? Have you already faced issues such as human papillomavirus, endometriosis or perimenopause? Knowing what your body requires will help you make smart choices now that will help you fight off temptation and remind you to treat yourself with TLC.

3 DON'T WAIT UNTIL YOU HAVE A PROBLEM. You may not have osteoporosis or heart disease yet, but protecting yourself now is the key to living better and longer. Also, take into account your family's medical history An increased awareness of what medical conditions have affected your ancestors will help you recognize what may or may not affect you. Once you identify the specific issues, you'll be more likely to stick to a smart-health program.

4 MONITOR HOW YOU FEEL. Dr. Reiss believes once you're armed with the right knowledge about how supplements work for you, from antioxidants to hormones, you're the best judge of whether or not they're working. Note how you feel when taking them and talk to your doctor to help you adjust dosages.

5 TRACK POSITIVE CHANGES. Monitoring developments in how you look and feel, such as increased energy, brighter skin and a happier mood, will help you stay in touch with the positive reasons you're making smart health choices. You'll also help keep your new commitment at the forefront of your mind.

6 NOTE NEGATIVE DIFFERENCES. Whenever you're changing your dose or adding a new supplement, note any side effects and talk to your doctor about reducing or stopping dosages.

A TYPICAL DAY FOLLOWING THE BEST BODY NOW HEALTH PROGRAM

Below is a compilation of the top supplements that work for women at any age. When customizing your Best Body Now health plan, you may take them all, those that apply to your specific health or family history or those that round out your nutritional needs. Talk to your doctor about which work best for you. These supplements are best taken with food.

MAGNESIUM GLYCINATE. Magnesium is one of the most abundant nutrients in your body and is responsible for many healthy functions, including regulating blood sugar, boosting your immune system and maintaining normal blood pressure. The glycinate form is more absorbable than other forms, making it more desirable for disease prevention. Take 1,000 mg daily, beginning with 400 mg and increasing daily in 100 mg increments, for hormone, cell and bone health.

VITAMIN D. It's challenging to get enough immunity-boosting, bone-strengthening and cancer-fighting vitamin D through food and sunlight, so it's important for many women to supplement their diet. Research published in the *American Journal of Clinical Nutrition* found that cancer rates in women after menopause declined by as much as 77 percent when they took 1,100 IU daily. Take 1,100 IU daily for calcium absorption from food and cancer prevention.

B COMPLEX. You will likely notice changes, such as greater energy, more radiant skin and hair, and less anxiety and stress, when you begin taking B vitamins. Take 25 to 100 mg daily for energy and adrenal function.

FISH OIL. This immune system booster has been associated with everything from cancer, depression and heart disease prevention to improving overall mood. Take 1,000 to 2,000 mg twice daily for heart health and disease prevention.

GREEN TEA EXTRACT. Another antioxidant that may help reduce cholesterol and fight a variety of cancers, including ovarian, breast and colorectal. Take 125 mg daily for heart health and cancer prevention.

VITAMIN K_2. A vitamin that's been shown to maintain and strengthen bones, as well as improve heart function. Take 75 to 150 mcg daily to build bone and boost heart health.

CURCUMIN. An anti-inflammatory, curcumin may be helpful in warding off diseases such as Alzheimer's, cancer, multiple sclerosis, arthritis and more. Take 600 mg daily to reduce your risk of cancer and boost your immune system.

COENZYME Q_{10}. This antiaging nutrient may boost your immune system, improve your energy levels, strengthen your workout performance and slow the aging process. Take 100 to 300 mg daily for energy and disease prevention.

N-ACETYL CYSTEINE (NAC). A powerful antioxidant, NAC helps detoxify the body and fight free radicals that cause heart, lung and autoimmune diseases. Take 500 to 1,000 mg twice daily for liver detoxification and disease prevention.

VITAMIN E COMPLEX. This complex may fight heart disease and build bone and strengthen cells. Take 400 to 800 IU daily for skin health and disease prevention.

R-ALPHA LIPOIC ACID. Many researchers believe this antioxidant can slow the aging process, improve metabolism and fight age-related illnesses. Take 150 mg twice daily for cancer and heart disease prevention.

POMEGRANATE EXTRACT. A study in the *Journal of Nutrition* showed that pomegranate juice reduces cholesterol and heart disease risk, while other studies suggest the antioxidant may help prevent osteoporosis. Take 100 mg to support heart health.

RESVERATROL. This wonder antiviral has been shown in studies, such as one published in the *Journal of Agricultural and Food Chemistry*, to stop tumor cell proliferation, and it may help prevent age-related diseases. Take 100 mg daily to protect against cancer, heart disease and inflammation.

BEST BODY NOW Health Benefits

What are some of the healthy head-to-toe differences you'll see from making smarter health choices?

- A heightened libido
- Younger-looking, more radiant skin
- Boundless energy
- A faster metabolism
- A strong immune system
- Few to no symptoms associated with PMS, perimenopause and menopause

TAILORED HEALTH GUIDELINES FOR EVERY AGE

WHILE THE FUNDAMENTAL TENETS OF THIS PLAN STAY THE SAME, your body changes over time. Start by taking a look at the daily recommendation of supplements just listed. Then read the following sections about how your health and hormone needs may be different in your thirties, forties, fifties and beyond and use those insights to create stronger, smarter health habits in each Best Body Now decade. Customize your personal plan with your doctor based on your nutrition, health, family history and lifestyle needs.

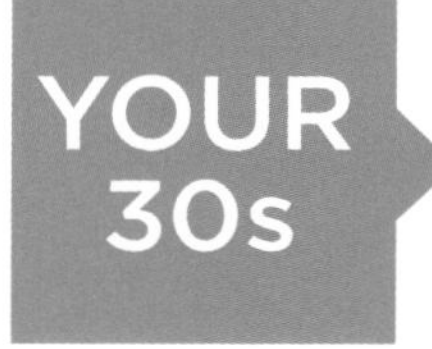

Start Disease-Fighting, Life-Enhancing Healthy Habits

In my thirties, the only real must-have daily requirements I thought I needed were a multivitamin and calcium pill. This reflected the sum total of my collective wisdom about healthy supplementation. I now know there is so much I could have done then to ward off problems that may not appear for another decade or two. Dr. Reiss explains that smart health habits can begin to change your chemistry immediately and work to prevent, treat or manage conditions no matter your age.

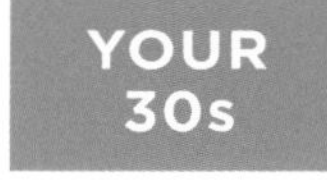

What's Happening in Your 30s That Impacts Your Health

By your thirties, you may be well acquainted with the symptoms of premenstrual syndrome, depending on your particular makeup. The side effects common with your monthly cycle can be managed with few to no issues if you arm yourself with the right supplements, combined with a healthy diet and exercise.

Many women start families in their thirties. This often comes with multitasking, overloaded schedules and forgetting or forgoing a health strategy. A busy life can

TOSCA TIDBIT

Keep your medical records completely organized and up-to-date, including your family's medical history. You'll help your doctor help you make smarter decisions about your health. Remember, you have a right to know what's in your file.

increase anxiety and impact hormone levels, which constantly fluctuate based on everything from your menstrual cycles to anxiety levels and more. It's important to set your body up so it's operating at peak health if or when you decide to have children, as well as staying energetic and strong while you raise them. It's not good enough to pick up bits and pieces of information about health while sitting in the waiting room at your beauty salon. We must have a more intelligent and informed strategy in place.

▶ Many women are on and off oral contraceptives during their thirties, stopping when they get pregnant and then using birth control pills or related contraceptive alternatives for protection again later between pregnancies.

▶ Your body begins to produce less and less estrogen and progesterone—the two sex hormones that ebb and flow during our monthly menstrual cycles—as you near forty, until you reach perimenopause.

▶ You're juggling everyone and everything all day long, which puts your body in that fight-or-flight stress state that causes adrenal glands to release cortisol to keep blood pressure and blood sugar levels in check. This hormone, however, was designed to be used in emergency situations only, so when it's overproduced because you're upset or worried, it can lead to problems including fatigue, weight gain and more. Chronic anxiety and cortisol also impact estrogen levels, causing them to drop, which can zap your libido, sleep cycle, memory, sensitivity, mood and appearance.

▶ Hectic on-the-go lifestyles can cause you to forget to take even the basics, including vitamins and heart-healthy fish oils, or not to use them properly. They can also trigger you to reach for processed foods that contain unhealthy, chemical ingredients, in both the food itself and its packaging, that impact the normal functioning of your hormones.

▶ Busy lives can have you reaching for anything to eat, including junk foods, empty-calorie snacks and quick-energy sugar fixes, which means you're depleted of the powerful nutrients you should be eating to keep the body and mind efficiently and effectively fueled.

▶ Bone density begins to drop in your thirties, and the rate eventually speeds up in your forties, which can lead to osteoporosis and fractures.

▶ Since you're so busy balancing your household, family and career, it can be tough to get in enough Zs. Adequate sleep keeps your body functioning properly, even if you feel as though you have enough energy with fewer hours of sleep. We need to rest every day in order to keep our immune systems, brain functions and bodies as a whole working as they should.

THE FIX? New Health Strategies for Your 30s:

> The brain and the body needs rest. Try to get seven or eight hours of sleep.

1 GET SEVEN HOURS OF SLEEP PER NIGHT TO KEEP ENERGY LEVELS HIGH. One thing I never skip is sleep. I don't operate at my best the next day if I shortchange myself when it comes to this important habit. After several days of sleep deprivation I am officially a mess. That's because the brain and body need rest, even if you feel energetic and alert sleeping just five hours a night. Try to get seven or eight hours of sleep. A minor caveat is that for the first couple of weeks, you'll potentially find yourself even more tired as your body readjusts to getting the right amount of sleep. Once you get past this stage, you'll start to see the benefits of getting enough sleep, such as improved memory, greater concentration and more energy than ever.

2 BATTLE PMS SYMPTOMS. B vitamins are potent anxiety relievers, and they also help reduce the symptoms of PMS, especially vitamin B_6. Unfortunately, vitamin B_6 taken alone suppresses the body's ability to absorb other B vitamins, so it's best to take this as a complex, which includes a range of other B vitamins. To start, take 100 mg of B complex twice a day with food to help battle PMS-related issues including depression, irritability, lack of motivation, fatigue and more. Even more, this dosage is a smart way to start heart disease prevention and lessen stress. Another option for battling PMS symptoms is 400 mg daily of highly absorbable magnesium glycinate. (Other forms of magnesium, including oxide and chloride, don't get absorbed by the body as well.) The reduction of PMS symptoms in the long run can be attributed to high doses of magnesium, along with calcium from food sources. And don't forget that factors including stress, exercise, alcohol and caffeine can also impact how you feel during this time of the month, so make sure you're also Eating Clean, exercising and taking time for yourself.

TOSCA TIDBIT

Consider your major stressors—a hefty work schedule, lack of downtime, an unhappy relationship—and take one small step today to resolve the issue. Add a weekly yoga class to put some calm on your agenda. Getting in touch with yourself is a wonderful way to nurture the person you are.

3 FIGHT ANXIETY AND STRESS. If you're feeling too much stress, consider adding in other anxiety reducers such as vitamin C in a dose of 1,000 mg and omega-3 fatty acids at about 1,000 to 2,000 mg a day with food. Of course, vitamin C and fish oil are best from food sources first, but supplements ensure you're as healthy as possible. If you're still feeling like your mind is racing during the day, another option for reducing anxiety is melatonin. This life-elongating hormone and antioxidant has incredible cardiovascular and breast cancer prevention properties and helps reduce stress levels. One study, published in the *Journal of Pineal Research*, showed melatonin supplements reduce stress and alleviate premenstrual symptoms. Start with the minimum daily dose of 1 mg, then gradually increase until your symptoms disappear. There's no overdose potential with melatonin, and your body will signal when the dose is too high for your system—some people find melatonin can make them feel overly sleepy or energetic or they wake up with a "sleep hangover" when taking too high a dose. If you notice any of these side effects, just reduce your dose by 0.5 mg.

4 ARM YOURSELF AGAINST THE SPREAD OF COMMON CANCERS. Human papillomavirus is a sexually transmitted disease that can cause cervical cancer when untreated and is becoming more common. Unfortunately, even if the virus leaves the body, which it does about 90 percent of the time on its own, it's been linked to the development of other cancers later in life. One way to help prevent cervical cancer is by eating cabbage as well as by taking supplements containing one of the phytochemicals found in it, a compound known as indole-3-carbinol (I3C). This compound is an anti-angiogenetic, meaning it stops the growth of new cancer cells, particularly ovarian and breast types. I3C works by increasing the levels of a beneficial hormone known as 2-hydroxy-estrogen that helps fight the disease. A study out of the University of Leicester and published in *Breast Cancer Research and Treatment* has shown that doses of 300 to 400 mg daily may kill breast cancer tumor cells. A *Journal of Nutrition* study confirms what Dr. Reiss's experience has shown: indole-3-carbinol can suppress the HPV virus' progression, as well as reverse the problems associated with the condition.

5 SUPPORT FLUCTUATING HORMONE LEVELS WITH BROCCOLI EXTRACT.

5 SUPPORT FLUCTUATING HORMONE LEVELS WITH BROCCOLI EXTRACT. As much as I love broccoli, sometimes I can't squeeze enough of it into my diet, but I need to. It contains a compound known as sulforaphane, which helps detoxify the liver and provides tremendous hormone support. It works by deactivating bad estrogens and increasing good estrogens such as 4-hydroxy-estrogen, which may help prevent breast cancer and reduce the negative side effects of birth control pills. Studies published in *Molecular Cancer Therapeutics* and *Toxicology and Applied Pharmacology* shows the substance inhibits growth and stops the proliferation of breast cancer cells. Sulforaphane comes in supplement form, and of course, it goes without saying you should also be eating the real deal as many times a week as possible.

6 STRENGTHEN YOUR IMMUNE SYSTEM FOR TODAY AND THE FUTURE. I travel quite a bit for my work, so I need a strong immune system. The antiviral known as humic acid was discovered in humus (the organic part of soil) but comes in forms safe for humans to use. Dr. Reiss recommends 500 mg daily to maintain optimal health and as much as 1,000 mg three times a day as treatment for everything from the flu to genital herpes to hepatitis C. He even uses it before getting on airplanes, in crowded spaces or after contact with someone who's sick.

7 INCREASE YOUR VITAMIN D INTAKE FOR CANCER PROTECTION AND PREGNANCY SUPPORT. One of the strongest antivirals is vitamin D, found in egg yolks, tuna, sardines and fortified cereals, but hardly any of us has enough of this nutrient in her diet. We should, though, because it boosts immunity and may ward off some types of cancers. Dr. Reiss recommends taking around 1,000 IU daily to begin warding off disease before it starts, but increases the dosage to 7,000 IU with pregnant patients to help with the baby's brain, organ and immune system development. There's also a tremendous amount of data showing the more antioxidants you're getting, the greater the benefits to pregnancy—pregnancy occurs more quickly, birth defects drop and fewer spontaneous abortions occur. Not only that, but vitamin D during pregnancy is said to benefit a child's health later in life. In research published in *Medical Hypotheses*, study author John McGrath hypothesizes that low prenatal and perinatal vitamin D levels may make children more susceptible to a variety of diseases later in life, including breast and colorectal cancer and multiple sclerosis. McGrath's other studies show links between prenatal vitamin D deficiency and problems in brain development, including schizophrenia. Check with your doctor to see what amount will work best for you; amounts over 1,000 mg should be taken under a doctor's supervision.

8 BOOST BONE HEALTH NOW TO PREVENT DISEASE LATER. Combat naturally occurring bone loss with a daily dose of vitamin K_2, which builds bone density and heart health. It's found in leafy greens, but Dr. Reiss also recommends 75 to 150 mcg daily as a supplement, so start with the lower 75 mcg dose in your thirties. The bonus? You'll be heightening your cardiovascular protection at the same time.

9 BOOST IMMUNITY WITH RESVERATROL AND PYCNOGENOL. Red wine contains numerous antioxidants, as well as a compound known as resveratrol, which the National Institutes of Health report protects against a variety of diseases, including endometriosis (a fairly common condition in women of childbearing age where cells normally found in the lining of the uterus implant on tissues elsewhere in the abdomen), breast cancer, heart disease and inflammation. To get the most benefits, start with a supplement that combines grape seed extracts, red wine extract and pure resveratrol in 100 mg doses. Also, studies such as the one published in the *Journal of Reproductive Medicine* have shown an extract from a tree found in Normandy, France, that is sold under the name Pycnogenol has immune-boosting effects and was successful in treating endometriosis. Doses range from 50 to 300 mg daily.

10 TAKE A DOSE OF CANCER-FIGHTING GINGKO. An unexpected benefit of oral contraceptives is that studies indicate they decrease the risk of ovarian cancer, but unfortunately they come with hormonal side effects. You can get a similar ovarian cancer prevention effect by taking gingko biloba supplements (for women in their thirties, Dr. Reiss recommends 120 mg doses two to three times daily with food).

11 INCREASE FERTILITY THROUGH NATURAL HORMONE SUPPLEMENTATION. The hormone pregnenolone supports the embryonic development process, from conception to the early stages of a baby's development, and helps keep your overall hormone environment functioning normally. Dr. Reiss uses it to help women who want to improve fertility by starting with 50 mg doses with food for best absorption, then increasing that dose to 100 mg after two weeks. The supplement also boosts memory, pain management, social confidence and alertness, and helps decrease cholesterol.

MINI ROAD BLOCKS

Most of the time the toughest issues around supplement changes are remembering to take your vitamins or managing what time to take them. We've got some simple Best Body Now strategies to help you stay on track.

1 I DON'T HAVE TIME TO MANAGE ALL THESE SUPPLEMENTS—IT'S OVERWHELMING.

THE BEST BODY NOW FIX: I say you don't have time not to. Figure out a system that makes it seamless. For example, spend fifteen minutes on Sunday nights dividing your vitamins for the week so you don't have to think about it every day. Some online companies have an automatic order refill system. Or buy two bottles of everything at once so you don't have to run to the store so often.

2 I CAN'T REMEMBER TO TAKE VITAMINS.

THE BEST BODY NOW FIX: If you can remember to take your kids to school, fix dinner, schedule your parents' appointments and so on. I know you can do this, too. Remember, you're the first item on your to-do list. Place your supplements in spots where you won't forget, such as your desk for lunch or your gym tote for evenings.

3 I CAN'T AFFORD IT.

THE BEST BODY NOW FIX: Supplements are an investment that pays off in quality of life and longevity. Talk to your doctor, pharmacist or other health care provider about less expensive, reputable brands on the market. Also, determine what you really need. By arming yourself with the most effective regimen, you'll not only have better results, you'll also streamline costs.

4 I DON'T LIKE TAKING PILLS.

THE BEST BODY NOW FIX: Many supplements and hormones are equally effective in capsule, powder, gel or cream form. Talk to your health care provider about options that are easier for you to take.

5 I FEEL FINE RIGHT NOW.

THE BEST BODY NOW FIX: Many of the problems we see develop later in life actually started in our twenties and thirties. Even if you feel fine now, arming yourself for the future is the key to antiaging. With the Best Body Now program, you combat problems before they even start.

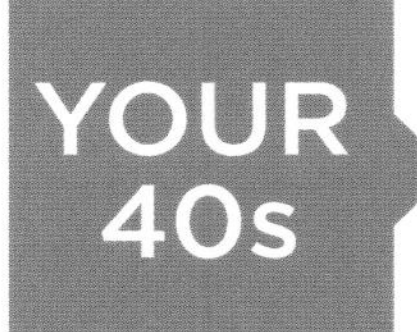

Protect Against Age-Related Health Risks and Diseases

I reached my forties in great stride, with momentum from Eating Clean and strength training, both of which provided me with the nutrients and energy levels necessary to reverse the symptoms of perimenopause. Dr. Reiss agrees that Eating Clean and working out provide a strong foundation for antiaging, but you also need to supplement your body with nutrients you're not getting from food or that are depleted because you're stressed out or not getting enough sleep.

As Dr. Reiss explains, the biggest mistake most women make is putting themselves last, especially in their forties. It's true—everyone depends on you, from your children to your aging parents—but if you don't take care of yourself first, you sacrifice the health and function of your family, too. It's something I've experienced firsthand.

> The biggest mistake most women make is putting themselves last.

Once again, though, just a few simple adjustments to your health plan in your forties can arm you for this decade. You'll also ward off some of the problems many women see in their fifties.

YOUR 40s What's Happening in Your 40s That Impacts Your Health

- Perimenopause begins. This is the time when our bodies produce smaller amounts of estrogen and progesterone, the hormones responsible for many bodily functions. Perimenopause typically comes with an onslaught of symptoms, including weight gain, irritability, mood changes, hot flashes, loss of interest in activities you used to care about, a loss in your natural caregiver mentality and more. Many women attempt to combat this weight gain by undereating. Unfortunately, when you don't eat enough or skip meals, you can slow your metabolism, which causes you to burn fewer calories and store more fat. Instead of lean muscles and beautiful curves, you'll either have an unhealthy, "skinny-fat" look or have trouble shedding those last few pounds.

- Heart disease risk and stroke risk in women increase with age. Heart disease is the leading cause of death for women—eight times as many women die from heart attacks than breast cancer, according to the National Coalition for Women with Heart Disease. It's happening to women in their thirties and forties and what's shocking is that under age fifty, heart attacks in women are twice as likely to be fatal as in men. Major risk factors include being overweight, high cholesterol and diabetes, all of which can be controlled through supplements and nutrition.

- Cancer risk increases with age. The average onset of the five most prevalent types in women—breast, lung, colorectal, uterine and ovarian—is in the forties. Breast cancer is the most common cancer for women. One in eight women who live to be eighty-five will be diagnosed with the disease, according to the American Cancer Society.

- Many women suffer with insomnia, often related to a decrease in the hormone estrogen, as well as high levels of stress.

- Many women also struggle with depression, also a symptom of perimenopause and related hormone fluctuations.

- Your rate of bone loss increases and your risk of osteoporosis climbs, which means you're at greater risk of a fracture. More than half of women over sixty-five have osteoporosis.

- As many as four out of five women may have uterine fibroids, which are benign growths that occur in the tissues of the uterus, according to the National Uterine Fibroids Foundation. By forty, nearly 40 percent of women have them, and by fifty, that figure rises to nearly 70 percent, according to research published in the *American Journal of Obstetrics and Gynecology*. Some of the symptoms are back, pelvis or leg pain, heavier bleeding during your periods and frequent urination.

- Stress gets worse, as many women in their forties are often taking care not only of their children but also aging parents in addition to a full plate of career, family life and the daily to-do list that comes from running a household.

THE FIX? New Health Strategies for Your 40s:

1 SUPPLEMENT WITH SLEEP INDUCERS IF YOU HAVE TROUBLE SLEEPING.

Hormone fluctuations and stress can make it difficult to sleep. Unfortunately, explains Dr. Reiss, lack of sleep in the long run can greatly impact your immune system, which can leave you vulnerable to sickness or disease. One remedy is magnesium glycinate. A dose taken at night will contribute calming effects. Start with 400 mg daily and increase by 100 mg increments until you find the dose that helps you sleep—there is no toxic dose of magnesium. You can also add a 1 mg starting dose of melatonin to your diet or increase your current dose in 0.5 mg increments.

2 INCREASE GOJI BERRY INTAKE FOR PERIMENOPAUSE SYMPTOM RELIEF. I love this wonder fruit that's packed with antioxidants. Originally from Asia, the berries are so fragile they must be dried in order for us on this continent to enjoy them. I keep dried berries in the pantry for a quick snack. Goji berry extract has been shown to increase estriol (one of three estrogens produced by the body). Estriol can improve bone density and boost cardiovascular strength by improving circulation and lowering cholesterol, as well as counter perimenopausal symptoms including hot flashes, vaginal dryness and urine leakage. The standard dose is 500 mg a few times a week with food.

3 INCREASE YOUR B-COMPLEX DOSAGE TO REDUCE STRESS AND BOOST HEART HEALTH. Hopefully you've been taking your B vitamins throughout your thirties to help reduce PMS symptoms, ease stress and boost cardiovascular health. Consider transitioning to a higher dose if you're still battling stress and depression or have a family history of heart disease.

4 PREVENT DISEASE LATER BY TAKING VITAMIN D NOW. The powerhouse disease fighter vitamin D is linked not only to cancer prevention but also to reducing hypertension, maintaining our body's calcium levels and boosting immunity, all important for women in their forties—and the National Institutes of Health reports that most of us aren't getting enough from foods that contain vitamin D, such as eggs, tuna and mackerel. Dr. Reiss recommends patients take between 1,000 IU and 3,000 IU daily, but because overdoses can be harmful, check with your doctor to find a dose that's right for your body.

5 IMPROVE BONE HEALTH AND SLEEP BETTER WITH MAGNESIUM SUPPLEMENTS. I was so surprised to read the latest medical studies indicating that taking calcium alone may not be the most efficient way to maintain healthy bone cells. For example, in an article published in the *Journal of Nutrition*, author and former Harvard professor Mark Hegsted discusses the high prevalence of hip fractures in people whose dairy consumption and calcium intake are high. As it turns out, your bones reach peak density by your mid-thirties. That, combined with the loss of your body's ability to absorb calcium as you reach your forties and fifties, means you need to take steps to stop bone loss. One solution is to gain the benefits associated with calcium by taking magnesium, the star nutrient that increases and maintains healthy bone cells in women. Magnesium directly supports the energy center of the cells, which is the main energy resource for many of the metabolic processes in the body. Dr. Reiss recommends up to 1,000 mg daily of magnesium glycinate, starting with around 400 mg and increasing the dose by 100 mg daily to minimize side effects including diarrhea and sleepiness. Start now to combat bone loss that may lead to osteoporosis in your fifties.

6 TAKE FISH OIL TO BOOST IMMUNITY AND HEART HEALTH. I eat tons of the smaller types of wild fish because they contain the most amounts of DHA and EPA, the two major types of heart-healthy omega-3 fatty acids. Compared to farmed fish, wild species have lower mercury levels and pack higher amounts of nutrients. In addition to eating fish a few times a week, I take 1,000 to 2,000 mg of fish oil twice a day with food to lower bad cholesterol, raise good cholesterol and reduce the risk of plaque building up in my arteries. Omega-3s may also prevent, treat and manage diseases such as multiple sclerosis and Parkinson's, thanks to their anti-inflammatory effects. (Normal inflammation is part of the body's healing process, but an overactive immune system, as in certain diseases such as multiple sclerosis or arthritis, can cause tissue to degrade.)

7 PROTECT BONES AND HEART HEALTH WITH VITAMIN K_2. By your forties, you may already be on a low-dose (75 mcg) regimen of bone-building, heart-healthy vitamin K_2 to start warding off osteoporosis and cardiovascular disease, which can begin developing during this decade, explains Dr. Reiss. If so, consider changing your dose to 100 mcg, as bone loss increases in our forties, as does our risk of heart problems, including heart attacks.

8 ELEVATE YOUR MOOD WITH NATURAL DEPRESSION FIGHTERS. Can you relate to the feeling of euphoria you get when you fall in love or even simply eat an amazing meal with friends? It is the result of a brain chemical called dopamine, which gives you feelings of pleasure and can motivate you to continue doing or start doing something you want to do, such as exercise, take a bath, or spend time with family. When dopamine levels drop, you can feel depressed, lethargic and unmotivated to do anything. There are natural ways to increase dopamine levels—ginkgo biloba, L-arginine, St. John's wort and Pycnogenol have all been shown in studies to raise this brain chemical naturally, explains Dr. Reiss. Increased amounts of this happiness trigger help combat the depression associated with perimenopause, as well as the side effects of stress. Gingko has also been shown to fight ovarian cancer and multiple sclerosis in studies. The typical dosage of gingko is 120 mg daily.

9 IMPROVE YOUR BRAIN FUNCTION AND PREVENT PROBLEMS LATER. Adaptogens are immune-boosting natural herbs that contain powerful antioxidants that combat stress, anxiety and fatigue, explains Dr. Reiss. The most well-known ones are gingko biloba, ginseng, holy basil, maca and licorice. Studies, such as those reported by the University of Maryland Medical Center, have shown these substances also boost memory and mood, presumably because you will be less stressed. If you try them, follow the recommendations printed on the bottle you purchase.

10 HELP YOUR BODY NATURALLY BURN POUNDS. L-carnitine is an amino acid that not only has amazing cardiovascular benefits but helps your body better oxidize fat and prevent weight gain related to perimenopause. Dr. Reiss recommends taking 1 to 6 grams added to water while exercising to also help in training and recovery.

11 INCREASE YOUR INTAKE OF TURMERIC FOR DISEASE PROTECTION. This main spice found in Indian curries actually does more than make a meal taste incredible. When eaten, turmeric signals more than 2,500 genes to work more efficiently, which is crucial to how our bodies grow, develop and function, explains Dr. Reiss. Turmeric has been linked to the prevention of everything from cancer to Alzheimer's to multiple sclerosis. Start now to prevent the onset of conditions beginning in your fifties. The typical recommended dose is 400 to 600 mg, taken two to three times daily, but check the packaging of the product you purchase for specific recommendations. Start at the lower dose now and increase your dose in your fifties. Remember to add turmeric to your cooking, too, since it is as effective when used as a spice in your food. It must, however, be cooked in order to be effective.

> When eaten, turmeric signals more than 2,500 genes to work more efficiently.

12 SAFEGUARD YOUR MEMORY WITH NATURAL HORMONES. Your brain function begins to decline in your forties but it doesn't have to be that way. Pregnenolone, a naturally occurring hormone, similar to estrogen, progesterone and DHEA, has been shown to increase memory, alertness, social skills and overall brain function. In a study published in *Progress in Neurobiology*, researchers discovered that pregnenolone may actually spur the growth of new nerve tissue, something that formerly was believed to be impossible. Dr. Reiss recommends starting with 50 mg with food at breakfast or lunch, then after two weeks upping the dose to 100 mg.

THE WORST HEALTH HABITS

Some health habits are unhealthy, and some are downright abysmal. I've listed five of the worst here.

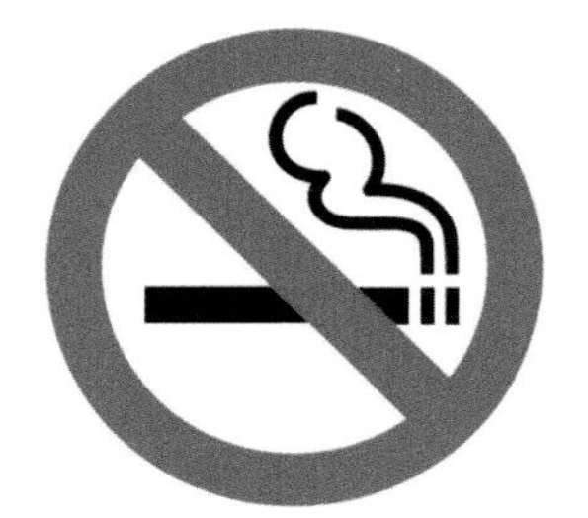

1 SMOKING. There's no controversy here. If you're still doing this, consult your doctor about ways to stop. Nothing you take in pill form can counter a daily pack-a-day habit.

2 SUCCUMBING TO STRESS. Burning your adrenals nonstop is a guaranteed way to deplete your immune system. Doing so in the long term, explains Dr. Reiss, may lead to numerous conditions including cancer, cardiovascular disease and more. Look for natural calming remedies such as magnesium, L-tryptophan and melatonin.

3 SKIPPING SLEEP. Getting fewer hours of sleep will seriously impact your longevity, explains Dr. Reiss. Less than seven or eight hours a night has been linked to obesity, shorter attention span, reduced memory and poor decision-making skills. Supplementing with magnesium, L-tryptophan and melatonin can help you sleep better.

4 AVOIDING CHECKUPS AND TESTS. The only real way to determine what your body needs is to be tested by your doctor. Make an appointment today and you're one step closer to your Best Body Now.

5 TREATING SYMPTOMS, NOT THE UNDERLYING PROBLEM. So many times when we take aspirin, antidepressants or other meds, we're just pushing the problem aside to get back to life. Most often, Dr. Reiss explains, our symptoms are related to hormones, and these problems can be repaired at the source rather than just temporarily mitigated.

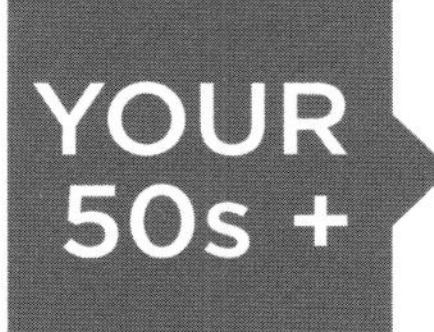

Strengthen Your Health Profile

My health approach for fifty mirrors what I did in my forties—I created a strong foundation of immune-boosting, age-proofing habits and made essential adjustments to help me prepare for the hormonal and age-related changes that come with this new decade. The focus during your fifties is improving brain function, cardiovascular protection, stress reduction, and managing and reducing the symptoms of menopause. As mentioned before, always check in with your doctor about specific issues related to your body's unique needs and requirements. The doses we give here are simply guidelines from Dr. Reiss's research, experience and practice, as well as that of the medical community.

> The focus during your fifties is improving brain function, cardiovascular protection, stress reduction, and managing and reducing the symptoms of menopause.

YOUR 50s +

What's Happening in Your 50s and Beyond That Impacts Your Health

- Menopause, which usually begins around your early fifties, marks the stopping of your period, as well as a significant drop in the hormone estrogen. When natural estrogen levels fall, you may begin to experience symptoms including migraines, insomnia, night sweats, hot flashes, vaginal dryness, depression and lack of interest in sex.

- Menopause brings with it cardiovascular issues: blood pressure and unhealthy LDL cholesterol begin rising and healthy HDL cholesterol decreases as a result of changing hormone levels. The risk of cardiovascular disease increases by 50 percent if you've got at least two risk factors such as high blood pressure, smoking, drinking and more.

- Brain function and memory start to decline more significantly, and women can begin experiencing problems with memory, learning and attention span. You also may start seeing early signs of dementia.

- Loss of bone density continues, with the National Osteoporosis Foundation reporting that one in two women over fifty will have at least one fracture from osteoporosis and, on average, can lose about 7 percent of their bone density during this decade.

DHEA: A POWERFUL HORMONE FOR YOUR BEST BODY NOW

DHEA, COMMONLY THOUGHT TO BE ONLY a male hormone or miscategorized as an anabolic steroid (a synthetic steroid often misused by athletes and bodybuilders to enhance performance) is actually the most prevalent hormone in a woman's body. Dr. Reiss has treated more than seven thousand women in his practice with bioidentical DHEA because of its powerful benefits and fountain-of-youth-like results. Some of those benefits include prevention of breast cancer, cardiovascular disease, diabetes, autoimmune disorders and depression, as well as improvement in memory, muscle and bone strength and sexuality. It also helps combat symptoms of menopause.

These positive effects have long been applauded in medical journals and scientific studies. However, because bioidentical DHEA has been confused with an anabolic steroid—again, it's not—many doctors today will try to deter patients from taking it, even though it's proven to be safe and highly effective. Dr. Reiss starts patients with 5 mg of pills or capsules taken daily for two weeks to establish dose level. If the initial dose is too high, side effects may include irritability, acne and some hair loss within four weeks. If that happens, the initial dose simply needs to be cut in half. If the dose causes no problems, increase by 5 mg daily for another two weeks. Most women top out at 10 to 15 mg without untoward side effects.

Decades of stress begin to take their toll. In this decade diseases including cancer, heart disease, multiple sclerosis, Parkinson's and more begin to take hold in the body. Even if you haven't started prevention yet, it's never too late to boost your immunity and begin a healthier, Best Body Now lifestyle in order to give yourself the best fighting chance against some of these crippling diseases. Cancers of the anus, bladder, mouth and esophagus occurring in our fifties have been linked to having had human papillomavirus in your thirties, even if treated.

> It's never too late to boost your immunity and begin a healthier, Best Body Now lifestyle.

THE FIX? New Health Strategies For Your 50s +:

1 PREVENT CANCER AND MEMORY PROBLEMS OCCURRING AT THIS AGE. Although vitamin E has valuable health benefits for women of all ages, it's particularly important in your fifties to consume more of this vitamin in order to help prevent cancer and Alzheimer's, as well as to enhance memory and brain function. Look for vitamin E complex, which contains all the disease-fighting forms of this nutrient, including tocopherols and tocotrienols. (Most over-the-counter supplements just contain alpha-tocopherol, so you need to double-check the label before buying in order to get the full spectrum of benefits.) If you're already taking a vitamin E complex, Dr. Reiss advises increasing the dose to the maximum 800 IU, along with an additional 100 mg of memory-boosting tocotrienols, taking both with food. Brown rice is a valuable food source of these potent forms of vitamin E.

2 ADD GOJI BERRY SUPPLEMENTS TO STRENGTHEN BONES AND SUPPORT HEART HEALTH. One of the newest fruits discovered to have very high antioxidant levels is a berry grown in Asia, called goji. It's been shown to improve bone density and is believed to ward off heart disease, thanks to its positive effects on estriol, one of the major types of the hormone estrogen that boosts bone and heart health. If you're already taking the standard supplement dose of 500 mg a few times a week, aim to take it daily. I also enjoy the dried berries in my hot oatmeal, smoothies and shakes.

3 INCREASE YOUR INTAKE OF B COMPLEX FOR MOOD HEALTH AND DISEASE PREVENTION. The family of B vitamins work together to combat stress, depression and cardiovascular disease, all common risks and diseases that become prevalent after menopause. According to Dr. Reiss, you can safely increase your dosage of B complex to 300 mg, especially if you're dealing with any of these issues.

4 BATTLE MEMORY, BONE AND IMMUNITY ISSUES WITH VITAMIN D. Even if your bones seem fine and your memory is sharp as ever, bone tissue and brain function have been deteriorating since your thirties and forties. The good news is you can combat brain and memory issues and ward off diseases such as multiple sclerosis, rheumatoid arthritis, Alzheimer's and osteoporosis with vitamin D, an antiviral that prevents the spread of viruses in your body. Talk to your doctor about an appropriate dose for you.

5 PROTECT YOUR HEART WITH COENZYME Q_{10}. Hopefully you're already taking this antioxidant as part of your basic Best Body Now health plan. If so, it's been helping to protect your cardiovascular system. If not, start now and you can still reap the heart benefits. It's especially important for women taking beta-blockers (used to control blood pressure), cholesterol medications and antidepressants, because as Dr. Reiss explains, these medications suppress coenzyme Q_{10} in the body. Supplement with 100 to 300 mg daily with food.

6 SUPPORT HEART AND BONE HEALTH WITH VITAMIN K_2. Vitamin K_2 is a powerhouse cardiovascular and bone supporter, explains Dr. Reiss. You can get the nutrient through greens and other vegetables as well as certain oils, such as olive and coconut oil. Still, supplementing in your fifties especially can do wonders for your heart and bones. Try for 75 mcg daily with food.

7 IMPROVE MEMORY WITH NATURAL BRAIN BOOSTERS. A hormone derivative of DHEA called 7-keto not only helps speed weight loss but also has been shown to have similar benefits as DHEA, including boosting memory, improving brain function and enhancing the immune system. Dr. Reiss recommends 200 mg a day for memory-boosting benefits. Pregnenolone, another hormone found naturally in the body, also supports memory function. If you've already started taking 50 to 100 mg in your forties, add 50 mg to see if you have improved results. The maximum daily dose he recommends is 300 mg daily.

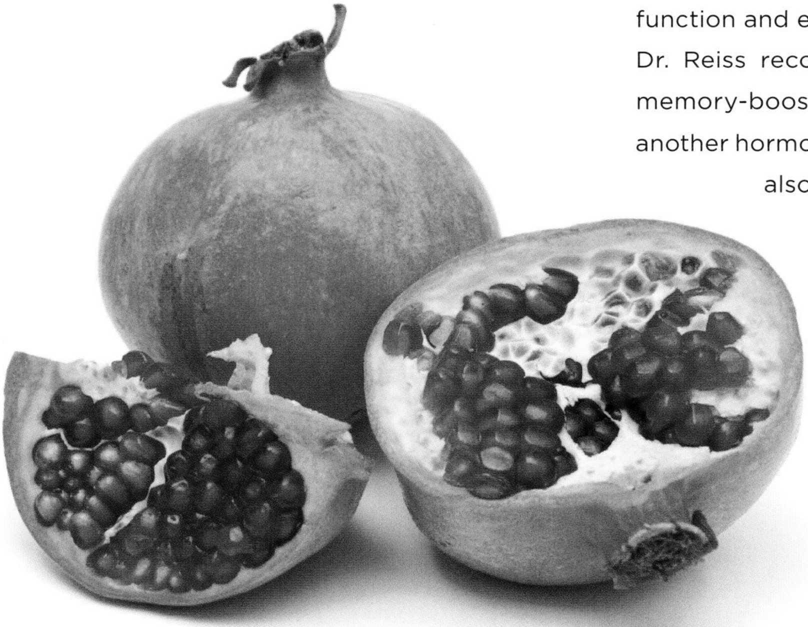

8 FIGHT DEPRESSION NATURALLY.

Even if your diet is rich in small, nutrient-dense wild fish, you likely still need to supplement with fish oil. This powerful anti-inflammatory contains omega-3 fatty acids that Best Body Now women in their fifties need more than ever to combat depression and bring on happiness. Dr. Reiss recommends 1,000 to 2,000 mg daily, so if you're already taking it, go for the maximum dosage. For a triple punch, make sure you're also getting enough vitamin D and magnesium glycinate, and your mood is sure to get a boost.

9 ADD ANTIOXIDANTS AND ANTI-VIRALS FOR POWERFUL DISEASE PREVENTION.

We've already listed them on your daily must-haves at the beginning of the chapter, but it's so important that it warrants this gentle reminder. Antioxidants and antivirals such as those found in pomegranate, green tea, red wine, curcumin and grape extract can strengthen immunity to help you fight years of less-than-perfect nutrition, stress and other lifestyle factors that often come back to haunt you in your fifties, explains Dr. Reiss. Refer to the basics of the program at the start of the chapter for specific doses. It's more important than ever in your fifties and the sooner you start, the more quickly your body will enjoy the healthy benefits.

10 TAKE MORE MAGNESIUM TO RELIEVE MENOPAUSAL SYMPTOMS.

This powerful nutrient should also be taken by women of all ages, but if you're in your fifties, consider the maximum dosage of 1,000 mg daily for relief of menopausal systems, cancer prevention, and bone and heart health. Magnesium has a calming effect, so I take my dose before bed to help me sleep.

> Hot flashes and night sweats may seem as though they're an inevitable part of menopause, but they don't have to be.

11 CONSIDER SUPPLEMENTING WITH ESTRIOL TO MANAGE MENOPAUSE SYMPTOMS. Hot flashes and night sweats may seem as though they're an inevitable part of menopause, but they don't have to be. One solution is estriol, one of the major types of estrogen offering numerous benefits to the body, especially after menopause, explains Dr. Reiss. He prescribes it in cream, gel, suppository and sublingual forms to reduce the risk of breast cancer, treat and prevent the progression of multiple sclerosis, lower inflammation in our bodies that can lead to disease, alleviate hot flashes, reduce night sweats and stop vaginal dryness. Talk to your doctor about a treatment plan for you.

12 REST BETTER AT NIGHT WITH NATURAL SLEEP AIDS. Treat every day as though it's Thanksgiving by supplementing with L-tryptophan, the amino acid in turkey that helps you get your post-meal nap. When taken, it increases serotonin levels. These are the hormones that calm your mood and help you fall asleep, Dr. Reiss explains. Increasing your intake can help fight depression, insomnia, lack of libido, migraines and sugar cravings. Follow the instructions found on the bottle you purchase—the typical dose ranges from 500 to 6,000 mg with no side effects.

The "H" Factor: A-List Proof That Life Gets Better at 40

The inimitable and ageless Goldie Hawn, sixty-three, doesn't ever seem to slow down. After decades of stardom and earning an Oscar, she started the Cosmic Production Company at fifty-eight. Other impressive milestones? She graced her first *Playboy* cover at thirty-nine and continues to be featured on celebrity hot lists and magazine covers, including a recent issue of AARP's magazine. If this is what the sixties look like, we're in good shape.

MY BEST BODY NOW

Triumph of the Not-So-Average Jane
Julie Van Acker's Journey

THEN
5'4", AGE 37
164 POUNDS

NOW
AGE 42
118 POUNDS

My life changes started at the urging of my doctor, after my weight climbed to nearly 165, my body fat rose to 32 percent and my cholesterol reached 214. It seemed my career in the processed food industry, including retail sales, in-store demos and new-product testing, had caught up with me. With my father, mother and sister all on lifelong meds, and for more than just high cholesterol, I decided now was the time to make a change in my life and get going with better eating habits, exercise and a more determined mind-set.

With my husband's encouragement, we hired a personal chef to teach us about meal planning, preparations, fresh ingredients and more, rather than prepackaged meals or dinner helpers. I also hired a personal trainer who introduced me to Tosca's program and books on Eating Clean. My biggest takeaway was to prepare, prepare, prepare. By planning you can avoid making bad choices. I learned to eat for fuel and not "just because." I acted as if everything I put in my mouth was either a step toward or away from my goals.

My metabolism began changing and the pounds dropped off. But that was just the beginning. My self-esteem skyrocketed in all areas, from my marriage to my career to my social life. In May 2008, I entered my first bodybuilding competition.

As I compete in these figure competitions I keep noticing that the older classes are the tougher classes. It's true, fifty is the new forty, forty is the new thirty, etc. Muscle maturity and having the confidence and knowledge that you've made a change in your life shows onstage. Younger women have come up to me asking how I got my physique. I love it.

I'm still in the processed foods industry, surrounded by unhealthy choices every day. But I stay on track by writing and tracking goals, surrounding myself with motivational quotes, finding new exercises to stay challenged and taking a cooler with healthy foods to work so I make smart food decisions. It is not selfish to eat every three hours and to make things that taste good and you enjoy. It is responsible to introduce to your family and friends a better way of eating, living and being a good role model. Teach others your newfound ways and they will catch on. They will tire of being the ones that are tired, overweight and unhappy about their clothes and athletic abilities.

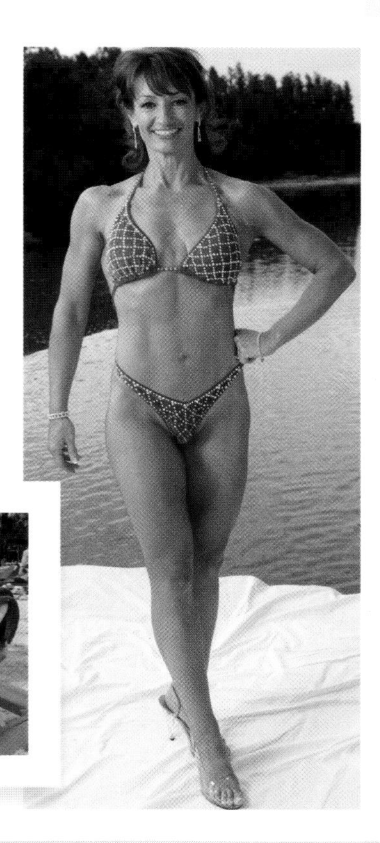

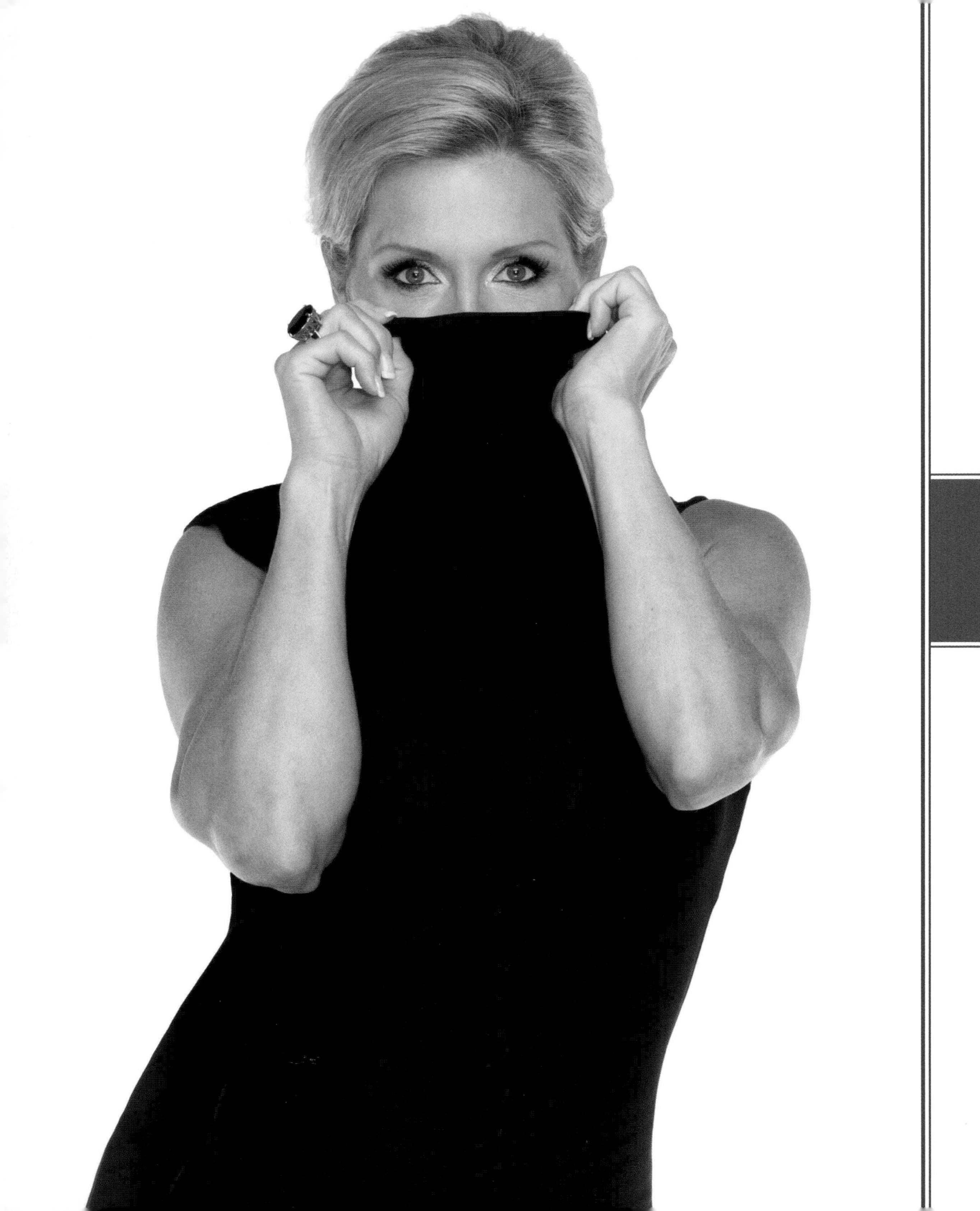

7 Best Body Now Beauty

THE BEST BODY NOW PHILOSOPHY IS ALL ABOUT CREATING health and beauty from the inside out. When I started Eating Clean and living the Best Body Now lifestyle, I didn't just lose weight and discover new muscle definition. When I took care of my body, my body responded with rejuvenated, smooth skin, strong nails and thick, shiny hair. I actually began to look younger and more beautiful! This chapter includes all of the essential beauty tips you need to put your most beautiful self forward, the Best Body Now way.

> When I took care of my body, I actually began to look younger and more beautiful!

In addition to the insider beauty secrets I've picked up over the years, the recommendations, advice and guidance in this chapter come from the very people I turned to myself: Dr. Trevor Born, a cosmetic dermatologist, and celebrity makeup artist Carol Shaw, two well-known and sought-after beauty experts. I first met Dr. Born while searching for ways to supplement my antiaging diet and exercise program with beauty treatments that achieved the same stunning results. I was impressed to learn that Dr. Born uses the latest technology and many advanced noninvasive treatments, combined with healthy lifestyle strategies, to deliver progressive antiaging solutions. By following his advice, I was able to achieve and maintain the youthful radiance I hadn't seen for years. Making improved nutrition choices and exercising brings you to a point where the body does look and feel more youthful, but there are numerous noninvasive methods one can explore to help keep age at bay. I sought not to cut and sew myself a new image but to work with what I had and what I was learning to enhance the process.

However, I knew that even the best skin care program can't undo years of beauty don'ts or erase fine lines and dark circles. That's where Carol Shaw, celebrity makeup artist and founder of Lorac Cosmetics, comes in. Her work regularly graces the red carpet and magazine covers. Although she works with numerous Hollywood clients, her trademark style is to create a gorgeous face that looks as if you aren't wearing much makeup at all, a philosophy that works with my hectic lifestyle. Her natural-is-best approach also resonates with my desire to be healthier in all areas of my life—her Lorac products are formulated with pure ingredients such as plant extracts, emollients and natural conditioners, and without irritants like fragrance and oil. In other words, she uses the same natural principles in her beauty products that I do in my Best Body Now program. And at fifty, Carol inspires me by being one more example of a woman who is sexier, healthier and better than ever—no matter her age.

TOSCA TIDBIT

Treat your Best Body Now journey as a privilege. Think of your hard work as a reward, not a chore, punishment or obligation. Remind yourself of how strong you feel after a powerful sweat session, a healthy meal or sharing active quality time with family—it's far more satisfying than a candy bar or a night of television. The joy of eating a chocolate chip cookie is short-lived compared to the pain of not being able to fit into your skinny jeans or a pretty dress.

Beauty Secrets to Keep You Turning Heads

ONE OF THE BIGGEST MISTAKES I MADE in my twenties and thirties was assuming that how I fueled and treated my body didn't impact my appearance, especially my skin and hair. When I started following the Best Body Now fitness and nutrition program, I looked and felt healthier than ever. I discovered that garbage foods, such as sugar- and salt-laden snacks, did not just make me feel twice my age, but also made me look it.

> Garbage foods, such as sugar- and salt-laden snacks, did not just make me feel twice my age, but also made me look it.

What I learned is that what's good for your body is also ideal for your beauty. Both Dr. Born and Carol see dramatic results in their celebrity clients who commit to lifestyle changes like exercising regularly and fueling their body with fresh produce, whole grains and lean, healthy proteins. We know that vitamins, particularly vitamin A, the B vitamins and vitamin C are potent immune system boosters, but as Dr. Born points out, they also promote smooth, even skin tone, create healthy cell tissue and prevent or minimize the signs of aging. Omega-3 fatty acids don't just improve your heart and brain health but also make your skin supple and your hair resilient, strong and shiny.

> What's good for your body is also ideal for your beauty.

Today, I focus not only on fueling my body through nutrition, fitness and smart supplements but also on nourishing my skin and treating myself to a daily beauty routine that makes me look and feel better. My glow comes from both my newfound confidence and my healthy, radiant skin—which got that way because I treated it correctly.

BEST BODY NOW Beauty Basics

DR. BORN'S PHILOSOPHY IS THAT AN everyday skin care system can be easy—it can take as few as three steps—but still give you healthy, youthful results. Carol agrees. Her philosophy of "beauty made simple" stems from her own struggles with sensitive skin, as well as those of her celebrity clients. She believes skin is the essence of beauty, so you should always start with great skin and then add color. Once you have a skin care routine that works for you, the makeup component isn't just about coverage; it's also about highlighting your own natural beauty and features.

Your basic beauty routine can take as little as ten minutes using as few as five products, explains Carol. It's a minimal amount of effort for maximum beauty results that will have you looking your best and feeling amazing about yourself. And if you invest in your skin by taking good care of it now, you will have beautiful, radiant skin for life.

> If you invest in your skin by taking good care of it now, you will have beautiful, radiant skin for life.

Here are your Best Body Now beauty basics, no matter what your age:

✔ **CLEANSE AND PREPARE YOUR SKIN FOR MAKEUP.** Cleansing and "resurfacing," or exfoliating, your skin sloughs off dead skin cells, cleans out pores and gives you a healthy, radiant glow, explains Dr. Born. You can do a gentle exfoliation with a scrub or mask every day, as well as use a cleansing tool such as the Clarisonic, which uses sonic technology to thoroughly clean pores and exfoliate skin, morning and night. Not only are you left with a youthful, rejuvenated complexion, but, as Carol explains, you'll have the perfect smooth surface for beginning your makeup application. Since I started using the Clarisonic on a daily basis for cleansing my skin I have noticed an improved radiance and brightness to my skin. I am certain this simple brushing tool is the reason why my skin is clearer and my pores, especially on my nose, are smaller. I am so happy to have found this tool because prior to this I was actually using my electric toothbrush on my face! Not quite the same thing.

✔ **HYDRATE YOUR SKIN.** Dr. Born recommends keeping skin hydrated by applying a moisturizer with active ingredients such as vitamin C immediately after you exfoliate every morning and evening. Not only is this an important step for the condition of your skin, but, as Carol explains, the combination of exfoliation and hydration creates a smooth surface that helps your makeup glide on for a more natural look.

> One of the most important antiaging tools for skin is UV protection.

USE SUNSCREEN DAILY. One of the most important antiaging tools for skin is UV protection, explains Dr. Born. Judicious use of a product with an SPF of 15 or higher every morning before you leave the house (and reapplying it throughout the day depending on your exposure to the sun) needs to become a daily skin protection habit. In the morning, apply at least 1 ounce—about a shot glass worth—of sunscreen to your body for complete protection against the sun's harmful UV rays. You'll also need another tablespoon for your face and neck. Dr. Born recommends using cosmetics with SPF 15 or higher already added, which saves time. Because reapplication throughout the day is important, Carol recommends foundation powders with SPF that allow you to touch up your UV protection midday without having to take off your makeup and reapply sunscreen; they're also easy to pack in your cosmetic case if you're on the go.

PERFECT YOUR SKIN TONE. Even women with great skin need to even out its texture and tone and protect it from future damage. Carol recommends finding the right foundation for your skin type, whether it's a powder for oilier skin, an antiaging formula or a tinted moisturizer for lighter coverage. The idea is to create a flawless finish—this means finding a foundation that looks natural, matches your skin tone and feels like you're wearing nothing at all. What's right for you may evolve as you age or even as the seasons change, both of which impact how oily or dry your skin is. The changing nature of your skin is why it is important to revise your skin care regimen frequently. I make changes in the winter and again in the summer each year.

MATCH FOUNDATION TO YOUR SKIN TONE. Unfortunately, we're all not born with perfect, poreless, evenly toned skin. How do you know if a foundation is the right shade? Smooth it into your jawline—it should disappear perfectly into your skin in natural light. And remember that the foundation color you need can change in response to changes in your skin color. For instance, in the summer months you may be slightly more tan than in the winter. And some women experience changes in skin color in response to hormonal changes, so be aware that one foundation may not work for you all year long.

ADD YOUTHFUL GLOW. A luminizing bronzer has light-reflecting particles that can make you look more radiant whether you're thirty or fifty. Look for shades that give you a natural bronze glow and avoid any that are too orange or dark. The result? You'll have a healthy glow and look younger in seconds. Sometimes I will just use a bronzer for my cheeks rather than a blush.

FINISH WITH BROWS. Carol finds that well-groomed eyebrows are a simple way to look put together in an instant—the right arch can transform your look and give you an instant eyelift. Go to a professional the first time and then maintain the shape on your own. Brush brows after makeup application and you'll look fresh before you greet your day. I am convinced this is one of those powerful celeb secrets well known to them and misunderstood by the rest of us. I confess I now have a habit of checking out people's eyebrows all the time.

APPLY BLUSH OR BRONZER FOR A YOUTHFUL LOOK. Since our natural coloring fades as we age, it's important to wear a subtle color in the appropriate places, particularly your cheeks. Estée Lauder had a saying: "Please, more blush." A brighter blush will help to enhance your face and give it a pop of color. Powder blush is the easiest formula to work with because it blends well and works on the majority of skin types. If you make a mistake such as using color that's too bold or bright, you can easily correct this by blending with a clean powder puff. If you have dry skin or like a dewy look, choose a cream blush, but stick to powder if you have uneven skin or are prone to breakouts.

BEST BODY NOW BENEFITS

WHAT ARE SOME OF THE BEAUTIFUL differences you'll see from incorporating smart beauty habits? A healthy glow is just the beginning of the positive changes you will notice, along with fewer wrinkles and fine lines and a clear, even complexion. Possibly the most significant result from your new skin care efforts is the intangible one—that certain something that can only be defined as the glow resulting from the knowledge that you look, well, *hot*!

The most significant result from your new skin care efforts is the intangible one—the glow resulting from the knowledge that you look, well, *hot!*

START YOUR BEST BODY NOW

BECAUSE I'M IN THE SPOTLIGHT AND IN front of the cameras so often, readers often ask how I manage to look so young. While great food and fitness habits are fundamental to looking youthful and radiant, we can all use a few tweaks to our routine. Here are some of Carol's quick tips that help me look my best.

1 **PURGE YOUR COSMETIC BAG, DRAWERS AND CLOSETS.** Old makeup can be contaminated with bacteria. Throw out opened products more than a year old—or three months for mascara. Most skin care products, such as night creams and sunscreen, have an expiration date on the packaging.

2 **CARRY YOUR ESSENTIALS.** Carol keeps her five basics in her bathroom, purse, travel bag and gym tote so she can easily transform in five minutes or less. Even just a swipe of gloss or mascara midday can rejuvenate how you look and feel. I buy duplicates of these five basics and stash one set in my purse, one in my home and one at the office.

3 **FIND AN ARTIST.** Carol recommends using the resources around you, which includes finding an expert at a beauty store or spa in your area. She can work with you to help you use products you have or teach you to apply what you've bought. All you need is one session and then you can go back seasonally for updates on new products, techniques, brushes or shades.

4 **START WITH WHAT YOU KNOW.** Most women have colors that resonate with them. If you're more comfortable with peach tones, start there because you're more likely to stick with a routine you're confident with. Also, rid your cosmetic bag of shades that no longer work for your skin tone or lifestyle. You can explore new shades or products once you're into a regular beauty habit you like.

5 INVEST IN A GOOD PALETTE. Many brands design their makeup palettes with the idea that the eye shadow and blush colors can be mixed and matched together for easy and coordinated application. Find one palette you like and experiment with the shades—it's a great place to start to feel more comfortable with trying new colors or techniques.

6 PERFECT A SMOKY EYE. Even though the smoky eye you see in movies and on television and in magazines seems unattainable, it can be really simple to do—and it's a great way to feel sexy at any age. It's easiest to start with a palette because your highlighter, lid shades and contour shades are all included. All you'll need in addition is liner and mascara. The easy how-to:

- Apply the lightest highlighter shade from brow to lash to create a canvas.
- Use the middle shade—whether smoke, taupe, brown or gray—over the eyelid, then blend it into the crease softly and then toward the outer corner. Softly wing out to elongate the eye.
- Smudge the darkest shade from halfway on the lid to the outer corner and out at the edge to add depth and darkness.
- Use the dark shade to smudge under lower lashes as liner.
- Line top lash line with black liner and smudge. Finish with mascara and light peach, pink or nude lips.

7 FIND THE PERFECT NATURAL LIP COLOR. Look for liners and lipsticks in colors no deeper than a shade darker than your own for the quintessential natural look. Carol loves this look with the smoky eye in the evenings, and it works for day when you need a touch of color.

TAILORED BEAUTY TIPS FOR EVERY AGE

YOUR BEST BODY NOW BEAUTY ROUTINE WON'T CHANGE MUCH going forward; however, you can expect to make minor adjustments as you age. The next sections outline the differences in our beauty needs in each Best Body Now decade and how you can beat the clock with proven antiaging strategies, from skin care treatments to makeup tricks.

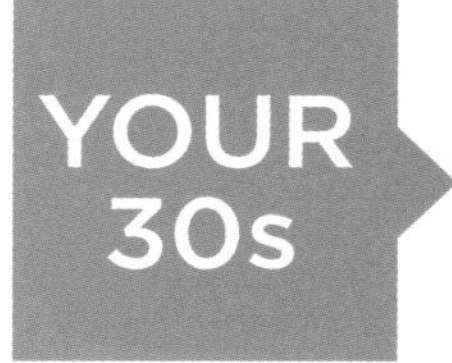

Start Confidence-Boosting, Age-Proofing Beauty Habits

In my thirties my beauty routine, which in effect wasn't a routine at all when I think about it, consisted of washing, drying and moisturizing my skin with no rhyme or reason and definitely no concern for specific products. I can remember a time when I was knee-deep in diapers and used baby products on my face because they were all over the house already. I thought this was enough. I didn't realize that exfoliating or using sunscreen daily, for example, would ultimately take years off my face and help me look more radiant. Not only did I have poor beauty habits, but I was also chronically dehydrated and fueling my body with sugar and fat. As a result, my skin looked tired, worn and grayish. It lacked the smooth, supple texture that I've since rediscovered. Since I changed my routine to the Best Body Now plan, fine lines and wrinkles, as well as droopy eyes and dark circles, have vanished. Pores the size of dinner plates have also disappeared and blemishes have been relegated to my adolescent days. I've realized firsthand that no matter when you start to take care of your skin and incorporate smart beauty habits, you will see results fast—you simply have to make a commitment to yourself that skin care matters.

Since I changed my routine to the Best Body Now plan, fine lines and wrinkles, as well as droopy eyes and dark circles, have vanished.

YOUR 30s What's Happening in Your 30s That Impacts Your Beauty

Significant life changes can elevate anxiety and stress levels, which in turn stimulate the stress response. The body has no recourse but to produce more of the stress response hormone cortisol, which experts believe causes an increase in oil production in the skin. Unfortunately, the result is not pretty. You can expect to see clogged pores, blemishes and even acne.

Changes in hormones can also cause adult acne in your thirties, explains Dr. Born. Some studies suggest as many as one in five women between twenty-five and forty deal with this condition. This can be challenging to manage, and if over-the-counter products aren't working, you may require prescription medication, such as Accutane or oral contraceptives. Don't anguish over these problems at home. Seek the help of a board-certified dermatologist to guide you through the treatment of such outbreaks.

Rosacea, an umbrella term for a skin condition causing the appearance of acne-like bumps and red, discolored skin, is prevalent in your thirties, often peaking by your forties and fifties. Again, a skin professional can be invaluable in solving these skin concerns.

Most women are juggling numerous responsibilities, from household to family to career. Being pressed for time can make you inclined to skip or skimp on important beauty steps. Carol knows that to stick with your beauty routine, it needs to be fast and easy.

Multitasking in your thirties can also mean stress. Whether you're getting married, starting a family or building a career, most women have numerous obligations during this decade. Dr. Born points to the presidents of the United States as an example—most of them age more quickly than the rest of us in response to the intense and relentless stress levels of the job. I have noticed an increase in President Obama's gray hair already!

Lack of sleep can also impact our beauty routine. Carol finds her clients often turn to caffeine or junk food or skip exercise if they don't get their Zs, all of which can wreak havoc on skin and compromise your Best Body Now beauty plan.

Sun exposure may be at an all-time high during this period, due to outdoor activities, exercise, vacations and more. Unfortunately, as Dr. Born explains, UV rays from the sun break down collagen (the protein that forms the structure for skin cells), damage skin cell DNA and cause signs of premature aging, such as wrinkles, fine lines, hyperpigmentation and uneven texture and tone.

Our outer layer of skin naturally sheds each day and is replaced with new skin cells, which helps create a youthful, radiant glow. This natural process of skin renewal slows in our twenties, and by our thirties we can begin to lose the healthy radiance we had in our teens and early twenties, explains Dr. Born.

Many of us begin to see the effects of loss of collagen in this decade, explains Dr. Born. By your late twenties and thirties, your skin begins to lose collagen and elastin, another protein that contributes to skin's elasticity.

In addition to loss of skin cells, you start to experience underlying bone and deep tissue changes by the time you hit thirty, as well as a natural loss of fat volume in the face. It is this loss of fat in the face that causes you to lose definition in your face, creating a look that most people describe as their face "falling" as they get older. All of this will begin to appear in your forties, explains Dr. Born, unless you take preventive measures in your thirties. This is not to say we cannot enjoy a beautiful face full of expression as it naturally ages, but the idea here is to head off unnecessary aging changes with helpful natural approaches to your skin care.

Skin discoloration, also known as hyperpigmentation, brown spots, sun spots or age spots, starts to appear in your thirties. According to Dr. Born, the most common cause is sun damage, but hormonal changes related to pregnancy or oral contraceptives may also play a role in causing unnecessary brown patches to appear on the skin.

Signs of aging due to a variety of issues, from sun damage to stress to lack of sleep, begin to appear in this decade in the form of fine lines, especially in the eye area. Expression lines may also appear around the lips and on the forehead.

TOSCA TIDBIT

A great way to infuse your life with passion is to do something you used to love when you were younger. Were you a dancer, a soccer player, an artist? It doesn't matter what your level of accomplishment was—find that old tutu, pick up the ball you used to kick around or dredge up those paintbrushes—and start again. Use this inspiration to fuel all areas of your world.

THE FIX? New Beauty Strategies for Your 30s:

1 START A CLEANSING HABIT TO FIGHT BREAKOUTS. As Dr. Born explains, a regular morning and evening cleansing routine is essential for warding off or controlling skin issues that can occur in your thirties, including adult acne or even PMS-related breakouts. Keeping skin clean is the simplest and least expensive step in creating beautiful skin.

2 CONSIDER CLEANSING FACIALS. While Dr. Born says no real antiaging benefits will come directly from these spa treatments, you will get the benefit of a deep cleanse, in addition to the restorative effects of relaxation, hydration and stress reduction. There are a variety of good options available from professionals, as well as through over-the-counter products.

3 USE RETINOIDS TO BANISH ACNE. Acne that isn't helped through daily cleansing or topical blemish-fighting products can often be treated through dermatologist-strength solutions, such as retinoids, as Dr. Born explains. Retinoids are vitamin A derivatives, such as Retin-A, Micro and Renova, that can be used to diminish the symptoms of acne common in your thirties. Retinoids are used topically in cream or gel form and are available from your dermatologist by prescription. Retoinic acids can also be used to diminish fine lines and wrinkles and smooth skin texture. If you have rosacea, you have to be cautious about using these products—be sure to consult with your doctor.

4 STIMULATE COLLAGEN PRODUCTION AND CELL TURNOVER TO COMBAT AGING. Retinoids and topical application of the antioxidant vitamin C are two proven techniques to stimulate collagen production and trigger cell turnover, explains Dr. Born. They can be used daily or weekly, either morning or night, depending on your skin's sensitivity, to dramatically improve skin texture and reverse sun damage. Your dermatologist can work with you on finding the right dosage and frequency. Since vitamin C is fairly unstable and can become oxidized and ineffective when exposed to air, Dr. Born advises finding products that are packaged in single applications.

5 TREAT EARLY SIGNS OF SUN DAMAGE. The effects of harmful UV rays accumulate over time, explains Dr. Born, and result in issues such as irregular skin texture and color and loss of volume, elasticity and collagen. There are numerous treatments for irregular pigmentation. Among them is the combination of the topical steroid hydroquinone and retinoic acid, which is available by prescription (Triluma). Dr. Born also points to a new tripeptide—amino acids that improve skin condition by stimulating collagen, smoothing appearance and stimulating cell renewal—called Lumixyl. This antiaging ingredient targets superficial pigmentation, which he combines with a microdermabrasion for best results.

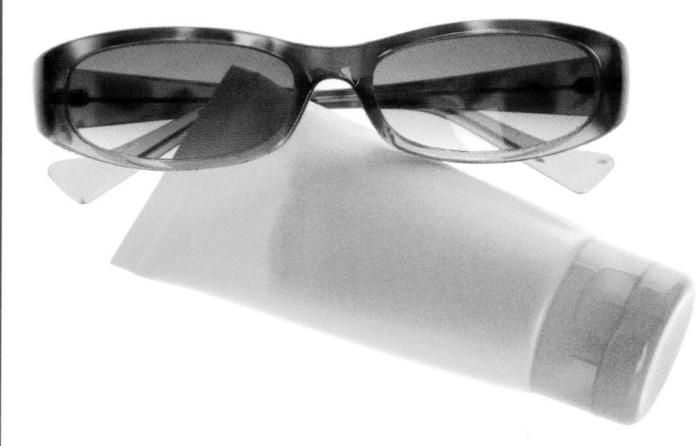

6 KEEP THE EYE AREA HYDRATED. Lack of hydration can cause fine lines and wrinkles to be more prominent, especially around your eyes. Look for moisturizing eye creams designed to help prevent signs of aging and fatigue, which are available both over the counter and through a dermatologist. Not only do you get antiaging benefits from morning and evening use, but as Carol explains, applying in the morning will help concealers and brighteners glide on and blend more easily.

Lack of hydration can cause fine lines and wrinkles to be more prominent, especially around your eyes.

7 FIND YOUR FIVE CORE MAKEUP PRODUCTS. Narrowing your essentials to the basics is the first step toward finding a simple routine you can master on a daily basis, as well as while you're on the go. Her top five skin care products for the thirties: (1) a foundation suited to your skin type, (2) concealer to cover skin imperfections and dark circles under the eyes, (3) blush or bronzer for a quick pop of color in a shade that complements your natural skin flush, (4) mascara to open up the eyes, and (5) a touch of lip gloss. A great way to test new options is to visit a store that allows you to try products in-store or offers take-home samples. In-store makeup artists can also help you determine what shades or formulas work best for your skin type.

8 IDENTIFY THE RIGHT FOUNDATION FOR YOUR SKIN TYPE. If you're prone to breakouts due to PMS, stress or the environment, consider switching to products designed for sensitive skin, explains Carol. These brands are formulated without irritating ingredients such as heavy oils, parabens and fragrance, and with ingredients such as natural antiaging peptides and essential oils. Because skin tends to be more hydrated naturally in our thirties, she adds, powder foundations may work for you instead of cream foundation, especially if your skin is oily.

9 MASTER THE ART OF CONCEALER. Even supermodels have blemishes, scars, imperfections and dark circles, so it's only natural that we do, too. The good news is that they're an easy fix, says Carol. Look for a concealer that matches your skin tone or is a shade lighter. Apply with a foundation brush, then use your fingers to blend for natural coverage. Top with powder.

10 USE BEAUTY PRODUCTS DESIGNED TO DO DOUBLE DUTY. Streamline your morning routine with beauty products created to do more than one thing, advises Carol. Foundations or moisturizers with SPF, for example, take away one extra step. Tinted moisturizers also cut down on application time and provide lighter coverage—they may be all you need in your thirties.

11 MASK LACK OF SLEEP WITH A SHIMMERY EYE SHADOW. A soft wash of shimmery eye shadow on the lids in a nude or pastel shade brightens the entire eye area for an instant fresh-faced glow, no matter how tired you are, explains Carol. It's a quick trick to look refreshed.

12 RECAPTURE A YOUTHFUL FLUSH WITH COLOR. A sweep of bronzer or brightly colored blush on your cheeks—right where you normally flush when exercising—will give you that fresh-faced, just-worked-out look, explains Carol. It's a fast way to perk up your face, mask fatigue and brighten your glow.

Make Everyday Products Multitask

Just because a product isn't designed to work overtime doesn't mean you can't get creative, says Carol. Her favorite time-saving trick? Take a swipe of blush or bronzer with your finger and place a dab on lids for eye shadow and a touch on cheeks for blush. All you need is gloss and you're ready to walk out the door. You don't have to be precise—your goal is to add color to perk up your look. It's an ideal everyday tip that can make you feel better in an instant.

STAY ON TRACK

THE GOOD THING ABOUT BEAUTY HABITS IS THAT THEY'RE FUN to incorporate. Who doesn't want to look her best? Here are some foolproof strategies that get quick results and make staying on track easier than ever. Trust me, you will love the beautiful results you see in the mirror.

1 SCHEDULE AN APPOINTMENT WITH YOUR DERMATOLOGIST. A professional consultation is an ideal way to learn about your options for antiaging treatments, including laser resurfacing or chemical peels, explains Dr. Born. Once you speak with a doctor and create a baseline for monitoring your skin changes, you'll be better able to track the results you get from products and treatments, as well as determine when to change your course of action.

2 GET A PROFESSIONAL TWEEZING. Get a good arch shape flattering to your face. Done properly, a professional tweezing can lift your features and make you appear years younger instantly. Then keep your tweezers handy and do your own touch-ups every couple of days to keep your arches looking groomed for longer.

3 CURL YOUR LASHES. This may seem like unnecessary primping, but it's not. Curled lashes are a fast way to create a youthful, wide-eyed look, no matter your age. I use an eyelash curler before putting on mascara every day—it literally takes a minute. Top with mascara to add a richness and volume that really opens your eyes.

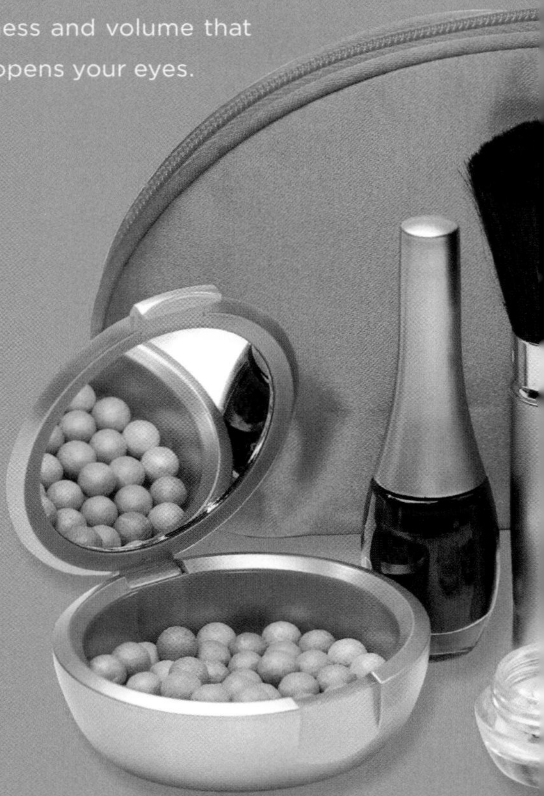

4 MASK GRAY HAIRS. One trick I learned is that you can easily mask a few stray grays with a mascara wand. (Just don't use it again on your eyes.) This is a good way to make a color treatment last if you've got darker hair.

5 USE SHINE SERUM. If your hair has lost its youthful luster, apply a shine serum before blow-drying. There are many great products available through your hair salon, beauty supply store or local drugstore.

6 APPLY BRONZER. Carol recommends using a bronzer on cheekbones for an instant pick-me-up. It's essential to get a shade that doesn't make you look orange or too dark, but more like you've got a touch of natural sunlight.

7 SWITCH TO A POWDER PUFF. Brushes take off the shine but don't necessarily add coverage. Instead of a flawless, finished look, you'll be prone to streaking and get zero coverage. Carol recommends using powder puffs instead; they are easy to find at any beauty supply store. Note: If you do use brushes, it is important to clean them regularly—at least once a week.

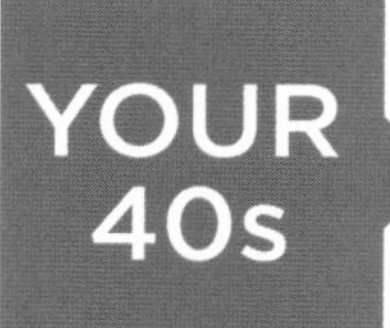

Age-Proof Yourself

In my forties, I'd just begun eating more healthfully and exercising regularly, which started my Best Body Now transformation. I looked and felt better than ever. Many of the signs of aging—dull skin, fine lines and wrinkles, and dark circles—began to disappear the better care I took of myself nutritionally and physically. My hair and nails also got stronger and healthier. As I started to embrace this new me, I incorporated more beauty principles and advice from experts such as Dr. Born and Carol to take better care of my skin. The results were incredible. No longer did I want to look like I did in my twenties—I was sexier and more radiant than ever!

The following section is designed to target the biggest skin challenges of this decade: changes in texture and tone, as well as loss of collagen and elasticity. In your thirties, your skin care and makeup routines are more focused on prevention, the forties are geared toward targeting specific issues.

> No longer did I want to look like I did in my twenties—I was sexier and more radiant than ever!

YOUR 40s What's Happening in Your 40s That Impacts Your Beauty

- Women in their forties can have dull skin, as natural skin cell turnover continues to slow down with age, explains Dr. Born. The process begins slowing in your twenties (who knew?), and by the forties skin can start to look decidedly lackluster.

- Hormonal changes during perimenopause and menopause can change skin's texture, tone and elasticity due to slowed elastin and collagen production. Also, the tapering off of the production of human growth hormone and estrogen, explains Dr. Born, affects skin volume and texture.

- In addition to loss of skin cells, the bone and deep tissue changes, as well as a loss of facial fat volume that began in your thirties, start to show in your forties, Dr. Born explains. This contributes to the lack of fullness and what is often described as your face "falling" as it ages.

- While many women's skin becomes drier as they age, causing fine lines and wrinkles, others experience adult-onset acne as a result of hormone changes during perimenopause.

- Fine lines and wrinkles, especially around the mouth and eyes, become more prevalent in this decade, thanks to a variety of factors. Effects of bad habits start to show in the face in the form of hyperpigmentation, uneven texture and tone, wrinkles and more.

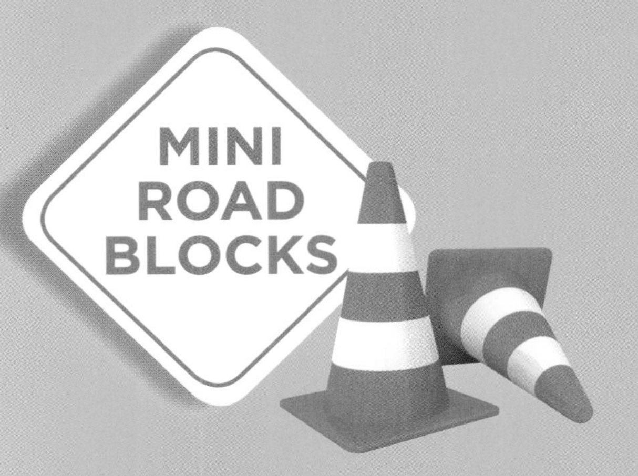

Pressed for time or struggle with sensitive skin? Dr. Born and Carol have Best Body Now fixes for all of your beauty roadblocks so you can look better than ever—no excuses.

1 I'M OVERWHELMED BY MAKEUP.

THE BEST BODY NOW FIX: If you're overwhelmed, find out how to do the basics and determine a few must-have products, then work from there, advises Carol. A good first step if you're starting fresh is to use a palette, which contains all the coordinating shades you'll need in a single component. How-to videos are available online or you can contact a makeup artist. The good news is you can create a very beautiful look with only a few different items. The right makeup can transform a woman. It takes very little time and effort yet generates an enormous increase in your self-esteem.

2 I'VE LOST THAT YOUTHFUL GLOW.

THE BEST BODY NOW FIX: Cleansing and exfoliating daily are the first steps toward achieving a natural glow. You can also fake a glow by adding luminizers, which contain light-reflecting particles, to your moisturizers, or using hydrators, foundations and powders that already contain luminizing ingredients.

3 I DON'T HAVE TIME.

THE BEST BODY NOW FIX: You only need the five basics: concealer, foundation, mascara, lip gloss and bronzer—to create a beautiful look quickly. Carol's routine takes just five to ten minutes a day. She also recommends using multitasking products including exfoliating cleansers, moisturizers with SPF, and so on.

4 MY SKIN IS SENSITIVE.

THE BEST BODY NOW FIX: Sensitive skin can be frustrating, but fortunately there are many products formulated without common irritants. Carol recommends looking for oil-free solutions that are not drying and don't contain fragrance or parabens. Natural ingredients, such as vitamins, minerals, botanicals and essential oils, help nourish and soothe skin. Some beauty supply stores allow you to sample the products before buying, which is smart if your skin is sensitive.

THE FIX? New Beauty Strategies for Your 40s:

1 INTEGRATE HUMAN GROWTH FACTORS INTO YOUR ANTIAGING REGIMEN. Human growth factors mimic naturally occurring hormones in the body that support and control cell growth and structure. As part of your beauty regimen, human growth factors can help stimulate collagen production and the creation of new skin cells, explains Dr. Born. They're available in cream form from your dermatologist and are good alternatives to vitamin C or retinoids, especially if you've got sensitive skin. Check with your physician.

2 EVEN SKIN TONE AND SOFTEN EXPRESSION LINES. Another option Dr. Born recommends for stimulating skin cell turnover is vitamin A derivatives, called retinoids. Most options, such as Renova, Micro and Retin-A, are available by prescription through your dermatologist. Like human growth factors and vitamin C, they smooth texture and tone, erase dark spots and minimize the look of fine lines and wrinkles. Because retinoids can irritate the skin, you'll need to work with your doctor on a dosage and frequency that works for you. Another powerful antiaging solution is the antioxidant Prevage MD with 1 percent idebenone, a wrinkle fighter that can help smooth lines and improve skin tone.

3 CONSIDER DAILY USE OF HIGHER-POTENCY AGE-PROOFING SERUMS. Age-proofing formulations with powerful, effective ingredients such as vitamin C work to smooth texture and even skin tone, explains Dr. Born. When used daily just after cleansing and before moisturizing, they can prevent or reverse hyperpigmentation and fine lines.

4 COMBAT ADULT ACNE WITH A MORE AGGRESSIVE TREATMENT. If you're already cleansing skin morning and evening and using topical drying agents and retinoic acids, Dr. Born recommends trying more aggressive treatments, such as a salicylic peel. It's a stronger form of the salicylic acid found over the counter in blemish creams and is designed to reduce oil, clear pores and control breakouts. You can also talk to your dermatologist about oral medications, such as tricyclics, or newer topical medications such as Clindoxyl, dapsone or isotretinoin that help clear skin.

5 TALK TO YOUR DOCTOR ABOUT SKIN-PERFECTING GLYCOLIC PEELS. If you're already exfoliating daily, you're already giving your skin a mild form of microdermabrasion. You can stimulate even more cell turnover and bring back radiant skin with glycolic acid peels, which use chemicals to remove a very thin top layer of damaged skin cells. Healthy new skin cells replace fine lines, discoloration and acne. You can also get milder peel effects from over-the-counter or spa facials with lower percentages of fruit acid, lactic acid, salicylic acid or glycolic acid.

6 REVERSE HYPERPIGMENTATION AND SUN SPOTS WITH PHOTO-REJUVENTATION. Some women have sun damage that's difficult to treat with over-the-counter or prescription creams. Dr. Born suggests trying a more advanced option. Intense pulsed light photorejuventation (IPL) or broadband light (BBL), a noninvasive broad-spectrum light, targets red and brown colors beneath the skin and stimulates collagen and cell turnover. Treatments last from thirty minutes to an hour. The procedure requires three to six sessions over the course of one month, but you'll see a reduction in wrinkles, freckles, rosacea, broken capillaries, acne and scars, and a marked improvement in your skin texture and tone.

7 OPT FOR AN ANTIAGING HYDRATING EYE CREAM. Combat fine lines and wrinkles with more than hydration. Look for treatments that combat signs of aging, including puffiness, dark circles, fine lines and drooping skin, while adding much-needed moisture. They'll include ingredients like vitamin C, peptides, hyaluronic acid and antioxidants such as coffeeberry and idebenone.

8 APPLY LUMINIZERS TO FAKE A NATURAL GLOW. To combat dryness and add a natural glow, Carol suggests using bronzers or luminizers that add a touch of radiance to the skin. They come in gel, serum, powder or liquid form and you can mix them into your foundation or dab onto cheekbones after you moisturize.

9 RETHINK YOUR FOUNDATION. Even if you've always had healthy skin, by the time you reach your forties, you'll likely begin to see changes in texture and tone. If you haven't been doing so, Carol recommends using foundation to help even out skin texture and create a flawless look. If you're already using it, consider switching your formula to one with antiaging properties. You may also need to consider whether your skin has changed during or after menopause—if it is oilier or more breakout-prone, you may want to try a powder. If your skin has become drier, hydrating foundations may help you add moisture and that all-important glow.

10 CONCEAL SIGNS OF FATIGUE AND AGING. Concealers are ideal for concealing dark undereye circles and blemishes. The mistake many women make, explains Carol, is they paint on the product, causing it to lay on the surface of the skin, particularly in the creases, defeating the purpose of trying to hide imperfections. She recommends applying concealer with a brush, then using your fingers to warm the product so it blends easily into the skin. This removes excess product and creates a more natural look with less creasing.

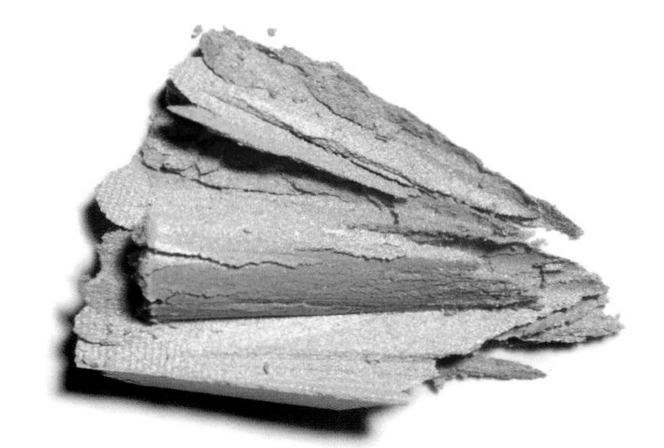

11 ADD A TOUCH OF CORAL OR PINK FOR YOUTHFULNESS. Don't worry if you don't have a natural flush of youthful color—you can fake it. Carol recommends a pop of coral or pink on your lips or cheeks. It will help you look pretty, healthy and youthful, and these shades work for nearly everyone.

12 PERFECT YOUR POUT WITH LINER. Give yourself an extra two minutes each morning to counter the natural thinning of the lips that happens in your forties. Carol's trick is to line the outside edge of your lip line without drawing outside the lip. This creates a natural but fuller-looking edge and helps color stay on longer.

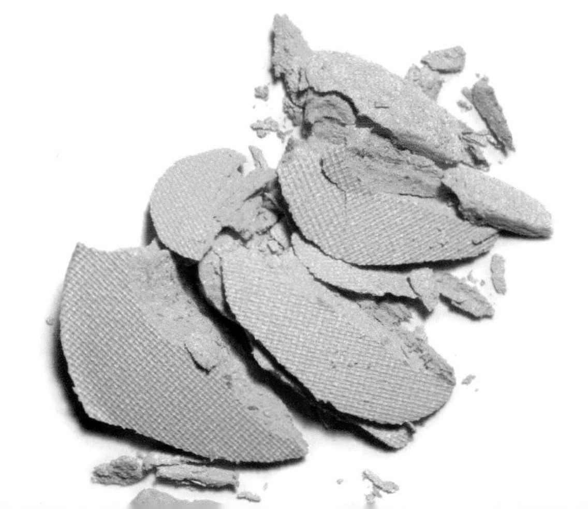

13 LIGHTEN DEEP-SET EYES OR DARK EYE AREAS. Darkness around eyes, which can cause you to appear older, typically happens as a result of genetics and skin tone, and can be exacerbated by fatigue. Brighten eyes by using a lighter highlighter or shimmery eye shadow on your lid, extended up to your brow, advises Carol. Add a light to medium taupe hue—depending on your skin tone—in the crease and smudge brown or black liner or shadow on the lash line, then top with mascara to open eyes.

14 AVOID OVERPLUCKING YOUR BROWS. Once you begin tweezing, the hair follicle becomes damaged, and over time the hair will stop growing back, explains Dr. Born. Unfortunately, thinner brows can make you appear older than you are. Creating a fuller, natural-looking brow with a brow pencil or powder is an easy trick Carol suggests for a more youthful look. Giving your brows a quick comb and shape before you leave the house is a fast way to get a finished look as well.

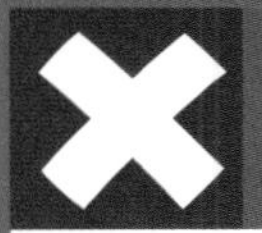

THE WORST BEAUTY HABITS

Let's face it—many of our habits, some seemingly harmless, wreak havoc on our skin and can make us look years older than we actually are, especially later in life. Dr. Born shares his nine worst skin care violations below.

1 SMOKING. Not only bad for your body, this habit is a quick way to add ten to twenty years to your face by depriving your skin cells of oxygen and nutrients and causing the breakdown of elastin. If you don't break the habit, you'll find wrinkles around your eyes and lips prematurely.

2 STRESS. Excessive worry can show up in your face over time in the form of worry lines and wrinkles. Dr. Born advises patients to reduce stress through activities such as meditation and yoga and to pinpoint stressors, from relationships to work environment, and minimize them. He also points to yogis as the perfect example of how a relaxed mind-set can make you look ageless.

3 ALCOHOL. Alcohol contributes to premature aging of the skin. It creates a red, flushed appearance due to damaged blood vessels that appear near the skin's surface.

4 TANNING OR FORGOING SUNSCREEN. UV rays damage skin cells and accelerate aging. Wear sunscreen daily for optimal protection and avoid tanning to keep skin looking younger, longer.

5 SLEEP DEPRIVATION. Not getting enough sleep robs your body of recharging REM (rapid eye movement) sleep, which prevents your brain and body from relaxing. In turn, this speeds the aging process. Fatigue can cause sagging skin, bags, dark circles and uneven skin tone.

6 LACK OF EXERCISE. Not only does exercise fuel your body, it also triggers human growth hormone production in your body, which is a proven age-proofing substance.

7 NOT CLEANSING BEFORE BED. Clean skin is an essential component of Your Best Body Now beauty routine. A twice-daily cleanse removes oil, impurities, dirt and more from your pores, prevents breakouts and can speed cell turnover.

8 TOUCHING BLEMISHES. Every time you touch an acne head you extend its life by five days, cautions Dr. Born. Daily cleansing, combined with a topical over-the-counter blemish fighter that dries the pimple, will help it clear up faster. For deeper, under-the-skin blemishes, talk to your dermatologist about a steroid injection.

9 UNPROFESSIONAL OR EXCESSIVE HAIR REMOVAL. Waxing, threading, plucking and lasering are all valid forms of hair removal. Dr. Born advises against overshaping brows, which can result in permanent hair loss. He also cautions those using retinoic acids to remove facial hair to be careful because they thin the skin—certain hair-removal procedures can cause tears, burns or even hyperpigmentation with at-home use if you're not careful.

My beauty approach for my fifth decade moves beyond makeup and skin care. It's firmly based on the head-to-toe Best Body Now approach to being my best self.

YOUR 50s + Recapture Youthful Beauty

My beauty approach for my fifth decade moves beyond makeup and skin care. It's firmly based on the head-to-toe Best Body Now approach to being my best self. In addition to the beauty tips and tricks listed below, I incorporate exercise, nutrition and wellness strategies for mind and body—that's because when I feel incredible, I look incredible, something plastic surgery or exaggerated makeup techniques cannot duplicate. That's probably one of the biggest beauty lessons I've experienced firsthand, and one Dr. Born and Carol believe in, too. They point to activities that reduce stress, such as exercise and meditation, as well as beauty tricks and strategies for looking your best in this decade. The next section includes all of the strategies you need to become truly ageless and let your natural beauty shine through, no matter how old you are.

When I feel incredible, I look incredible, something plastic surgery or exaggerated makeup techniques cannot duplicate.

YOUR 50s + What's Happening in Your 50s and Beyond That Impacts Your Beauty

By the time you reach your fifties, you will start to lose definition in your eyes, jaw, lips and neck, explains Dr. Born. Changes in your eye area may be more drastic because the skin in this area is naturally thinner and shows signs of aging more quickly than the rest of your face.

Menopause, officially defined as the point when you haven't had a period for an entire year, usually occurs in this decade. It causes fluctuations in hormones (see Chapter 6 for more details), which can dramatically impact collagen production. According to Dr. Born, loss of collagen and slowed production can result in uneven texture, lessened elasticity and changes in facial volume.

Hormone fluctuations can also cause changes in the skin, causing it to become drier or oilier, explains Dr. Born—it varies by person. Researchers believe dryness may be related to your body's decreased production of oil and a reduced ability to retain hydration. On the other hand, some women may have an increase in oil production, due to increases of hormones like DHEA and testosterone (see Chapter 6 for more information on hormones). This increase in oil, combined with a reduction in skin cell turnover, can lead to clogged pores and acne.

▶ While rosacea is most common in women in their thirties and forties, the problem is most often diagnosed during menopause, according to the National Rosacea Society. That's likely because hot flashes can exacerbate the symptoms.

▶ Hyperpigmentation, or discoloration of the skin, often caused by sun damage in your childhood, teens, twenties and thirties, begins to appear more prominently in your fifties, explains Dr. Born. Hormone fluctuations, due to menopause, can also cause an increase in age spots.

▶ Insomnia, a common side effect of menopause, can cause issues such as dark circles and wrinkles to become more apparent.

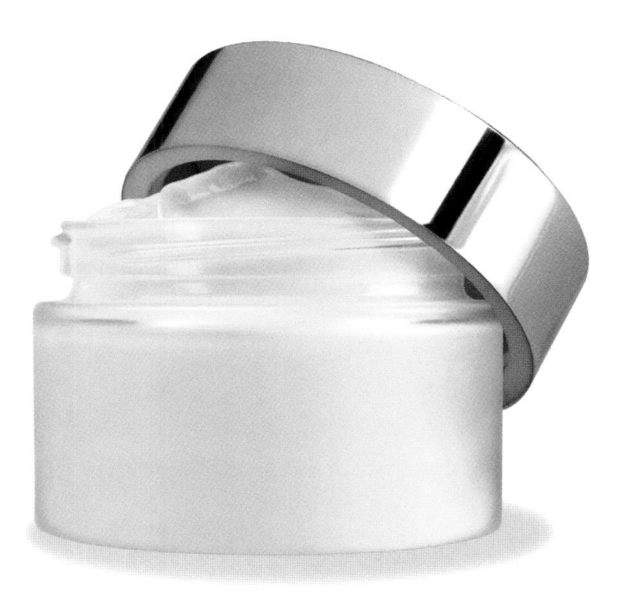

THE FIX? New Beauty Strategies for Your 50s +:

1 STAY HYDRATED BY DRINKING TEN 8-OUNCE GLASSES OF WATER A DAY. Water intake is an important component of the Best Body Now diet (see Chapter 4). Drinking plenty of water is particularly important as you age, because it helps fuel healthy cells and keeps skin hydrated.

2 TREAT CROW'S FEET IN THE EYE AREA. If you're not already using a hydrating eye cream to target fine lines and wrinkles, Dr. Born advises switching to one now. Look for high-potency over-the-counter products with active ingredients such as botanicals, antioxidants, vitamin C or niacin. Or talk to your dermatologist about prescription formulas right for you.

3 INTEGRATE HUMAN GROWTH FACTORS INTO YOUR ANTIAGING REGIMEN. Human growth factors mimic your natural hormones to support cell growth and stimulate collagen and cell turnover. If you haven't been using human growth factors, consider doing so now to counter deep wrinkles and lines. The substances are available in cream form from your dermatologist (in brands like SkinMedica) and are good alternatives to vitamin C or retinoic acids if your skin is easily irritated.

4 RESTORE SKIN ELASTICITY TO PREVENT AND DIMINISH WRINKLES WITH LED LIGHT. Laser skin rejuvenation can eliminate signs of aging, including wrinkles and fine lines. Dr. Born uses a procedure called Gentle Waves Skin Therapy, which uses LED lights to trigger skin cells to produce more elastin and collagen. The device is used twice a week for four to five weeks, along with an enzyme mask, to improve skin elasticity, smooth wrinkles and minimize scars. Another wrinkle-fighting alternative is a noninvasive skin-rejuvenating procedure called Thermage that tightens skin and triggers collagen production in a one-hour-long treatment. Improvements can be seen immediately and last two to three years.

5 TREAT DRY SKIN TO A THICKER HYDRATING CREAM. Many women notice that their skin becomes less hydrated after menopause. You can counter this by switching from a nightly moisturizer to a more intense hydrating cream or oil. Effective products are available both over the counter or through your dermatologist. I like to use products that contain as many natural ingredients as possible, in keeping with the Best Body Now philosophy of eating minimally processed foods. Believe me, our cosmetics and skin care products do find their way into our systems.

6 REMOVE HYPERPIGMENTATION AND DISCOLORATION WITH FRACTIONATED LASER RESURFACING. Dr. Born has seen impressive results with this in-office procedure that uses laser light to pierce small holes in the skin and eliminate the dark pigment beneath the surface. As the damaged skin heals, healthy new tissue forms to replace it. You'll usually have about eight days' recovery time, but it can really help remove scars and brown spots.

7 SWITCH TO A POTENT AGE-FIGHTING SERUM TO REVERSE SIGNS OF AGING. If you're already using formulations to smooth texture, even tone and hydrate, look for more advanced products designed to diminish deeper lines and wrinkles. The results won't be as dramatic as a treatment like laser skin rejuvenation, but you'll likely see creases diminish at least visually.

8 USE LUMINIZERS TO FAKE A NATURAL GLOW. Luminizers contain light-refracting particles capable of masking fine lines and wrinkles. Carol suggests looking for products naturally enhanced with luminizing ingredients, such as blush, bronzer, foundation, powder or tinted moisturizers. You can also add cream or gel luminizers to your moisturizer or foundation to instantly give your skin a hydrated look.

9 MASK SIGNS OF AGING AROUND THE EYES. One of Carol's favorite celebrity tricks for brightening the eye area is to add luminizer to concealer. The concealer covers dark circles while the luminizer reflects light and masks both darkness and fine lines. This magic combination can be used anywhere you want to smooth skin and hide shadows, and works well for expression lines and wrinkles. Place the concealer on the crease to lighten the area, then use the luminizer to diminish and diffuse their appearance. Top with a bit of powder to hold. Skin will appear smoother, as well as more youthful and radiant.

10 CONSIDER SWITCHING TO AN ANTIAGING FOUNDATION. Many liquid foundations contain ingredients designed to counter, minimize or prevent fine lines and wrinkles. If you're not already using such a product, Carol suggests making a change, especially because skin at this age is often drier and has begun to show signs of aging.

11 USE LINER FOR AN INSTANT EYE LIFT. If you've got smaller eyes or are losing definition on your lids, liner is one way to visually counter the effects. Carol's technique is to use thinner liner along the lash line beginning on the inside of the eye toward the nose and gradually get thicker as you move toward the outer edge of the eye. The line lifts up and out, so eyes appear larger and more defined.

12 COUNTER DROOPING LIDS WITH SHIMMERY SHADOWS. Loss of eye definition is normal as we age and often manifests in drooping lids or crow's feet. You can draw attention away from these areas and create the illusion of brighter, more open eyes by using a light-colored, shimmery shadow, explains Carol. Look for sophisticated, luxe shades such as champagne, taupe, bronze or light gray. For even more definition, add dark liner and top with mascara for a modern but "age-appropriate," beautiful look. Contrary to what you may think, more makeup is not better. Apply carefully with a light hand to make the most of what you have.

13 GROW FULLER, MORE YOUTHFUL LASHES. Full, thick lashes can give the appearance of that wide-eyed, youthful look and can help make up for loss of eye definition as you age. Both over-the-counter brands and dermatologist-recommended solutions, such as Latisse, are viable options for you to consider. Be cautioned, however, that there are some side effects with these eyelash serums, so seek the advice of a doctor or dermatologist before using.

14 CREATE FULL, YOUTHFUL BROWS.

Many women struggle with thinning brows because hair naturally thins with age, and a lifetime of overplucking can stop eyebrows from growing. To correct, Carol advises using a brow pencil or powder to shape and enhance your arches. Don't overdraw or create radically filled-in brows, which look unnatural. Simply shade in holes or elongate them to make them more noticeable and prominent. The trick is to match the color of your brows to your hair. Hair-growth serums, available over the counter or through your dermatologist, can also help regrow sparse brows. Products designed to help create fuller eyelashes can also create fuller arches. I find there are always a few pesky eyebrow hairs that want to grow longer than others, and I have to trim them with a pair of eyebrow scissors. Keep a lookout for these! Here is where a magnifying mirror can be your best friend.

15 USE LIP LINER TO KEEP LIPSTICK IN PLACE.

Fine lines and wrinkles in the mouth area can cause lipsticks and glosses to bleed a bit. Carol's easy remedy is to use a lip liner one or two shades darker than your natural lip color. Apply after your lipstick, following your lip line, to define your lips and make the color last. Avoid the temptation to draw a harsh line outside your lips, which looks unnatural. It also helps to keep lips resurfaced and moist through daily exfoliation—you can exfoliate your lips while you exfoliate your face.

16 FAKE A YOUTHFUL SMILE.

Although lips become thinner naturally as we age, they don't have to look that way. Carol's easy fix: line your lips in a shade that matches your natural lip color, then top with gloss for a fuller look. You can also top your lipstick with gloss. Another insider trick is to whiten teeth—whiter teeth will brighten your smile.

The "H" factor: A-list proof that life gets better at 40

No one can deny the seductive power of Kim Cattrall, who is still turning heads in her early fifties. What's ironic is that she truly became known as a sex symbol during her role as a fortysomething vixen on *Sex and the City*—not the typical age for such a role, but honestly, I don't think anyone could sizzle on-screen like she did.

MY BEST BODY NOW

Triumph of the Not-So-Average Jane
Debi Straley's Journey

THEN
5'7", AGE 40
142 POUNDS

NOW
AGE 42
125 POUNDS

My Best Body Now came as the result of a summer gone bad: About two years ago, I completely let myself go, eating whatever I wanted and enjoying a cool Smirnoff Ice on every hot summer night. When the season ended, I couldn't fit into my jeans or skirts, despite always being fit and in shape in the past. My body slipped out of control!

I committed to being in the best shape of my life and began with Eating Clean, combined with lifting weights five days a week. My biggest temptation was nighttime, when I wanted to snack. Instead, I surfed fitness sites on the Internet to keep my mind focused on keeping a sexy, lean body and off grabbing a handful of Doritos.

I use simple tips like writing down my food and fitness results daily so I stay on track and motivated. Your family sometimes won't always understand why you won't have a glass of wine or a brownie. That's okay. You have to commit to your Best Body Now for yourself and no one else. My kids fully support me and are learning great lessons on how to eat to fuel their bodies, rather than just filling up with junk.

I proved to myself that I could do what I set out to do. It wasn't easy, but it certainly wasn't as difficult as I thought it was going to be. You'll find that as you go through your journey, you will set a good example for others to follow. It's a great feeling to have someone tell you that you've motivated them to live a healthier life.

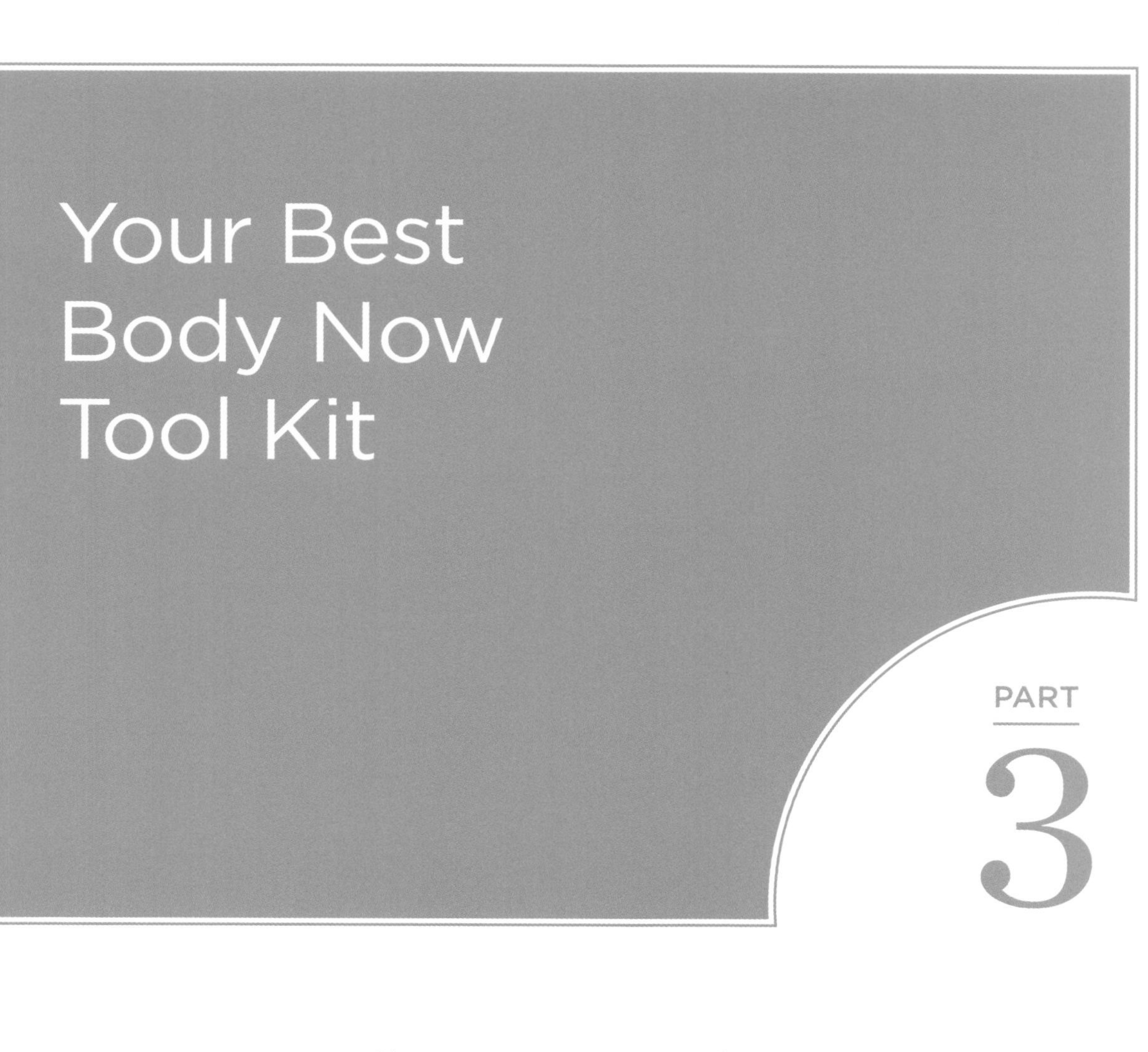

Your Best Body Now Tool Kit

PART

3

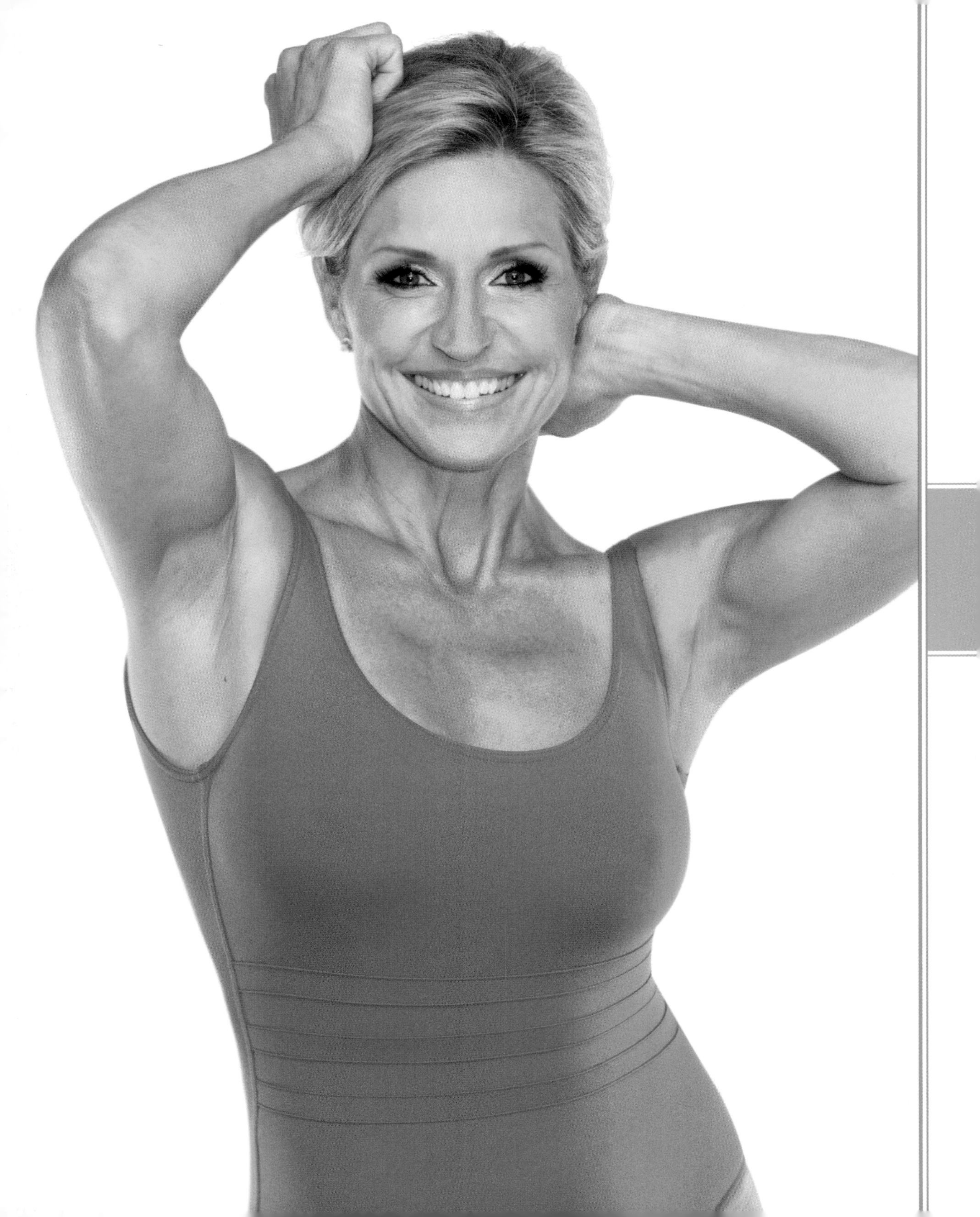

Best Body Now Inspiration 8

RETRAINING YOUR BRAIN TO THINK POSITIVE, EMPOWERING thoughts guaranteeing Best Body Now success may be a challenging process, particularly for those of you who are caregivers and unaccustomed to putting yourself first. Yet I know you will love the results. Why? Because changing your inner dialogue not only feels empowering but is also the fuel that will drive this transformational Best Body Now journey. Don't you want to meet the best possible version of yourself? To me that is the juice that drives the process.

Changing your inner dialogue not only feels empowering, but is also the fuel that will drive this transformational Best Body Now journey.

To help create the Best Body Now inspiration plan, I turned to the recommendations, advice and guidance of San Francisco-based psychologist Dr. Michelle Gannon. I admire her because she not only is fitness- and nutrition-focused personally but also uses many of the principles of the Best Body Now plan in her private practice. Her specialties include body image, relationships, intimacy and sexuality, pregnancy, infertility, transition to motherhood, parenting, work/life balance, perimenopause, friendships and self-esteem—all of the issues you may be dealing with now and as you begin your transformation. Dr. Gannon also helps individuals and couples live more authentic, empowered and healthy lives in their thirties, forties and fifties. A working mother with two young sons, she deeply appreciates the importance of balancing caring for others while taking care of herself. She understands the Best Body Now journey because she applies the same principles in her life.

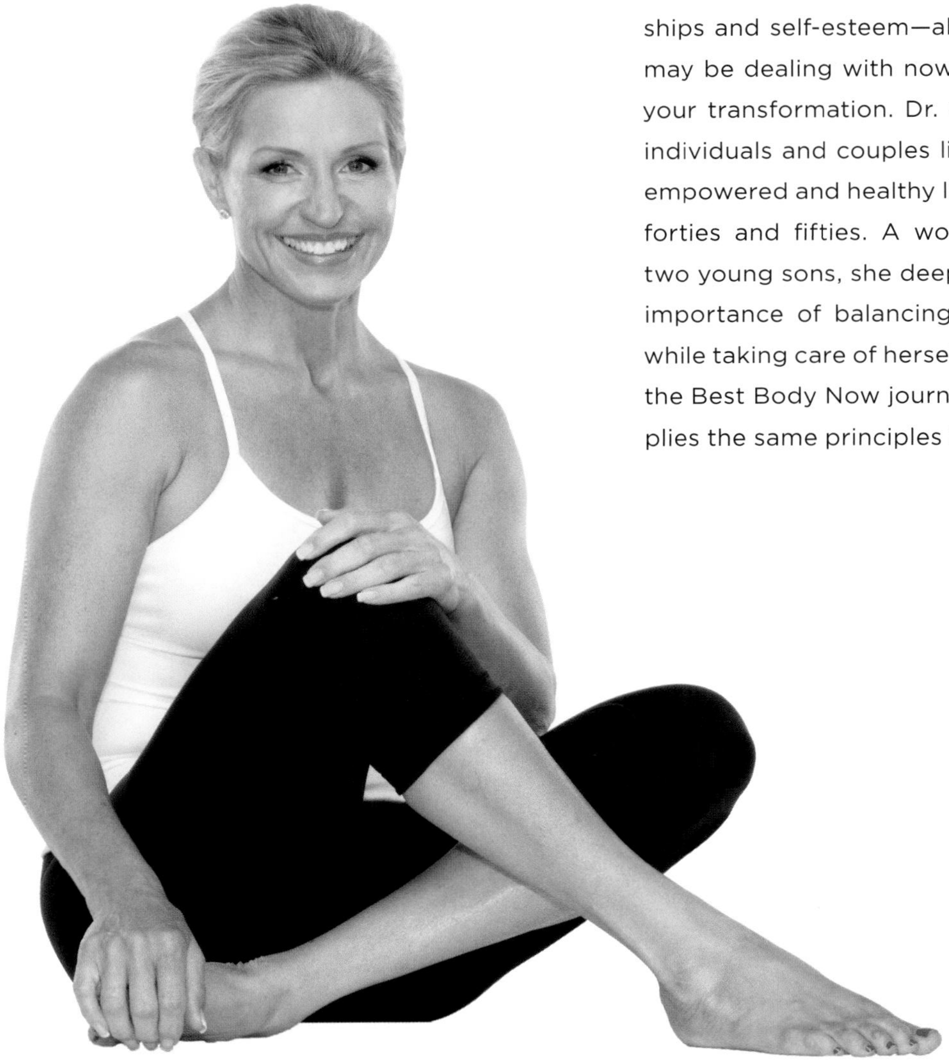

TOSCA'S MOOD MAKEOVER

A tough mental attitude is all about making day-by-day, minute-by-minute choices, and understanding that some situations are bigger challenges than others. Here's what I keep handy to keep my head and heart positive, focused and dedicated to my Best Body Now success.

JOURNAL. To record daily successes, big and small.

INSPIRATIONAL NOTES. Placed anywhere and everywhere I need them.

OLD PHOTOS. Seeing how far I've come gives me an instant mind-shift.

DREAMBOARD. Post your dreams on a bulletin board, canvas, poster or wall—you'll become what you believe.

OLD JEANS. My plus-size jeans still hang in my closet for an immediate visual attitude check.

A BOOK OF QUOTES. For quick reminders, I carry a mini notepad that lists my favorite inspirational quotes. I add meaningful or motivational thoughts as they occur to me to remind myself that a positive attitude is a personal choice. It only takes a second to change a negative outlook to an optimistic one.

UPDATED MUSIC. I'm always looking for new songs to keep my energy up. I often ask for the latest tunes from my younger and much cooler daughters! What a playlist I now have on my iPod!

NOTES FROM MY GIRLS. They warm my heart and remind me of why I embarked on this journey. I look at them when I need a reminder that what I'm doing is worth it. Each of us needs a hero in life.

A FAVORITE OUTFIT. I know what I feel sexiest wearing and put it on when I need extra confidence.

DATES WITH MYSELF. On my calendar, once a month, I give myself a reward day. Whatever I want to do, that time is mine.

BOOKS ON MY DESK. I keep a beautiful book propped up on my desk each month. Right now the book is *Diana: The Portrait* by Rosalind Coward. Last month it was *Women of Our Time* by Frederick S. Voss. I find them inspirational and they push me to keep reaching higher with my own life.

Inspirational Insights That Arm You for Best Body Now Success

THE TECHNIQUES I USE TO KEEP A positive attitude and stay motivated are quick and simple, but essential to achieving your goals. In this chapter, Dr. Gannon has outlined all of the tools you need to take charge of your emotional state of mind and commit to happiness. These are the same strategies she has used to help patients transform their lives for twenty years—and they've helped me change my life, too.

> Mood is something I am personally in charge of and can actually change.

You may not believe you can fundamentally change who you are or how you speak to yourself, but I have learned from personal experience that you can—and I have spoken to thousands of women on this same path who have also successfully made these changes.

The big lesson for me over the past decade has been that mood is something I am personally in charge of and can actually change. It's all too easy to get stuck in a mood rut and slip into a state of self-pity, sadness, hopelessness and depression. After a while, you unknowingly start to live like a negative, unhappy and unmotivated person. Conversely, you can live life like a motivated, joyful and fulfilled person by *acting* like one and making healthy Best Body Now changes in your life.

Positive change starts with self-reflection. Ask yourself today: "Am I the person I want to be?" "Am I living the life I want?" and "What kind of life do I want to be living?" If you're not quite there yet, you are not alone. Many women feel like you do—I know because I did, too. Unfortunately, your life isn't "practice" for the time when you arrive at a happier, healthier place. Every day you wake up is a new opportunity for you to become the strong, vibrant, sexy and confident woman you want to be, and intentionally live the way you deserve to live. This is your life, and the right time to start your Best Body Now journey is *now*.

> Every day is a new opportunity for you to become the strong, vibrant, sexy and confident woman you want to be.

While learning to allow yourself to live more fully, it is important to make changes—even small ones—on every level, Dr. Gannon explains, from eating nutritious foods and exercising more to improving your happiness and strengthening your relationships.

> This is your life, and the right time to start your Best Body Now journey is *now.*

Even the smallest of positive decisions contributes to eventual success. Every choice you make toward putting yourself as the top priority will work toward improving your overall mental and emotional health. The end result is a happy, fulfilling and joyful life: the goal of your Best Body Now transformation. From this day forward, decide to live your life with purpose. Your Best Body Now is within your reach—you can do it!

BEST BODY NOW Inspiration Basics

TAKE AN HONEST LOOK AT YOUR LIFE. In order to get the greatest results from the Best Body Now journey, start by assessing where you are today, advises Dr. Gannon. How happy and content are you with your life? How do you feel about your body? How do you feel about your health? How is your relationship with your partner, children, parents, siblings, coworkers or friends? Do you like who you are? Are you the person you want to be? Are you living the life you desire? Are you frustrated because you feel something is missing in your life but can't work out what it is? If your answers are negative, then ask yourself what you need to change in order to make yourself happier, healthier and more confident.

Write down the answers to these questions and use them as a starting point for your journey. This is the perfect time to put down this book for a moment and pick up a pen. Find some paper and begin to write down all of your thoughts relating to these questions. A hard copy of where you stand right now emotionally will help you create a foundation upon which to build and transform your life. Look at what you have written each morning to help motivate you for the day, and then read it again before bed to remind yourself that you're creating a happier life. Positive affirmations such as these are an incredible way to ensure you inspire and celebrate success every day, as well as track your progress.

According to Zig Ziglar, the powerful motivational speaker, creating positive affirmations is guaranteed 100 percent to bring about change in your life. That is not a number to doubt!

START YOUR BEST BODY NOW

CHANGING YOUR MIND-SET MAY TAKE a few tries—you're only human. In this case, however, practicing healthy emotional habits can be just as life-altering, attitude-adjusting and happiness-inducing as being naturally joyful and positive. Try these tricks for taking the first steps to embracing your Best Body Now.

1 CREATE A DREAMBOARD. Corkboard, canvas, an old poster, the wall of your workout room—it doesn't matter what surface you use. The idea is to use this space for images of the new reality you're creating. Maybe it's a photo of you in your best shape, an exotic vacation you're planning as a reward for achieving your goal weight, or a pair of skinny jeans you're determined to wear again. Whatever your motivation, pin it on the board. Stick it where you'll see it every day.

2 LIST YOUR BEST BODY NOW COMMANDMENTS. Here are some of mine: I will not speak negatively about myself at any time, no matter what. I will praise myself just for trying, and I will double the praise when I reach my goal. Make ten or so to start—you can change them or add more later. Refer to them daily to remind yourself of the commitment you're making to you.

3 FIND A PERSONAL MANTRA. The mantra "Yes I can!" is never far from my mind. I repeat it several times daily. I especially repeat it when I am in the gym lifting weights that I could only have dreamed about lifting years ago. "Oh yes I can!" If anyone says I can't, then look out!

4 REMIND YOURSELF TO STAY TRUE TO YOUR NEW MIND-SET. Don't let others knock you off the Best Body Now path—no matter what anyone does or says, they can't take away the work you've done for yourself. I always remind myself to never lose my posture, even when a situation or person becomes challenging. I won't step into the gutter with someone else. I always take the high road and remind myself of who I am and how far I've come.

5 SHARE YOUR DREAMS WITH PEOPLE YOU LOVE. Once you tell your friends and family about a goal, you're suddenly more committed to achieving it. I've also learned there's great satisfaction in not only sharing your intention to reach an objective but also your results. It feels incredible to celebrate success with others who care.

6 USE SUCCESS TO FUEL EVEN GREATER ACHIEVEMENTS. Once you real a goal, such as losing 5 pounds or running three miles, channel that energy into another goal or a new challenge. The momentum from reaching one milestone will help fuel your energy to reach another.

7 CREATE A POSITIVE AFFIRMATION CARD. This is one of my favorite tricks for keeping myself on track and reinforcing a personal message to myself. I keep stacks of index cards on hand for just this purpose. When I need an extra push while in the process of accomplishing something challenging, I write positive words to myself on the index card and carry it with me. Often I create three cards saying the same thing so one can go in my purse, one in my gym bag and another near my computer. Studies have shown that by doing this, you are virtually guaranteed to accomplish the task. My current motivational message says, "Tosca, you can push harder and become a better motivational speaker." I also have another one for my training: "Ten more minutes, a few more miles, a little faster, girl!"

8 CELEBRATE YOUR SUCCESSES. Celebrate even the small successes as they validate your progress. Eating breakfast today is a reason to smile if you have not done so in the past. Each small positive change adds up to something big!

✔ STOP COMPARING YOURSELF TO OTHERS. One of the easiest changes you can make right now, advises Dr. Gannon, is to recognize that this is *your* journey, not someone else's. Do not let others' successes intimidate you or make you envious. Everyone has a different path as well as her own set of obstacles and challenges. If you stick to the Best Body Now plan and focus on improving *your* life, incredible change will happen for you, too.

> The addition of just one activity that you find uplifting or inspiring can make you happier on a daily basis.

✔ CONSIDER WHEN YOU WERE THE HAPPIEST. By thinking about times when you were joyful and fulfilled, you can find keys to improve your current levels of happiness. Do you need to spend more time with friends or loved ones? Do you need more quiet time or outlets for your creativity? Are you inspired when you are learning or exploring? Are you most empowered when you feel healthy and strong? Are you more energetic and positive on days when you're well rested? Do you have enough fun in your life now? Romance? Laughter? Identify what is missing in your life now, suggests Dr. Gannon, and add that back into your routine. The addition of just one activity that you find uplifting or inspiring, such as a Sunday evening bath or a family activity night, can make you happier on a daily basis.

Someone once told me if you have trouble identifying what makes you happy, think about the thing that, when you do it, takes you completely away from the current situation, from the here and now. For me this happens when I train or write and even when I paint or draw. For you it could be when you sing or when you work with others.

✔ REPRIORITIZE YOU. It is common for many women to believe that in order to be a good wife, mother, employee or friend they need to be self-sacrificing. I know I did and was often the last thing on my own to-do list. But the truth is that strategy doesn't work. To take care of others, you need to first focus on yourself; this is a clear indicator of emotional health. Starting now, give yourself permission to make *you* the priority in your life for a change. By nurturing yourself, you will become a better partner, mother, friend, worker and more—guaranteed.

> Give yourself permission to make *you* the priority in your life for a change.

✔ MAKE GOALS MANAGEABLE. Break down your goals into very specific, manageable baby steps in order to make them less intimidating and more achievable. For example, rather than trying to "drink more water," focus on the actionable goal of refilling your water bottle two times per day. Get more sleep by getting into bed thirty minutes earlier each night. Get more

> You can create lasting changes in your daily life by using normal everyday habits to reinforce and reward new behaviors.

exercise by scheduling a hiking date with a friend once a week. Read one novel a month to get your creative juices flowing. Take one continuing education class to challenge your mind. Go on a date with your partner one time per month. Dr. Gannon recommends starting with one or two small changes like these, because these successes will inspire you to make even more positive changes in your life. Another strategy that works? Be realistic about your goals and frame them as "I am going to be happier and more confident one step at a time."

When I began to make improved nutrition decisions, that was when the rest of me realized, "Hey! She means business! She does care about this body and this mind." Taking better care of yourself is a concrete sign that you are healing emotionally. Give yourself all the physical clues you can in order to remain successful in your efforts to become your best self now.

DOCUMENT YOUR PROGRESS. Noting the positive changes you're making in your life—either by sharing them with loved ones or by writing them down—will help ensure your success. If you're extroverted—you are outgoing and get energy from being with others—share your progress in an exercise class or online support group. Why? Because many extroverts feel their successes only "count" when they are shared with others. However, if you are more introverted—you get energy from being alone—keep notes in a journal or use downtime for self-reflection. The process of documenting your progress works because it makes you feel more responsible to your goals, which increases your odds of success.

TRY THE PREMACK PRINCIPLE. There are simple tricks for ensuring that your new Best Body Now habits stick. The Premack Principle, developed by David Premack, is based on the idea that you can create lasting changes in your daily life by using normal everyday habits to reinforce and reward new behaviors you'd like to embrace in the long term, such as Best Body Now habits. For example, Dr. Gannon suggests thinking about a ritual you perform every day that you enjoy—such as reading your favorite blog or newspaper, phoning a friend or taking a leisurely morning shower. Now, commit to doing the new behavior (eating a clean breakfast or strength training, for instance) *first,* and then reward yourself with what you really love to do. This means if you want to enjoy your favorite newspaper, you have to exercise *before* reading. Studies have found we are more likely to do undesirable or challenging new behaviors when we reward ourselves for doing them with everyday activities we love.

> Your new Best Body Now mind-set leaves no room for being mean to yourself. Be your own best friend.

BE A FRIEND TO YOURSELF. If a friend spoke to you about her challenges, you would likely be supportive and constructive in a loving, respectful way. Now think about how you speak to yourself. Are you just as kind and compassionate? Or are you harsh and critical? Your new Best Body Now mind-set leaves no room for being mean to yourself—no exceptions, no matter what. Treat yourself as you would a close friend trying to make difficult changes in her life, Dr. Gannon advises. Remember, every choice you make and every step you take—even just walking after dinner rather than watching television—deserves recognition. If a friend told you she chose exercise over TV, you would probably say, "Good for you! Way to go!" Be your own best friend and shower yourself with the same enthusiasm and support you generously offer to others.

SPRING-CLEAN YOUR NEGATIVE INFLUENCES. Just as you clean out your pantry or refrigerator of unhealthy foods for the Best Body Now program, Dr. Gannon recommends doing the same with unhealthy relationships. She points to research by Dr. John Gottman, founder of the Gottman Institute, which revealed that successful relationships have a 5-to-1 ratio of positive to negative interactions. This means every negative interaction (a disagreement, a misunderstanding or hurt feelings) needs to be counterbalanced with five positive interactions (being caring, loving or playful, for instance) to keep a relationship healthy and balanced. Consider all of your relationships. Which ones would benefit from more positive exchanges and which ones need stronger boundaries? To create and maintain lasting Best Body Now changes, give your relationships a makeover, too. This opens up your life to people who support rather than sabotage your journey. My strong support system has been an incredible influence on my transformation and continues to help me stay motivated and on track as I challenge myself with new goals.

CREATE HAPPINESS DAILY BY CREATING POSITIVE EXPERIENCES. Happy experiences help create even more happiness. When you fill your life with positive experiences, you are actively creating a

TOSCA TIDBIT

Reward yourself for achievements, no matter how small: a week of Eating Clean with no cheating, increasing your weight levels at the gym, getting eight hours of sleep. The only rule? Treat yourself with nonfood rewards.

joyful life. Think about it—if your day is filled with events that make you feel inspired, confident and satisfied, you naturally begin to feel happier. How incredible is that? Start with baby steps, Dr. Gannon suggests, such as taking a bit of time out of the day to do something you like: enjoy nature and the outdoors, spend time with a friend who makes you laugh, read an inspirational book, listen to uplifting music, take a lavender bath. Give yourself permission to enjoy your life—you deserve it. The upside is that when you enjoy your life more, your friends and loved ones benefit, too. Add just one activity you love to your day today and watch it blossom into other positive events.

CELEBRATE YOUR SUCCESS WITH OTHERS. I never would have been so successful with my Best Body Now transformation if it weren't for the positive reinforcement I had from my support network. It's natural for women to feel empowered when they share changes and achievements in their lives with friends. Having a support network can be extremely inspiring, Dr. Gannon says, especially when others share your enthusiasm and appreciate your achievements. Conversely, it can be dangerous to your success if you surround yourself with negative individuals who would rather take you down. To create your own support network, look for friends, loved ones, a therapist or even a trainer who can be proud and enthusiastic with you and encourage you to stick to your Best Body Now goals. I check in with my training partners and friends frequently to discuss everything from minor speed bumps to seemingly small victories—they help put life into perspective and are truly happy when I reach a goal. Online communities are also great resources for trading challenges and celebrating achievements with women who are going through the same journey as you.

> I never would have been so successful with my Best Body Now transformation if it weren't for the positive reinforcement I had from my support network.

SHOW GRATITUDE FOR WHAT YOU HAVE. Once I learned to focus on being happy with what I have, rather than concentrating on how far I have to go or how much I don't have, my entire perspective shifted. I became someone who was fortunate, rather than someone who lived without. Consider whether you look at the glass half empty or half full. Research, including studies from both the Mayo Clinic and National Institutes of Health, has found that optimistic people are happier, more peaceful and less stressed. The good news is that even if you're not naturally optimistic, you can learn to be more so. Here is what works for Dr. Gannon's clients. Start with this simple goal: at the end of each day, write down one thing you are grateful for. It can be

> Optimistic people are happier, more peaceful and less stressed.

as simple as "I am grateful heirloom tomatoes are in season," "I am grateful I walked my dog today," or even "I am grateful my favorite trainer is leading my exercise class." By tracking what you appreciate in a journal, you will learn to find something wonderful in every day and feel happier on a daily basis. Sometimes happiness is as simple as realizing you are happy and have that one little thing in your life that reinforces it. Work your way up to feeling grateful that your clothes fit better, your cholesterol level went down, you found a new gym partner or you feel happier—and your Best Body Now success will happen.

KEEP THE BIG PICTURE IN MIND. Right now you may be focusing on your weight-loss, fitness and health issues on a daily basis, but remember that life is a marathon, not a sprint. Keep in mind how the changes you are making right now can help you in the future, advises Dr. Gannon. Instead of focusing on how stressed, busy or even overwhelmed you feel, imagine a time when you will feel confident, optimistic and happy—that is possible even if you don't feel completely fulfilled today or even tomorrow, because you're making small steps that result in a bigger transformation over time. There is also much to be learned from the journey. You don't want to arrive at success ill-prepared. Living in the moment, as everyone's favorite TV host, Oprah, reminds us and teaches us to be fully present right now and thankful for what that moment brings. In ten years you will be a decade older, no matter what. But you have the power to make changes today that will guarantee your happiness in the future. When I started my Best Body Now journey I kept in mind who I ultimately wanted to be and how I wanted to live, which helped me stay focused and on track. I reminded myself I was excited to meet the person I was destined to become and that I had been asleep for many years prior. This is my time and this is your time.

> You have the power to make changes today that will guarantee your happiness in the future.

BEST BODY NOW INSPIRATION BENEFITS

WHAT ARE SOME OF THE BEST BODY Now differences you will see from making empowering changes for yourself? New levels of confidence, unshakable self-esteem, happier moods, less stress, a greater sense of fulfillment, closer relationships with family and friends and even improved health will be the result. By clearing out negative habits that don't work for you, you'll open yourself up for abundance on all levels.

STAY ON TRACK

TRY THESE STRATEGIES FOR STAYING FOCUSED AND MOTIVATED— they're the same ones I've used throughout my Best Body Now journey.

1 CREATE A SUCCESS BOARD. List your achievements and goals, add photos, attach mantras—anything and everything that will spur your success. Post it where you will see it every day.

2 MAKE YOURSELF UNCOMFORTABLE. Keep yourself challenged and inspired by living outside of your comfort zone. You'll be extra satisfied when you achieve something that isn't in your normal skill set, routine or habit.

3 CREATE INTERIM SUCCESSES. I love any opportunity I can get to celebrate my achievements. It's essential to staying motivated and happy along the way.

4 NOTICE HOW INCREDIBLE YOU FEEL. On days when I feel challenged, sluggish or unmotivated, I remind myself how healthy, confident and sexy I feel when I follow the Best Body Now program. It helps keep me inspired.

5 TRACK YOUR ACHIEVEMENTS. Big or small, I note every objective I reach. I love reviewing it at the end of the day to keep me fired up for the next day's challenges.

6 REACH OUT TO SOMEONE WHO NEEDS YOUR HELP. Nothing is more motivating than helping someone else live her life a little better.

TAILORED INSPIRATIONAL TOOLS FOR EVERY AGE

WHILE THE PRINCIPLES OF THIS BEST BODY NOW CONFIDENCE PLAN won't change, your life does as you age. Let's take a look at how your emotional needs differ in your thirties, forties, fifties and beyond and how to leverage happiness-boosting habits in each decade.

YOUR 30s Start Inspirational, Empowering Habits

During my thirties I spent much more time worrying about the well-being of my daughters and other family members than about how I was doing—I felt like nothing more than crumbs on a plate. If I was feeling sad or lonely, I would often ignore the pain. There were many times when I did feel incredibly lonely—I was a young mother with three small children who had to constantly uproot myself in order to follow my husband's career. I threw myself into decorating each new home we moved into and taking care of the daily needs of a growing family. Although I explored interests, including sewing, gardening, interior design, antiques hunting, going to school and volunteering at the children's school, I was never really fulfilled. I know now I was simply distracting myself from the real issue—that I was slowly losing the real me.

> The Best Body Now inspiration plan is about becoming the real you—the strongest, most confident woman you can be.

Sadness and isolation ultimately led to fatigue, boredom, depression and more. Luckily, I had something burning inside that told me I deserved more than that and had more to accomplish in this rich world. That's what the Best Body Now inspiration plan is all about—helping you champion becoming the real you. The strongest, most confident woman you can be is the inevitable result.

If you have started changing your eating and fitness habits already, you are off to an incredible start—food and exercise play essential roles in managing emotions (read Chapters 4 and 5 for more information). A February 2009 article from the Mayo

Clinic reported that physical exercise thirty minutes five days per week reduced depression, stress, fatigue, self-doubt and irritability. Dr. Gannon's practice has also shown that those who exercise are also more likely to stay committed to their eating plan and feel better about themselves. Fitness is also a powerful way to reduce cortisol, the stress hormone that can weaken the immune system if overtriggered.

> By reading this book, you've already started taking positive steps toward changing your life.

And when you put the advice into action and begin creating a healthy lifestyle, eating nutritious foods, exercising daily and applying these practical happiness principles, you'll quickly begin to feel more confident, energetic and empowered.

The following sections combine the latest research with Dr. Gannon's proven strategies to help you increase motivation, raise self-esteem and strengthen confidence to create the happy, healthy life you deserve. I've done it and I know you can, too!

YOUR 30s What's Happening in Your 30s That Impacts Your Emotions

- Many women in this decade are juggling multiple roles—wife, mother, friend, colleague, sister, daughter and more—and trying to prove themselves in all areas of life from work to home to relationships. Unfortunately, Dr. Gannon cautions that the challenge of constantly multitasking can take a toll on your emotional and physical health. And because most women have a difficult time setting boundaries and limits, they end up giving and giving at their own expense, often to the point of exhaustion.

- Even if you were athletic or outdoorsy in your twenties, by the time you reach your thirties you may feel as though you've got no time for physical activities. That makes sense: many women are handling everything from grocery shopping to laundry to the family schedule plus supporting a family, which leaves no time for exercise, even though studies show it makes us feel happier and more energetic. A busy life also means you are more likely to sleep less, eat out of frustration, drink more caffeine and rely on quick pick-me-up sugar fixes, all of which can contribute to moodiness.

- Hormone changes related to PMS can make you irritable and more emotional. PMS intensifies or exacerbates feelings you already have. Often women don't feel validated when having premenstrual mood

> This chronic "squeezing in" leads to feelings of being overwhelmed, stressed and irritable, as well as to exhaustion.

swings, Dr. Gannon says, nor do they know how to overcome the underlying feelings of stress and frustration that are heightened during this time. In my previous marriage, PMS was the butt of all jokes and was trundled out in front of the family as a kind of hilarious disease. It's horrible to be at the mercy of someone who doesn't understand this hormonal and often emotional time.

▸ When their schedules are overloaded, men are able to say "No" or "I'm too busy, not now." Women, however, have a harder time setting healthy boundaries like this, and instead respond, "Yes, I'm busy, but I'll squeeze it in." The downside, says Dr. Gannon, is that this chronic "squeezing in" leads to feelings of being overwhelmed, stressed and irritable, as well as to exhaustion. In my case making promises to do everything simply led to more depression because I couldn't do it all, at least not well, which further contributed to my feelings of inadequacy.

▸ In your thirties, it's natural to feel the pressure of trying to be perfect at home or on the job. But in the quest to really have it all—career, relationships, children, social lives—many women still feel unhappy with or guilty about the choices they make, Dr. Gannon says. Women with full-time careers often feel guilty for not spending enough time with their families. Those who stay home full-time can feel unfulfilled. Research has found that the happiest moms work part-time outside the home, but finding a career or job permitting limited hours and earning enough money can be challenging.

▸ Decisions about having children are also common in this age group. Some women feel like they are running out of time because they've postponed having children for their careers or they feel upset because they are not in relationships; if they want to become mothers, they feel pressure to do so quickly. Others are dealing with fertility issues, which heighten stress levels.

▸ Media stereotypes of beauty, combined with society's do-it-all expectations of women, leave many of us feeling like we

TOSCA TIDBIT

Consider a change in plans (a late night at work, a sick child, a rainy day) as an opportunity to test your resilience and motivation. Don't quit, skip workouts or cave in to pressure. I am always surprised at how often an "unpleasant" situation has a pleasant silver lining. Just give it a chance.

should look better, do more, be skinnier and so on.

- Significant life changes—such as marriage, divorce, pregnancy, new children, relocations and career advancement—can elevate our anxiety levels, leading to fatigue, sadness, irritability, anger and other negative symptoms and side effects.

- On-the-go lifestyles often mean you're stretched in too many directions, with not enough time for you, let alone quality time with the people you love. This can lead to feelings of loneliness, sadness or isolation, especially if you're entirely focused on other people's needs, rather than your own.

Women raising young children tend to sacrifice their own needs to take care of their families. Pushing aside your own desires and not making time for yourself can sabotage your self-esteem and cause you to question your contributions to society—which is exactly what happened to me. It wasn't until I started Eating Clean and making myself a priority that I was able to create my Best Body Now and find true happiness and fulfillment.

> When you realize trying to be perfect is really overrated—and, frankly, impossible—you will discover happiness

THE FIX? Inspirational Strategies for Your 30s:

1 ADJUST YOUR PERSONAL EXPECTATIONS. What would happen if you decided that you no longer wanted or needed to strive for perfection? What if you decided that being "good enough" was fabulous? Could you feel successful in your life without the extra pressure of making it be flawless? Dr. Gannon has found when women adjust their personal expectations to more reasonable standards they become more self-accepting and can find happiness and joy in their lives. When you realize trying to be perfect is really overrated—and, frankly, impossible—you will discover happiness is attainable. I call this an exercise in lowering the bar!

2 LEARN EACH OTHER'S LANGUAGE OF LOVE. As Dr. Gary Chapman explains in his book *The Five Love Languages*, most of us respond more powerfully to one of these five expressions of love: (1) words of appreciation, (2) physical touch, (3) gifts, (4) acts of service or (5) quality time. Rather than try to give every one to your family and friends all the time, Dr. Gannon recommends learning their preferred language of love—and having them learn yours, too. You will become a more efficient and effective caretaker when you speak their language. At the same time, ensuring that they know your love language, too, will help you receive the same appreciation and support you require.

> You alone hold the power over your emotions.

3 DELEGATE TO STREAMLINE YOUR LIFE AND REDUCE STRESS. It's normal to need help, especially as you make Best Body Now changes in your life, so don't be afraid to ask for it. Dr. Gannon advises asking your partner to handle more responsibilities, getting your friends to help you rally on days when you feel less motivated or delegating work to your team at the office. Doing so will help you feel less overwhelmed and more inspired because others are sharing in making your dreams come true. I have realized it takes courage, but ultimately we do need to ask others for help. The better care we take of ourselves—sometimes with help from others—the happier we will be. Asking for help also teaches others that they don't have to have all the answers, either, and that it is not a sign of weakness but rather a sign of strength to ask for help.

> It is not a sign of weakness but rather a sign of strength to ask for help.

4 LOOK FOR HAPPINESS WITHIN YOURSELF. In my late thirties, I finally learned it was up to me—not my husband, kids or anyone else—to ensure my happiness. Once you realize that you alone hold the power over your emotions, you can take responsibility for your life. Start by identifying what specifically makes you happy, Dr. Gannon advises, then find a way to make it happen. For me, it's nutritious foods, a powerful sweat session, feeling productive and purposeful, and quality time with family. I infuse those into my life every day.

> Stick to the commitment you have made to yourself.

5 SCHEDULE YOURSELF FIRST TO ENSURE YOUR NEEDS ARE MET. It feels normal to fill your calendar with commitments for others—work, family, friends, household chores or financial responsibilities. Instead of carving out time for everyone else, start with *you*. For example, schedule your exercise plan first. The motto in Dr. Gannon's household is the same as in mine: "When Mom exercises and is happy, the entire family is happy." You may get complaints at first as loved ones adjust to a different lifestyle, but stick to the commitment you have made to yourself. It works, and above all, you deserve it.

6 DON'T FORGET TO BREATHE.

Even if you don't have time for a yoga or meditation practice, you always have time to breathe—it's essential for helping you reduce stress and anxiety. When tension strikes, Dr. Gannon advises, sit quietly a few times a day with your eyes closed and breathe deeply for a minute. Inhale and exhale slowly while imagining a safe, relaxed place. Your heart rate will lower quickly as your anxiety lessens.

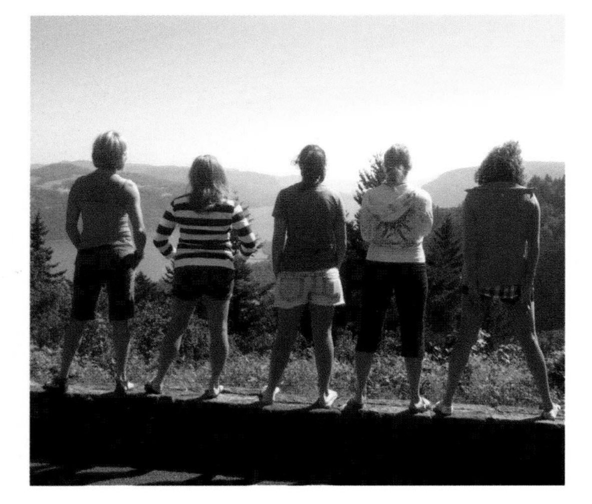

> When you have reached a milestone with the support of your husband, kids or close friends, invite them to share in the celebration.

7 REWARD YOURSELF *AND* YOUR FAMILY WITH YOUR SUCCESS.

Studies have shown that shared experiences such as day trips or movie nights lead to greater happiness than receiving tangible gifts. When you have reached a milestone with the support of your husband, kids or close friends, invite them to share in the celebration with a mini getaway or afternoon out. They will feel more involved, and you'll get to thank them for cheering you on while rewarding yourself for success. In the process you will also be creating lifelong memories. It's a win-win for everyone.

> Staying present is essential for enjoying your life to the fullest.

8 ENJOY THE JOURNEY.

Staying present in your life and in the moments happening right now is probably one of the most challenging mental habits to practice, but it is essential for enjoying your life to the fullest. Push aside worries and stress on a daily basis by focusing on staying present and noticing the things that bring you joy, peace and feelings of gratitude, Dr. Gannon suggests. When you focus on what brings you pleasure in any given moment, there is no room left to concentrate on negativity, anxiety or your to-do list.

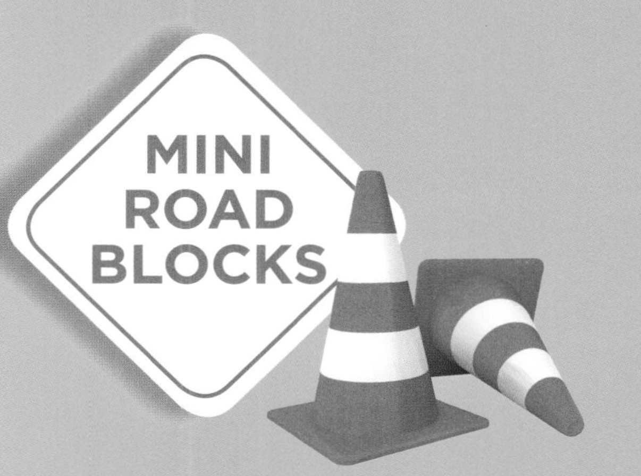

Most readers ask me how to stay motivated, especially in the beginning of your journey when new, healthier ways of thinking are still starting to become habits. Once you learn how to manage and stick to positive emotional changes, they'll become easier to incorporate into your life naturally. As your attitude changes, along with your health, nutrition and body, the move to confidence, self-esteem and happiness will be seamless because you feel and look so incredible. I've listed some of the most common Best Body Now challenges here, plus Dr. Gannon's advice on how to sidestep them.

1 I DON'T KNOW HOW TO SILENCE MY INNER CRITIC.

THE BEST BODY NOW FIX: Imagine what you would say to a friend who was overly critical or putting herself down, advises Dr. Gannon. Would you encourage the criticism? Or would you be caring, compassionate and constructive? Your goal is to help her become the person she wants to be, one step at a time. Imagine that you are this friend. When you consider that the friend is you, you're more likely to be understanding and inspirational, rather than judgmental. Treat your inner critic with love and compassion when she shows up, Dr. Gannon explains, and remind her that you don't have to be perfect.

2 I'M NOT NATURALLY HAPPY OR OPTIMISTIC.

THE BEST BODY NOW FIX: Some women are fortunate enough to be naturally happy or optimistic. Most likely, Dr. Gannon notes, this is because they grew up with families that taught them to look at life through a positive lens. Fortunately, even if you didn't grow up that way, by following the mood-boosting advice in this chapter, it is possible to learn to be happy. A good place to start is with a gratitude journal. When you challenge yourself to find the good in your day, you'll not only realize that wonderful things happen all the time, you'll also naturally start to seek it out all day long.

3 I HAVE A REALLY LONG ROAD AHEAD.

THE BEST BODY NOW FIX: It depends on how you define the road. Are you too focused on the end game rather than the incredible and often surprising milestones along the way? In your quest for your Best Body Now, Dr. Gannon recommends focusing on your success as you progress to keep you present and joyful in the journey. No one is ever fulfilled ▶

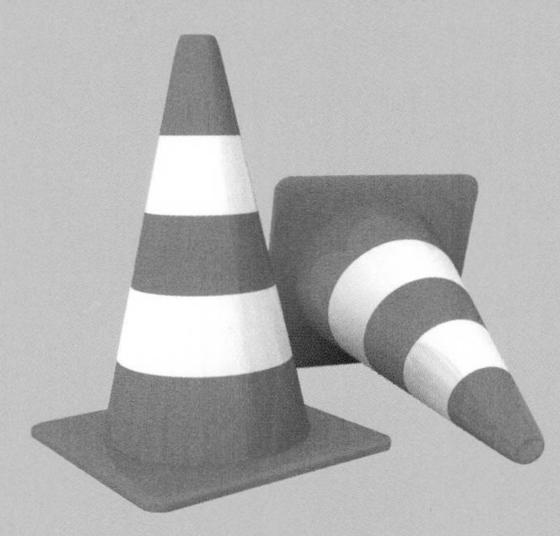

when she believes she will only be happy if she reaches a certain distant goal.

4 I KEEP FALLING OFF THE WAGON.

THE BEST BODY NOW FIX: Each new moment is another opportunity to start fresh. Just because you fell off the wagon at ten this morning doesn't mean you have to stay off it come noon today. So you didn't make it to your exercise class today; can you take a walk after dinner instead? If you skip breakfast, recommit to Eating Clean the rest of the day. Did you let a negative friend get you down? Pick yourself back up—call someone else who does inspire you. Consider what might be getting in your way, advises Dr. Gannon, and think about how to adjust your lifestyle to make Best Body Now habits stick. In the meantime, change your inner dialogue from "I keep falling off the wagon" to "Here's how I'm going to stick to my goals." That simple mind-set shift changes your perspective from the negative to the positive, which is far more empowering. A true success story is a person who has fought adversity and risen above it despite the test.

5 I FEEL OVERWHELMED.

THE BEST BODY NOW FIX: It's natural to feel like you've got a long road ahead, which can be daunting, but consider that in six months you can be living like you are living now or you can be six months into your Best Body Now journey. That means you are six months closer to a happier, healthier, stronger and sexier you. All you have to do is start. Use the advice in this chapter to help you create short- and long-term goals as well as strategies to stay on track. Even if you hit an obstacle or two along the way, ask yourself what's the worst that will happen, says Dr. Gannon. It's natural to run into roadblocks along the way, so you might as well expect them and be ready. Be gentle with yourself and start again tomorrow. This is your life, and you are in charge of what success means to you. For me, it means all the little choices I make in a day to keep me on my Best Body Now journey. A handful of successes can help you reach your long-term goals when you put yourself first and take small steps every day toward your dreams.

With forty years of life experience under your belt, now is the perfect opportunity to focus on *you*.

YOUR 40s Mood-Proof Yourself

I realized in my forties that each success I achieved helped fuel me to greater heights. Even during times when I felt particularly challenged, a positive attitude, combined with small goals and their resultant successes, kept me focused, happy and confident. The Best Body Now program takes effort, but positive emotional changes and newfound self-esteem will ensure you stop self-defeating, negative behaviors and focus on empowering thoughts that help you create the life you want. If you're in your forties and wondering whether it's too late to make changes, ask yourself if you're the happiest you can be in all areas of your life. If the answer is no, consider whether you're okay living the rest of your life the way it is today. To me, that question is a no-brainer. It's never too late to become the person you were meant to be, whether you're forty or sixty. Start now and your Best Body Now will be closer than ever!

It's never too late to become the person you were meant to be.

YOUR 40s What's Happening in Your 40s That Impacts Your Emotions

- Many women finally start to care less about what others think of them. While it's emotionally healthy to care what some people think about us some of the time, Dr. Gannon counsels that it's unhealthy to worry about everyone's opinion all of the time. With forty years of life experience under your belt, now is the perfect opportunity to focus on *you*.

- Changing hormones due to perimenopause, the time period that marks the transition to menopause, can lead to depression and irritability, as well as low energy, fatigue and more, all of which can wreak havoc on your emotions.

- By the time women hit their forties, many have had children. Some who are in their second marriages may be raising very young children as well as teens in the same household, which can add a whole new multitasking challenge to family life.

- Many women in their forties have put themselves last on their family's priority list and been living vicariously through their children for years, rather than achieving their goals and ambitions, too. This can damage your self-esteem and sense of worth, especially as children get older and start to create fulfilling lives for themselves. Fortunately, it's never too late to begin living out your own dreams and passions.

- It's common for women in their forties to find themselves at a crossroads where they're wondering whether they're truly living the life they had hoped to live. Many have children and have postponed prioritizing themselves until now, when their children are better able to care for themselves or are going off to college.

- Other women are taking care of young children and aging parents at the same time, trying to manage the double burden of what Dr. Gannon describes as the "sandwich generation." These many conflicting and evolving demands mean we need to be extra sensitive to our own needs.

- Research shows the average perimenopausal woman gains 10 pounds without changing her eating or exercise habits. This change in how you look can impact your emotions, suggests Dr. Gannon, causing you to feel uncomfortable with your body and unsure of how to lose the extra pounds. Experiencing these negative symptoms can make you feel even more isolated and lonely.

- Thanks to busy family schedules and career demands, by the time they reach their forties, many women discover that they have fallen out of touch with friends or let go of their own personal interests over time. Dr. Gannon finds that many of her forty-something clients feel they no longer have enough hobbies, interests or time with girlfriends and question whether their lives are as meaningful as they could be.

THE FIX? Inspirational Strategies for Your 40s:

1 RECOGNIZE THAT YOU *CAN* FEEL BETTER. It's normal for women to face emotional challenges during perimenopause, but Dr. Gannon stresses it is also important to realize that you have the power to help yourself feel stronger, happier and healthier. This mind-set change is essential to moving your perspective from "No I can't" to "Yes I can!" Following the Best Body Now nutrition and fitness plans will make an incredible difference in how you feel and look, which will begin to strengthen your self-confidence and self-esteem. Notice progress you're making in the plan—for instance, you moved from three push-ups to five—which will empower you to move past emotional issues common in this decade. Next, talk to girlfriends about how you feel. Dr. Gannon recommends surrounding yourself with those who empathize with you and truly care about your success, which will help you feel understood. This can also lessen the pressure you feel from yourself and the outside world. One caveat: when sharing with friends, make sure you keep each other optimistic and focused on the positive to ensure you stay on track.

2 STAY UPBEAT BY SURROUNDING YOURSELF WITH LIKE-MINDED PEOPLE. One of the greatest changes I made for myself is prioritizing time with my girlfriends who support my Best Body Now journey. Dr. Gannon advises her clients to do the same. That's because when you encourage each other to take risks, try new things and embrace life, you create a built-in support system of like-minded people who care deeply about you and your success. Being older also brings a heightened level of life experience and wisdom—many women describe themselves as having greater self-acceptance and a higher level of self-esteem at this age, Dr. Gannon adds. Sharing with friends can deepen the experience.

> Success breeds even more success.

3 ESTABLISH SHORT-TERM OBJECTIVES TO FUEL CONFIDENCE. It is easier to stay motivated when you've already tasted success—weight loss, an improved state of mind, younger-looking skin, the ability to run three miles and so on. Dr. Gannon notes this is because our self-esteem increases when we create opportunities to challenge ourselves and break old paradigms about what we can and can't do. It's true. I love to push myself and I've noticed in my own experience that success breeds even more success. Dr. Gannon advises starting by listing all the accomplishments you'd love to achieve, big or small—everyone will have something unique on her list. For example, I first wanted to compete on the physique stage. Once I accomplished that goal, I wanted an *Oxygen* cover. Next, I was determined to compete in swimsuit and modeling competitions. Finally, I wanted to write a book and then more books. Your list will likely look much different from mine because it's about what *you* envision for yourself. It's so much easier to set new challenges when you feel your life is full of possibilities rather than drudgery, and realize that the sheer volume of opportunity is boundless.

After you've created your list, ensure you stay on track by keeping long-term goals in mind. A new study in the *Journal of Consumer Research* shows you have more self-control when it comes to making healthy decisions (such as exercising or eating well) when you keep your focus on future objectives. If you start to feel swayed by temptation, don't think about the current situation, such as having an extra slice of pizza or forgoing your workout for a movie with friends. Instead, turn your attention to your bigger plan to drop 10 pounds by the summer. This will prevent you from buckling under pressure and ensure you stick to your path to success.

4 CELEBRATE WHAT YOU LIKE ABOUT YOURSELF. Noting your strengths and appreciating them will help you build self-esteem, self-acceptance and happiness. Consider your successes, Dr. Gannon recommends, and allow yourself to feel proud, the same way you would encourage a friend or loved one. Dr. Gannon also recommends starting by listing what you love about yourself: Are you a good friend? Do you listen well? Are you creative, musically talented or good at expressing your feelings? Make a list of ten of your positive attributes (that list will change as you progress in your journey). Find opportunities to celebrate one of them each day and use that energy to inspire your Best Body Now transformation.

5 FUEL YOUR OWN PRODUCTIVITY. Everyone has the same twenty-four hours in a day, but some of us are much more productive than others. Ever notice that tasks always get assigned to the busy person because she knows how to prioritize and get things done? When you make yourself your top priority, you'll be more productive and have more time for your family and friends, too. It's the only way to do a good job. Not doing so will only make you unhappy and resentful, and you'll need much more effort to accomplish everything you need to do.

6 CREATE A MORE MEANINGFUL LIFE. I'm motivated by reading biographies of purposeful, successful people who have lived meaningful purposeful lives. I'm also tremendously inspired by reading stories from people who've changed their lives after following my *Eat-Clean Diet*® books. This reminds me of the responsibility I have to them and others to do my best, so that they, too, can experience a fuller life. I also derive a great deal of motivation from my daughters—I owe it to them to take care of myself in every way possible and lead by example. All of these inspirations give my life meaning and help drive me forward.

To ensure you're living your most meaningful life, Dr. Gannon suggests asking yourself: If you have children, do you think they're proud of you? Are you setting a good example of living a healthy, productive, happy life? Are you showing them you can be positive and joyful even when life is busy and stressful? Consider how living a Best Body Now lifestyle can help you become more fulfilled and live a more meaningful life for you and your family.

Allow yourself to feel proud.

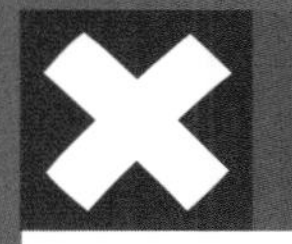

THE WORST ANTI-HAPPINESS HABITS

Don't let negativity or self-criticism sabotage your success. Read the following ways your attitude may be holding you back, plus how to change your mind-set so you can achieve your Best Body Now.

1 DOWNPLAYING COMPLIMENTS. Instead of pushing aside positive feedback, Dr. Gannon suggests letting yourself really feel and own compliments you receive.

2 FEARING SUCCESS. It's normal for many of us to fear success even more than we fear failure. What do you think will happen to your life if you actually do become fit and healthy? Will your family approve? Will your friends be jealous? What's more important than worrying about how others may react to your new life, Dr. Gannon says, is making yourself a priority. If a relationship changes because someone doesn't support you, that's okay—your new mind-set and lifestyle don't have room for anyone who stops you from becoming the best you can be.

3 SURROUNDING YOURSELF WITH NEGATIVE PEOPLE. Many of us have friends or loved ones in our lives who aren't as supportive, optimistic and empowering as they could be. When making changes, it's essential to be around those who empower you rather than attempt to hold you back. Consider joining online communities or social networks with those making the same sort of life changes. See "Spring Clean Your Negative Influences" earlier in the chapter for advice on how to surround yourself with more positive influences instead.

4 LETTING EXCUSES HOLD YOU BACK. When you reach a speed bump or obstacle in your life, simply acknowledge it as a pause in your plan, rather than something that prevents you from reaching your goals, advises Dr. Gannon. It's easy to fall into a victim mindset and get off track. It's best to expect a certain number of bumps in the road; that way you won't be totally thrown off track when you face one. Instead, jump back on the Best Body Now path right where you left off.

5 GETTING OVERWHELMED BY THE PROCESS. It can be daunting to consider where you're at today compared to where you want to be tomorrow, so it's important to remind yourself to enjoy the journey and that worthwhile efforts do take time. Make specific goals, recomends Dr. Gannon, and reward and celebrate yourself as you hit each milestone along the way. When you act the way you want to feel, she adds, you'll prevent yourself from being overwhelmed. Why? Because you're focused on what's bringing you happiness and change in the moment, rather than what is causing you stress.

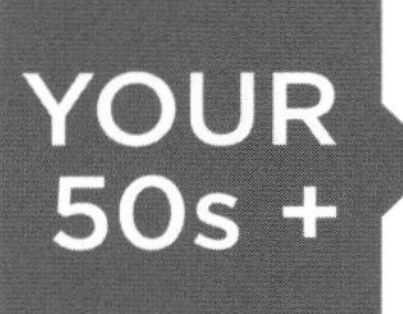

Create Happiness and Mental Toughness

I'm fortunate because I am finding that my fifties are not really that much different from my forties—with the exception that I feel happier and more alive than ever! I've entered a point in my life where I've gained such confidence in who I am and what I can do that things can only get better from here.

I started with small steps and created momentum, backed by strategies to help me stay focused and on track. What I've learned from sharing my secrets with women of all ages and walks of life is that it is possible to make changes no matter how old you are. You can retrain yourself to think empowering thoughts. To do so, Dr. Gannon suggests you start by setting goals and taking small steps to make them happen.

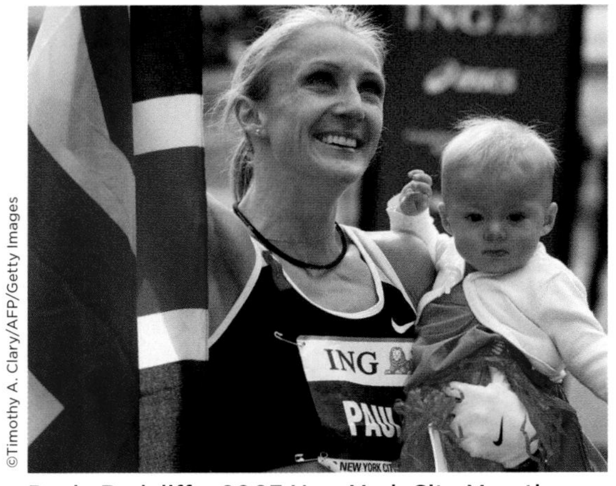

©Timothy A. Clary/AFP/Getty Images

Paula Radcliffe, 2007 New York City Marathon winner, with her daughter

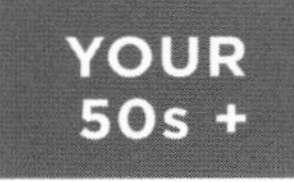

What's Happening in Your 50s and Beyond That Impacts Your Emotions

Changing hormones can stack weight around the midsection and make it more difficult to lose weight (see Chapters 4 and 5). Extra pounds can make you feel less confident and sexy.

Many women in their fifties are often at very different stages of life. Dr. Gannon sees this commonly in her practice. Some women have passed through perimenopause to menopause. Many have children who are grown up and have left the home, while others are still raising children and adolescents. While some of you might be thinking ahead to retirement, others are launching new businesses, hobbies and interests. Each of these milestones—becoming an empty nester, retiring, starting a new job, handling hormonal changes—brings with it its own set of emotional challenges, from added stress to a changing sense of self.

> Those who live their lives fully or reinvent themselves in their fifties feel the greatest self-esteem and happiness.

During this decade, many women are facing opportunities to rethink who they are and who they want to be. Dr. Gannon finds those who live their lives fully or reinvent themselves in their fifties feel the greatest self-esteem and happiness. They refuse to settle for stereotypes about middle age and embrace life more than ever.

With older children going off on their own or starting to take care of themselves, many women in this decade find themselves with an empty home or time on their hands, which can lead to feelings of boredom, isolation, uselessness and loneliness.

I feel sexier than ever.

Sexuality and confidence tend to peak at this age, despite women being older or dealing with symptoms of menopause. That has been my personal experience—I feel sexier than ever. Dr. Gannon says she often hears clients in their forties and fifties express that they're the most comfortable and confident with their sexuality than they've ever been. As Gail Sheehy writes in her book *Sex and the Seasoned Woman: Pursuing the Passionate Life*, "A seasoned woman is spicy. She has been marinated in life experience.... She knows who she is. She...is committed to living fully and passionately in the second half of life." Her research shows that many women in midlife are open to sex, love, new dreams, exploring spirituality and revitalizing their marriages as never before. Even if you are just beginning your Best Body Now journey, feel confident knowing these things and more are possible for you. Isn't it exciting to be part of this?

THE FIX? New Mood Strategies for Your 50s +:

1 REMEMBER THAT AGE IS JUST A NUMBER. Be positive and enthusiastic in your fifties by staying in the game—that's what I do. Dr. Gannon's philosophy, and mine, is that your age is just a number and not a reflection of how active, engaged and passionate you are (or should be) about life. Changing your perspective is easier said than done, especially if you've never made yourself a priority. However, once I began my Best Body Now transformation, I felt an enormous urge to discover more about myself, my talents and life than I had previously dared. Once you start to look at life in terms of how active, involved and enthusiastic you are, rather than how old you are, your happiness, energy levels and vitality will increase.

Look at life in terms of how active, involved and enthusiastic you are, rather than how old you are.

2 IDENTIFY WHAT MIGHT BE HOLDING YOU BACK. While making a large life transformation can be challenging, nothing is impossible no matter how old you are. It's essential to put your current situation in perspective to help you move past fear. Dr. Gannon's advice: discover the reasons that you just can't live the way you have been. Be specific, such as pinpointing high cholesterol, problems in your marriage or how you can't walk up a flight of stairs without being breathless. Then use that issue to gather the courage to make changes. Begin making adjustments to your life little by little so you ensure success, including removing unhealthy food from your pantry, scheduling workouts for the coming week and talking to a close friend about a goal. Every small step will move you forward in your Best Body Now journey and help you overcome what has been holding you back in the past.

> Every small step will move you forward in your Best Body Now journey.

3 MAKE NEW HABITS STICK BY CELEBRATING STEPS, NOT JUST GOALS. It *is* possible to teach an old dog new tricks. Instead of only celebrating yourself each time you reach a goal, celebrate each step of progress you make, advises Dr. Gannon. For example, be proud you have created a menu plan for the week and bought healthy foods, all steps in the process of Eating Clean all week. By acknowledging the little shifts on your way to achieving goals, you will create moments of pride and joy throughout the day and reinforce the new habits you're developing.

4 REDISCOVER YOUR CHILDHOOD CURIOSITIES. Throughout the many transitions of midlife, women doubt themselves as they age and begin to question their worth—I know I certainly did. However, I also felt I couldn't continue living a life without purpose. As you send your kids off to college or start to shift gears in your career, Dr. Gannon notes, doubts are common. A good place to start revitalizing your life is to unleash the curious little girl inside you. That's what I have done, and today I look for answers, insights and new information everywhere, a process of discovery that inspires me in new ways. Once you commit to your true self again—your passions, dreams and goals—all the magic and wonder of discovery you had as a child comes rushing back full force and helps give you the confidence, courage and motivation to make yourself happy. I am now back to that fully alive person I once was, overjoyed at where I've come and open to life.

5 SIDESTEP BOREDOM WITH SIMPLE STRATEGIES. Whenever my daughters complained they were bored, I always told them to go use their imagination. It's their responsibility to find what engages and inspires them. But as an adult, I dreaded boredom because it meant that I, too, had to confront myself, take responsibility for my life and self-motivate. What's interesting is that most people who are bored often turn to television and technology to engage them, Dr. Gannon reports—a strategy that only works in the short term. That's because it simply numbs us and allows us to check out. Instead of zoning out, determine what you can do to be more fully present and engaged in your life, advises Dr. Gannon. Read great books, travel, try new recipes, strengthen your relationships, meet new people, connect with old friends, brush up on a skill or even master something different. Make a list of all the experiences you want to have and do one thing every day toward making them happen. Soon enough you won't have time to be bored, only happy.

6 **LEARN TO RELAX.** Some women have the opposite problem of boredom—their schedules are more filled than ever, so relaxing doesn't seem like an option. Even getting enough restorative sleep can be a challenge. But fatigue and exhaustion can have a negative impact on your mood, says Dr. Gannon, making you grumpier and more prone to anxiety and depression. Research from the National Institutes of Health suggests that sleep gives brain neurons the chance to shut down and repair in order to function better while you're awake. When you're sleep-deprived, your brain doesn't work as efficiently and you begin to see changes in memory, mood and physical abilities. Other studies show that creating an evening ritual, such as taking a bath, journaling or reading a book, can help your body relax so you fall asleep more quickly and stay sleeping. One of my favorite bedtime rituals is curling up with an inspiring autobiography of one of my heroes. Some of my favorite reads include those about Lady Diana, Martha Stewart, Donald Trump, Julia Child, the Dutch athlete Fanny Blankers-Koen and famous artists including Andy Warhol and Pablo Picasso. When I first started making significant changes in my life, this helped me realize that other people had overcome much greater challenges, and I could do the same.

7 **APPRECIATE YOUR WISDOM.** One of the great gifts of aging, explains Dr. Gannon, is the security and comfort that comes from knowing who you are. Use

TOSCA TIDBIT

Your Best Body Now life has no room for regrets or unmet dreams. If you've always wanted to be a drummer but never tried, take a class, buy a CD or start reading inspirational books by famous musicians. Getting your creative juices flowing can increase your energy levels and put you in the positive mindset to beat any fears or challenges. Somehow exploring these untapped dreams helps to make you look younger, too.

> I'm not perfect, but now I realize that I don't really want or need to be.

your insights to boost your confidence, self-esteem and self-empowerment. As I closed the door on my forties I realized most of that decade had been spent learning to love, respect and develop who I really am. I now enjoy the experience of being a wise woman and feel freer to speak my mind. My zest for life is still burning strong. I now have the life experience to say confidently and wisely, "Bring it on!"

8 CHAMPION *YOU* AND INCREASE YOUR SELF-ACCEPTANCE. As a woman in her fifties, I like who I am. I'm not perfect, but now I realize I don't really want or need to be. Fifty is a reason to love yourself and be confident in who you are and all that you've already achieved, explains Dr. Gannon. The sexiest thing about any woman is her level of confidence. When you feel comfortable and confident in your skin, you literally shine. It all starts with accepting who you are, where you're at now and what you need to do to live a Best Body Now life. Are you eating well, taking care of your needs, speaking to yourself kindly, exercising? Once you realize that you are a strong, beautiful woman who is doing her best, nothing is too daunting or challenging for you to overcome. And even if the challenge is significant, you will have the emotional muscle to tackle it!

> The sexiest thing about any woman is her level of confidence.

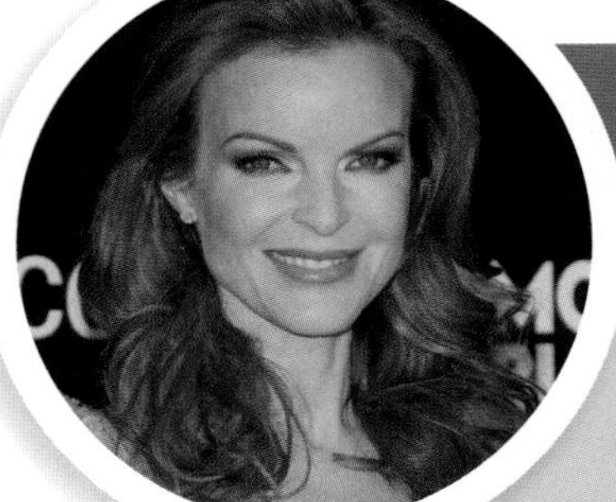

The "H" Factor: A-List Proof That Life Gets Better at 40

Award-winning television star and über-sexy forty-seven-year-old Marcia Cross got married for the first time at forty-two and had her first child at forty-four, all while starring in *Desperate Housewives*, one of the hottest television shows on the air. A mix of beauty and brains, Marcia left her hit show *Melrose Place* in her mid-thirties to complete a master's degree in psychology, showing that you can be and do anything at any time when you choose to do so. Thanks for the reminder, Marcia!

MY BEST BODY NOW

Triumph of the Not-So-Average Jane
Tammy Cardy's Journey

THEN
5'7", AGE 39
178 POUNDS

NOW
AGE 42
138 POUNDS

Before I discovered the Best Body Now program I was at a very unhappy point in my life. I was tired all the time and I was completely stressed at work and at home. I had little patience for my two small children. I would even go as far as to say that I felt borderline depressed. I hated how I looked and hated shopping for any clothes. I hated looking at myself in the mirror. I was round everywhere: my hips and thighs had expanded to the point that even my lounge-around-the-house baggies were tight and uncomfortable. My face had chunked out and I could no longer see any definition. I was still battling acne in my forties. My hair was very dry and a bit frizzy and difficult to style. I weighed 178 pounds and was miserable.

I ate a lot of fruit and veggies at meals, but it was the snacks and binges that were killing me. I always felt like I needed a nap by two o'clock each afternoon and would buy some sugary snack to get me through. The more sugary things I ate, the more I craved and the more I binged.

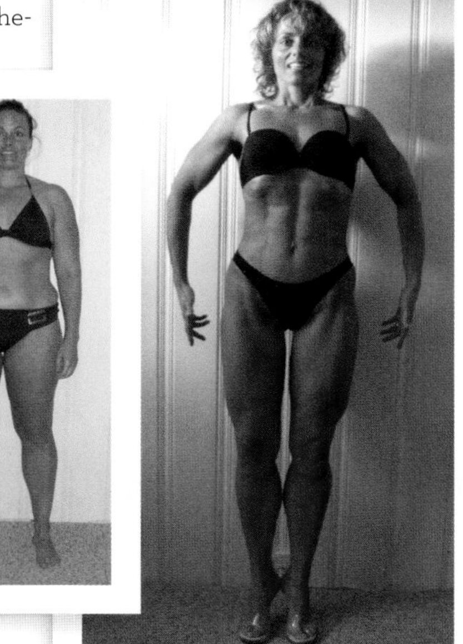

In 2006 my marriage was on the brink of separation and I made a last-ditch effort to help us get our life back on track. It just ended up causing more problems. Even when I made a conscious effort to be healthier, the stress of my job and collapsing marriage always won out and I would resort back to the emotional eating.

In December 2007, after a particularly unhealthy holiday season, I read about Tosca's program in *Oxygen*. I'd always had a desire to do a figure competition and I kept this in the back of my mind when I first began the Best Body Now journey. Before too long, I became less tired and my skin started to clear up. My afternoon nods were a thing of the past. I was Eating Clean and diligently working out four to five times a week.

By the three-month mark I was convinced I could do a competition that spring. Seven weeks away from the competition, I still had 15 pounds to lose. I signed up with a pro fitness competitor to get training by e-mail. The progress came fast. I felt great emotionally and was physically stronger than I had ever been in my life. I stepped onstage seven weeks later—just five months after first starting the program—at 138 pounds and placed second in the masters category.

Unfortunately, the stress of my marriage and work didn't let up. I resigned from my job and separated from my husband. Thanks to the Best Body Now plan, I'd become so strong over the previous year that I had the emotional strength to persevere. I've learned that when life isn't a bunch of roses you don't have to eat your way through the stress—by Eating Clean and sticking to the Best Body Now plan, I know I can conquer anything!

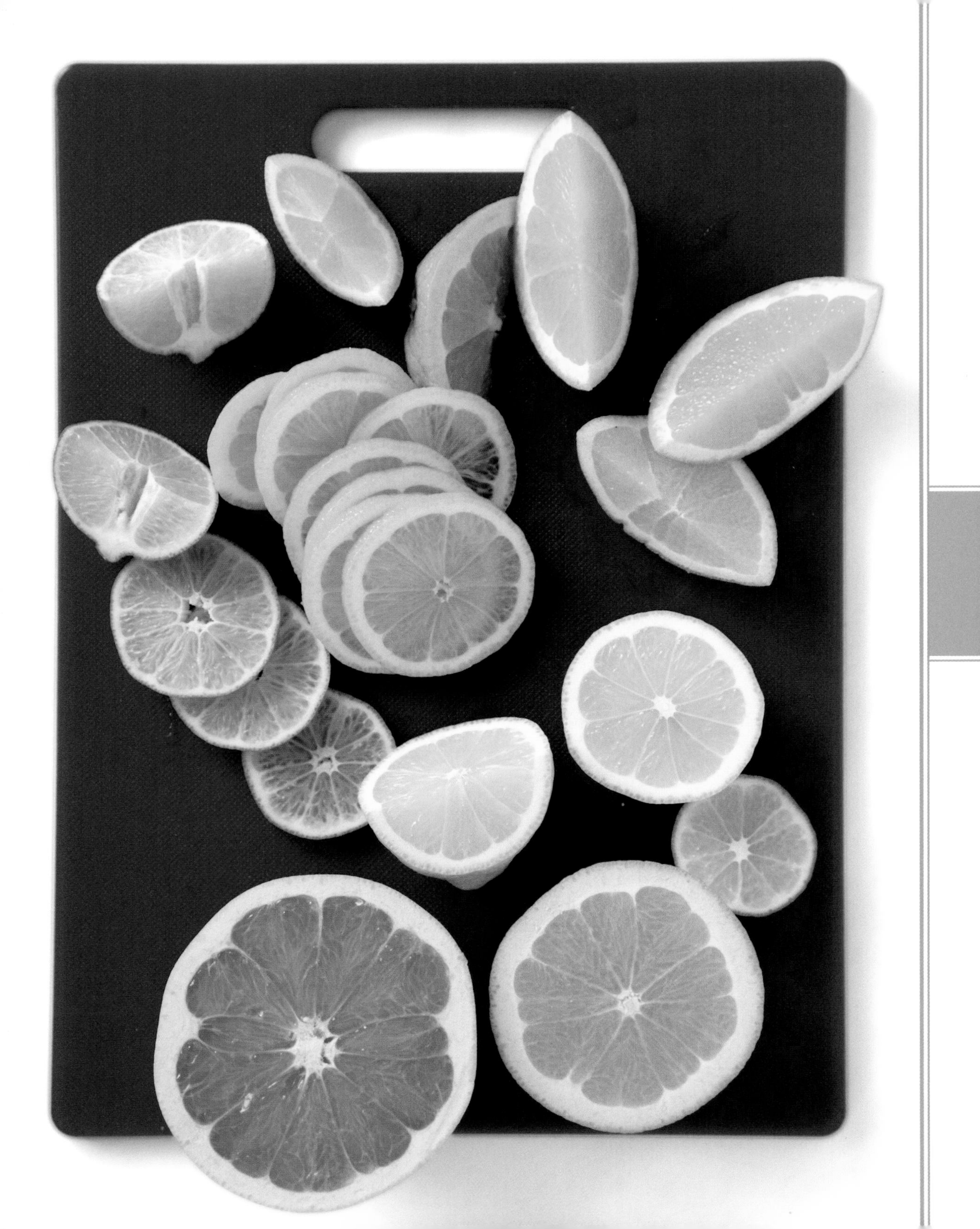

Best Body Now Recipes

9

ONE OF THE SECRETS TO BEST BODY NOW SUCCESS IS ARMING yourself with the right tools. This includes an arsenal of Eating Clean recipes that are delicious, nutritious and easy to prepare. I've created all the recipes in this chapter around the principles outlined in Chapter 4, so when you eat them, you can feel confident that you're following the Best Body Now plan. These are the very same dishes I make for myself and my family. Enjoy!

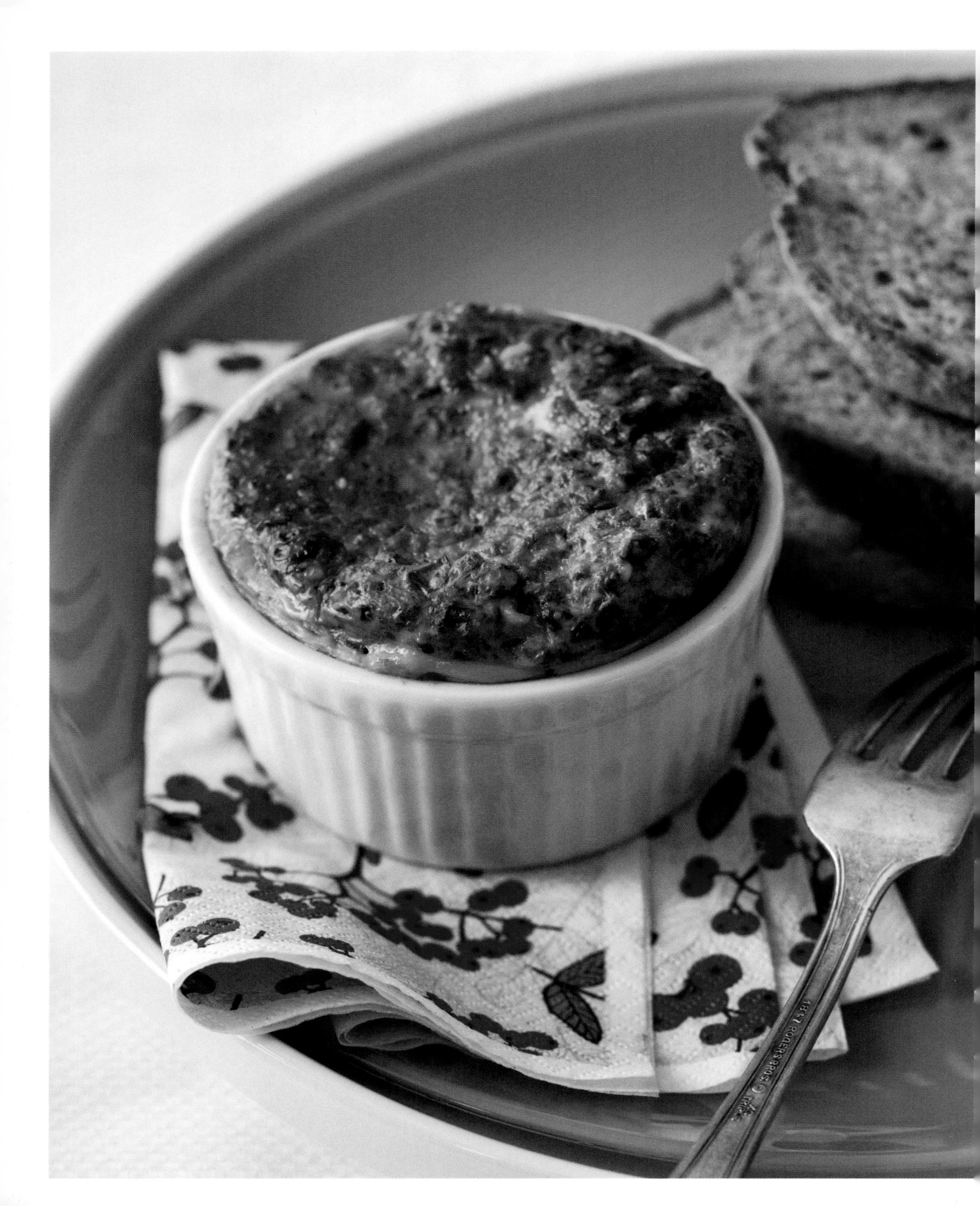
1847 ROGERS BROS.

GREEN EGG FRITTATA

BREAKFAST

PREP TIME: **10 MINUTES** COOK TIME: **35–40 MINUTES** YIELD: **8 SERVINGS**

This recipe can be prepared using a lasagna dish or ramekins.

INGREDIENTS

Olive oil to coat lasagna dish

10 egg whites plus 4 yolks

¾ cup skim milk

¼ teaspoon thyme

Simple Spinach Pesto
(see page 279)

DIRECTIONS

1 Preheat oven to 350 degrees. Lightly coat 9-by-13-inch lasagna dish with olive oil.

2 In a large bowl whisk eggs, milk and thyme. Add 1 cup of Spinach Pesto and whisk until well combined.

3 Pour egg mixture into lasagna dish and place on baking sheet in oven. Bake for 35–40 minutes, until egg is set. It will begin to crack on the top and brown on the edges.

4 Serve over toast or in a wrap.

NUTRITION INFORMATION PER SERVING: Calories: 166, Calories from Fat: 117, Protein: 10 g, Carbs: 5 g, Dietary Fiber: 2 g, Sugars: 2 g, Fat: 13 g, Sodium: 409 mg

TOSCA'S HOT OR COLD CEREAL MIX

BREAKFAST

COLD CEREAL MIX

PREP TIME: **5–10 MINUTES**
YIELD: **10 SERVINGS**

INGREDIENTS

2 cups oats

2 cups quinoa flakes

½ cup oat bran

½ cup flaxseed

½ cup wheat germ

DIRECTIONS

Combine all ingredients in a large bowl and transfer to an airtight container. This mix can be portioned as desired on top of cereal or yogurt, or served hot.

NUTRITIONAL VALUE FOR ½ CUP SERVING, NO MILK: Calories: 270, Calories from Fat: 63, Protein: 10 g, Carbs: 53 g, Dietary Fiber: 10 g, Sugars: 2 g, Fat: 7 g, Sodium: 5 mg

HOT CEREAL MIX

PREP TIME: **2 MINUTES**
COOK TIME: **10 MINUTES**
YIELD: **1 SERVING**

INGREDIENTS

½ cup cereal mix

1 cup skim or soy milk or water

1 teaspoon cinnamon

1 tablespoon honey

½ teaspoon vanilla extract

DIRECTIONS

1 In a saucepan, heat cereal mix and milk or liquid of your choice over medium heat, stirring occasionally. After 2 minutes add the remaining ingredients.

2 Cook for another 3–5 minutes depending on how thick you want your cereal to be.

3 Serve warm, topped with fresh or dried fruit.

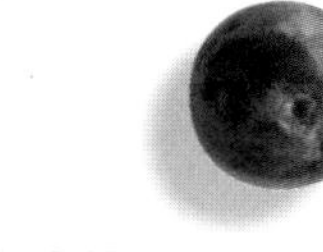

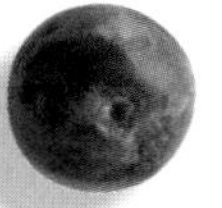

NUTRITIONAL VALUE PER SERVING: Calories: 426, Calories from Fat: 63, Protein: 19 g, Carbs: 85 g, Dietary Fiber: 11 g, Sugars: 32 g, Fat: 7 g, Sodium: 132 mg

EGG IN THE HOLE

BREAKFAST

PREP TIME: **10 MINUTES** COOK TIME: **10 MINUTES** YIELD: **4 ONE-SLICE SERVINGS OR 2 TWO-SLICE SERVINGS**

INGREDIENTS

2 cups spinach or kale

4 thick slices whole-grain bread

½ teaspoon sea salt

1 teaspoon pepper

3 tablespoons olive oil plus 2 teaspoons for pan

4 eggs whites plus 2 yolks

DIRECTIONS

1 Bring a medium pot of water to boil over high heat. Add spinach or kale. Cook for 2–3 minutes until tender. Transfer greens to a plate and set aside to cool.

2 Prepare bread by cutting a 1-inch hole in the center of each slice using a bottle cap, cookie cutter or knife. In a small bowl combine salt, pepper, and 3 tablespoons oil. Brush each side of bread with seasoned oil mixture.

3 Place a thin layer of cooled greens around the hole of each slice of bread.

4 In a separate bowl, whisk eggs.

5 Heat a large pan with remaining oil over medium heat. Place bread in pan green side up. Pour ¼ of whisked egg in hole of each slice of bread, allowing egg to top greens. Cook for 2–3 minutes, flip and cook for another 2 minutes.
Serve hot.

TIP: This is a fun way to serve greens and protein for kids. Keep in mind it doesn't have to look perfect. Think of it as a healthy French toast.

NUTRITIONAL VALUE PER TWO-SLICE SERVING: Calories: 430, Calories from Fat: 260, Protein: 18 g, Carbs: 27 g, Dietary Fiber: 5 g, Sugars: 4 g, Fat: 29 g, Sodium: 872 mg

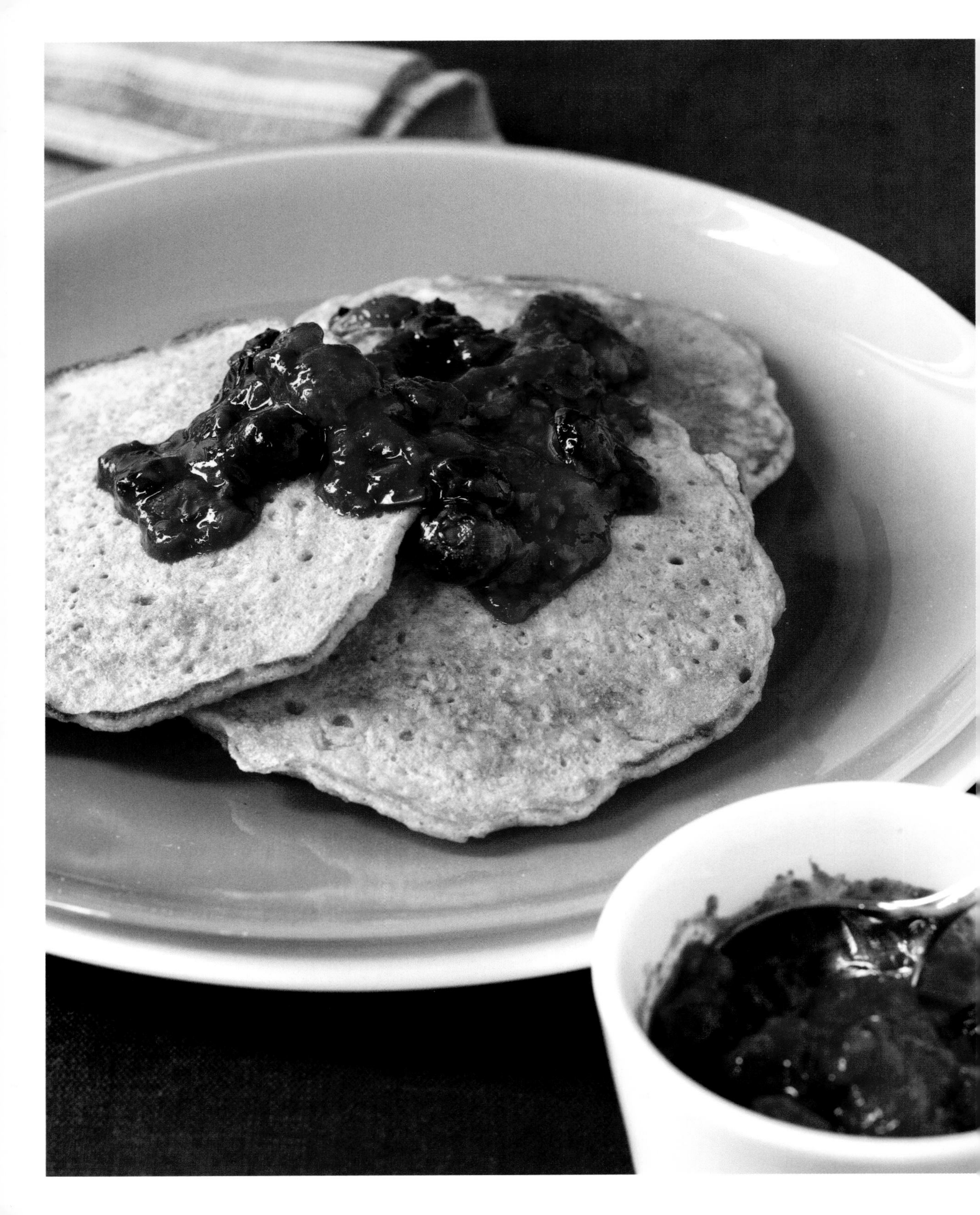

OAT PANCAKES AND STEWED FRUIT TOPPING

BREAKFAST

PREP TIME: **5 MINUTES** COOK TIME: **3 MINUTES EACH PANCAKE** YIELD: **4–6 SERVINGS**

INGREDIENTS

1 cup rolled oats

1/4 cup oat bran

3/4 spelt or whole-wheat flour

3 tablespoons sucanat

1 1/2 teaspoons baking powder

1/2 teaspoon salt

1 1/2 cups skim or soy milk

3 tablespoons melted coconut oil

2 egg whites plus 1 yolk

1/2 teaspoon vanilla

DIRECTIONS

1 Whisk dry ingredients together in a large bowl.

2 In a separate bowl, combine wet ingredients.

3 Add the wet ingredients to dry and whisk gently until just combined.

4 Lightly grease a large nonstick pan or griddle and heat over medium-low heat. Pour 1/3 cup of batter in pan. Cook until bubbles form, flip and cook until lightly brown. Continue making pancakes one at a time until all batter is used.

5 Serve immediately or keep warm in a 200-degree oven. Top with stewed fruit topping.

STEWED FRUIT TOPPING

INGREDIENTS

3 cups peeled and pitted peaches, apples, berries or any combination

1/2 cup water

2 cinnamon sticks

DIRECTIONS

Place all ingredients in a small saucepan. Bring to a boil, reduce heat to low and simmer for 20 minutes or until thickened. Serve hot.

NUTRITIONAL VALUE PER SERVING (WITH FRUIT): Calories: 400, Calories from Fat: 120, Protein: 14 g, Carbs: 60 g, Dietary Fiber: 8 g, Sugars: 24 g, Fat: 14 g, Sodium: 330 mg

GARLIC SOUP

PREP TIME: **10 MINUTES** COOK TIME: **1 ½ HOURS** YIELD: **6 SERVINGS**

INGREDIENTS

3 tablespoons olive oil, plus more for pan

9 heads of garlic, halved horizontally, with skins intact

4 cups low-sodium chicken stock

2 cups water

1 tablespoon thyme

1 tablespoon basil

½ tablespoon sea salt

½ tablespoon pepper

DIRECTIONS

1 Preheat oven to 350 degrees. Coat the bottom of a large ovenproof pan or Dutch oven with olive oil. Place garlic cut side down in prepared pan.

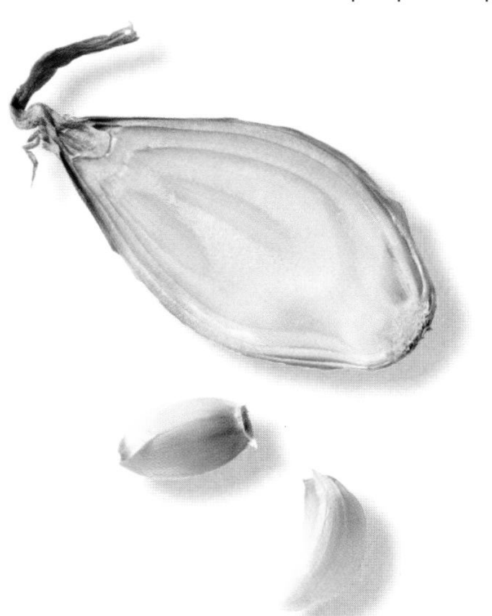

2 Roast the garlic for 1 hour, until soft and tender. Garlic should be golden brown and mushy to the touch.

3 Lift the skin from the garlic and discard; the garlic cloves will stick to the pan. Scrape garlic into a large pot or keep in Dutch oven for next steps.

4 Add stock and water, thyme, basil, salt and pepper to pot or Dutch oven and heat over medium-high heat. Bring soup to a boil, then simmer on low for 30 minutes.

NUTRITIONAL VALUE PER SERVING: Calories: 142, Calories from Fat: 66, Protein: 4 g, Carbs: 16 g, Dietary Fiber: 2 g, Sugars: 1 g, Fat: 7 g, Sodium: 96 mg

MEXICAN TOMATO CHICKEN SOUP

PREP TIME: **15 MINUTES** COOK TIME: **90 MINUTES** YIELD: **8 SERVINGS**

INGREDIENTS

4 plum tomatoes

2 carrots, peeled and chopped

2 small shallots

4 garlic cloves

4 green or red peppers, cored and cut into quarters

1 ½ tablespoons olive oil

1 ¼ pounds boneless, skinless chicken breast halves

1 cup chopped cilantro, plus 2 tablespoons for garnish

2 cups low-sodium chicken stock

3 cups water

1 teaspoon sea salt

1 teaspoon chili powder

1 teaspoon cinnamon

1 ¼ cups fresh or frozen corn kernels

1 cup rinsed, drained canned chickpeas

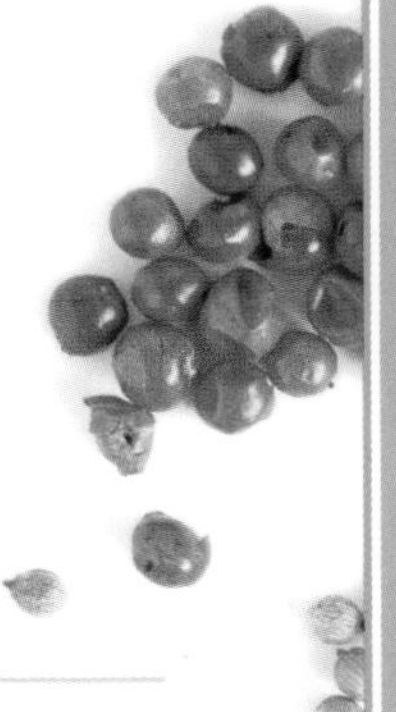

DIRECTIONS

1 Preheat oven to 400 degrees. Toss tomatoes, carrots, shallots, garlic and peppers in olive oil on a baking sheet lined with aluminum foil. Bake for 45 minutes.

2 Meanwhile, in a large pot, bring chicken, 2 cups cilantro, 1 ½ cups stock and water to a boil. Reduce heat to low and simmer gently until chicken is just cooked through, about 10 minutes.

3 Remove cooked chicken from soup and let cool. Dice into ½-inch cubes.

4 Strain broth through a colander to separate vegetables from broth. Reserve broth.

5 Let vegetables cool slightly. Place vegetables in food processor or blender with ½ cup reserved broth; blend until smooth. Transfer to pot.

6 Cook over medium heat for 5–10 minutes to thicken.

7 Add reserved broth, salt, chili powder, cinnamon, corn, chickpeas and cubed chicken. Simmer on low for 30 minutes. Top with remaining cilantro.

TIP: Top with avocado for extra nutritional value.

NUTRITIONAL VALUE PER SERVING: Calories: 131, Calories from Fat: 36, Protein: 7 g, Carbs: 20 g, Dietary Fiber: 5 g, Sugars: 2 g, Fat: 4 g, Sodium: 485 mg

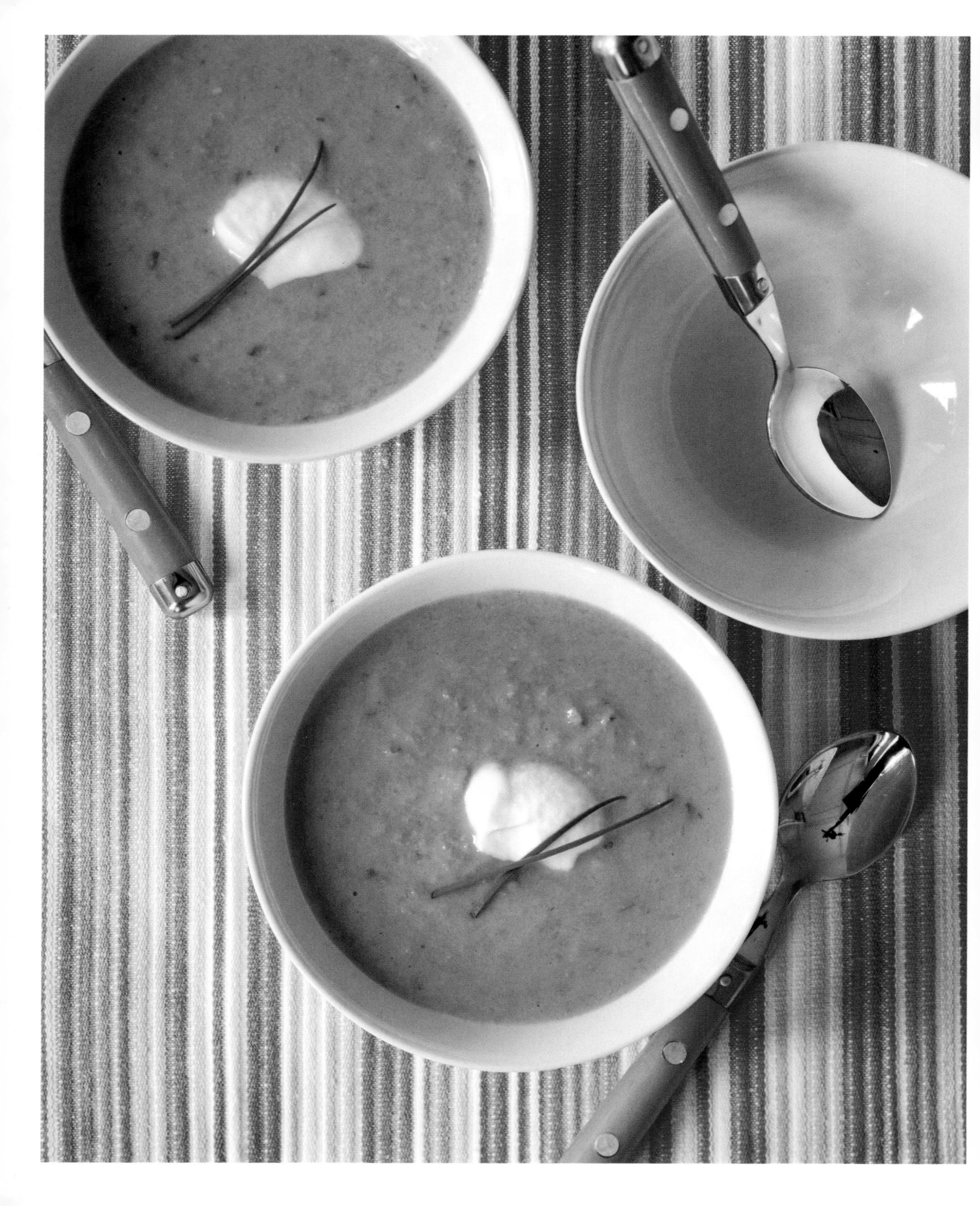

McNEILL HOUSE SUMMER PEA AND MINT SOUP

PREP TIME: **15 MINUTES** COOK TIME: **20–30 MINUTES** YIELD: **6 SERVINGS**

Prepare Yogurt Cheese before proceeding with recipe (see below).

INGREDIENTS

2 tablespoons olive oil

2 cups chopped leeks (whites only)

1 large white onion, chopped

4 cups low-sodium chicken stock

5 cups fresh or frozen peas

⅔ cup chopped fresh mint

Salt and pepper to taste

½ cup yogurt cheese

½ cup chopped fresh chives

DIRECTIONS

1 Heat oil in a large saucepan. Add leeks and onions. Gently cook over medium-low heat for 5–10 minutes until tender.

2 Add chicken stock and raise heat to medium. Bring to a boil.

3 Add the peas and cook for 2–4 minutes (if using frozen peas, cook for at least 3–5 minutes). Do not allow them to get mushy and overcooked.

4 Remove from heat and add mint, salt and pepper.

5 Allow the mixture to cool for 5 minutes. Do not strain. Puree in batches in the food processor.

6 Gently reheat pureed soup and stir in yogurt cheese. Garnish with chives to serve.

YOGURT CHEESE

Place four layers of damp cheesecloth in a fine-mesh sieve or colander. Place the colander over a bowl. Add 2 quarts low-fat plain yogurt and let drain overnight in the refrigerator. The result of the draining process will leave you with a soft, creamy cheese-like product. It is lower in calories than cream cheese but can be used in its place. It is also low in lactose, higher in protein and lower in sodium than cream cheese. The best part is that it is all natural.

TIP: You can also serve this soup cold. Make the soup 1 day in advance to fully chill. Serve in a wineglass with a whole-wheat bread stick for an elegant presentation.

TIP: Freezes well in sealable plastic bags.

NUTRITION INFORMATION PER SERVING: Calories: 179, Calories from Fat: 45, Protein: 9 g, Carbs: 26 g, Dietary Fiber: 7 g, Sugars: 8 g, Fat: 5 g, Sodium: 144 mg

ENSALADA MARACAIBO

PREP TIME: **15 MINUTES** YIELD: **8 SERVINGS**

INGREDIENTS

3 cups fresh or frozen corn kernels

4 cups red beans (about 2 cans), drained and rinsed

4 cups black beans (about 2 cans), drained and rinsed

1 red pepper, seeded and deveined, diced

¼ cup finely chopped cilantro

3 stalks celery, chopped

1 teaspoon chopped chilies

½ cup pear vinegar

¼ cup balsamic vinegar

¼ cup extra-virgin olive oil

2 small onions, finely chopped

2 tablespoons chopped scallions

Salt and pepper to taste

DIRECTIONS

1 Combine all ingredients in a large bowl, chill and serve.

NOTE: Chickpeas are a great substitute for the black or red beans. This can be used not only as a salad, but also as a great salsa or over meat.

NUTRITIONAL VALUE PER SERVING: Calories: 360, Calories from Fat: 72, Protein: 16 g, Carbs: 59 g, Dietary Fiber: 17 g, Sugars: 7 g, Fat: 8 g, Sodium: 350 mg

POT STICKERS IN SAUCE

PREP TIME: **25 MINUTES** COOK TIME: **20 MINUTES** YIELD: **24 SERVINGS**

INGREDIENTS

3 cups finely shredded cabbage

1 egg white, lightly beaten

1 tablespoon low-sodium soy sauce

1 tablespoon five-spice powder (recipe follows)

4 tablespoons minced scallions

2 cups shredded carrot

¼ pound ground lean chicken breast, cooked and drained

24 wonton wrappers, at room temperature

½ cup water

1 tablespoon oyster sauce

½ teaspoon honey

⅛ teaspoon crushed red pepper flakes

2 teaspoons lemon zest

1 tablespoon peanut oil

DIRECTIONS

1 Steam cabbage for 5–10 minutes. Cool to room temperature and squeeze out any excess moisture; set aside.

2 Filling: combine egg white, soy sauce, five-spice powder and scallions in a large bowl. Stir in cabbage, carrot and chicken. Combine lightly but do not overmix.

3 To prepare pot stickers, place 1 tablespoon filling in center of 1 wonton wrapper. Gather edges around filling, pressing firmly at top to seal. Repeat with remaining wrappers.

4 Place pot stickers on large baking sheet and refrigerate 1 hour or until cold.

5 Meanwhile, to prepare sauce, combine remaining ingredients except oil in small bowl; mix well.

6 Heat oil in large nonstick skillet over high heat. Add pot stickers and cook until bottoms are golden brown.

7 Add sauce to pan and cover. Cook for 3 minutes, uncover and cook until all liquid has been absorbed. (You can also steam the pot stickers for 5–10 minutes.)

FIVE-SPICE POWDER

INGREDIENTS

1 tablespoon anise seed

1 tablespoon ginger root

1 tablespoon fennel seed

1 tablespoon pepper

½ tablespoon ground cloves

DIRECTIONS

Grind all ingredients in spice grinder or food processor.

NUTRITION VALUE PER SINGLE POT STICKER, DIPPED IN SAUCE: Calories: 48, Calories from Fat: 14, Protein: 2 g, Carbs: 7 g, Dietary Fiber: 1 g, Sugars: 1 g, Fat: 2 g, Sodium: 92 mg

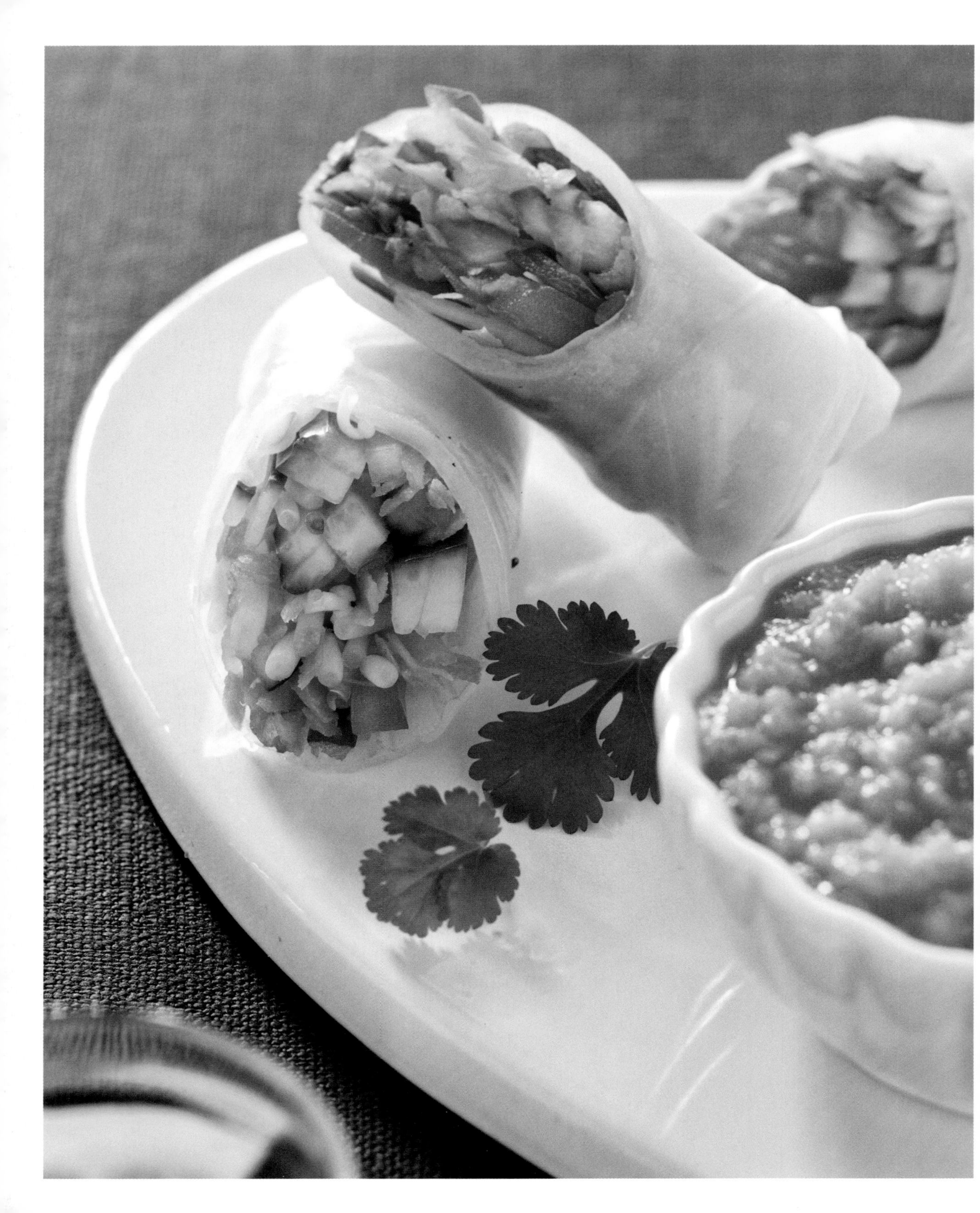

GARDEN SPRING ROLLS AND DIPPING SAUCE

PREP TIME: **30 MINUTES** YIELD: **5 SERVINGS**

SPRING ROLL

INGREDIENTS

2 packages rice-paper spring roll wrappers (20 wrappers)

1 cup grated carrot

1/4 cup bean sprouts

1 cucumber, julienned

1 red bell pepper, stem and seeds removed, julienned

4 green onions finely chopped, use only the green part

1 large bowl hot water

DIRECTIONS

1 Soak one rice-paper wrapper in a large bowl of hot water until softened.

2 Place a pinch each of carrots, sprouts, cucumber, bell pepper and green onion on the wrapper toward the bottom third of the rice paper.

3 Fold ends in and roll tightly to enclose filling.

4 Repeat with remaining wrappers. Chill before serving.

DIPPING SAUCE

INGREDIENTS

1 clove garlic

2 medium carrots, chopped

2 tablespoons coarsely grated peeled fresh ginger

1/4 cup rice wine vinegar (not seasoned)

2 tablespoons low-sodium soy sauce

1/4 teaspoon toasted sesame oil

Pinch each of coarse salt and freshly ground black pepper

1/2 teaspoon red pepper flakes

3 tablespoons vegetable oil

3 tablespoons water

DIRECTIONS

1 Combine garlic, carrot, ginger, vinegar, soy sauce, sesame oil, salt and both types of pepper in a food processor and blend until smooth.

2 With machine running, add vegetable oil and then water through the feed tube in a slow, steady stream.

3 Chill and serve sauce with spring rolls.

TIP: Rice paper is tricky to work with, but remember if it rips you can often enclose the tear. Keep trying! The dipping sauce is fabulous with almost anything. I like to use it as a refreshing alternative to hummus.

NUTRITION INFORMATION PER SERVING: Calories: 202, Calories from Fat: 81, Protein: 3 g, Carbs: 29 g, Dietary Fiber: 3 g, Sugars: 3 g, Fat: 9 g, Sodium: 470 mg

MEXICAN CHIPOTLE-MARINATED PORK TENDERLOIN

PREP TIME: **10 MINUTES PLUS MARINATING TIME** COOK TIME: **30 MINUTES** YIELD: **4 SERVINGS**

INGREDIENTS

1 can chipotle chili in adobo sauce

3 garlic cloves

½ cup coarsely chopped white onion (about 1 medium onion)

2 tablespoons lime juice

1 teaspoon sherry vinegar

1 teaspoon dried oregano

1 teaspoon sea salt

1 teaspoon black pepper

1 tablespoon olive oil

1 pound pork tenderloin, trimmed of fat

DIRECTIONS

1 Process chili, garlic, onion, lime juice, sherry vinegar, oregano, salt and pepper in a blender or food processor. Add olive oil and blend until smooth.

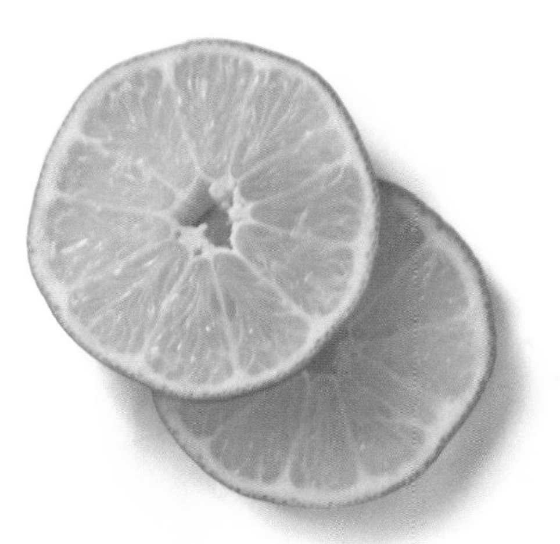

2 Place marinade and pork in a zippered plastic bag and toss to coat. Refrigerate for at least 1 hour or overnight.

3 Preheat oven to 350 degrees.

4 Heat a grill pan over high heat. Sear pork on all sides, about 2 minutes per side, until brown. Transfer pan to the oven and cook for 20–25 minutes.

5 Allow pork to rest before slicing, 5–10 minutes. This pork is beautiful by itself or topped with Simple Salsa (see page 279).

NUTRITIONAL VALUE PER SERVING: Calories: 248, Calories from Fat: 99, Protein: 32 g, Carbs: 5 g, Dietary Fiber: 1 g, Sugars: 1 g, Fat: 11 g, Sodium: 651 mg

HEARTY BRAISED PENNE

MEAT DISHES

PREP TIME: **20 MINUTES** COOK TIME: **2 HOURS** YIELD: **8 SERVINGS**

INGREDIENTS

4 pounds beef short ribs or skinless turkey legs

1 teaspoon sea salt

1 teaspoon pepper

¼ cup olive oil

1 large onion, diced

2 celery stalks, sliced

2 large carrots peeled and sliced

3 cloves garlic, coarsely chopped

5 Roma tomatoes, cut into eighths

1 cup red wine

1 teaspoon dried basil

3 tablespoons Dijon mustard

2 cups low-sodium beef or chicken broth

1 pound whole-wheat or spelt penne

4 cups fresh baby spinach

¼ cup freshly grated Parmesan (optional)

DIRECTIONS

1 Preheat the oven to 350 degrees.

2 Season meat with salt and pepper. Heat oil in a Dutch oven over medium heat. Brown meat on all sides, about 8–10 minutes. Remove meat to a plate.

3 Add the onion, celery, carrot and garlic to the Dutch oven and cook, stirring frequently until onions are tender and browned.

4 Add the tomatoes, wine, basil and mustard; bring to a boil; scrape the bottom of the pan to remove drippings. Return meat to the pan.

5 Add the broth, cover and place in the oven for 2 hours until the meat is very tender.

6 Remove meat from the cooking liquid. Transfer liquid to food processor or blender. Process until the mixture is smooth. Return to pan over low heat.

7 Bring a large pot of salted water to a boil, add pasta and cook 8–10 minutes until tender. Drain and place into a serving bowl.

8 Add spinach to sauce; stir occasionally.

9 Meanwhile, shred meat into small pieces using 2 forks or a knife. Discard bones. Stir the shredded meat into the sauce.

10 Toss sauce with pasta.

11 Sprinkle the pasta with Parmesan cheese if desired.

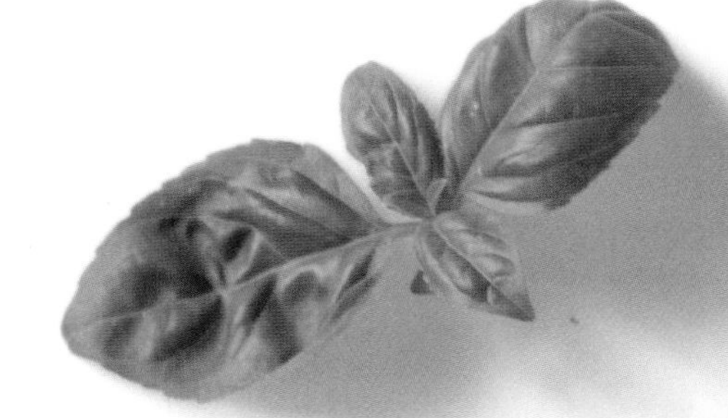

NUTRITIONAL VALUE FOR RECIPE MADE WITH BEEF SHORT RIBS: Calories: 643, Calories from Fat: 225, Protein: 54 g, Carbs: 49 g, Dietary Fiber: 7 g, Sugars: 1 g, Fat: 25 g, Sodium: 717 mg

NUTRITIONAL VALUE FOR RECIPE MADE WITH TURKEY: Calories: 363, Calories from Fat: 99, Protein: 19 g, Carbs: 49 g, Dietary Fiber: 8 g, Sugars: 2 g, Fat: 11 g, Sodium: 608 mg

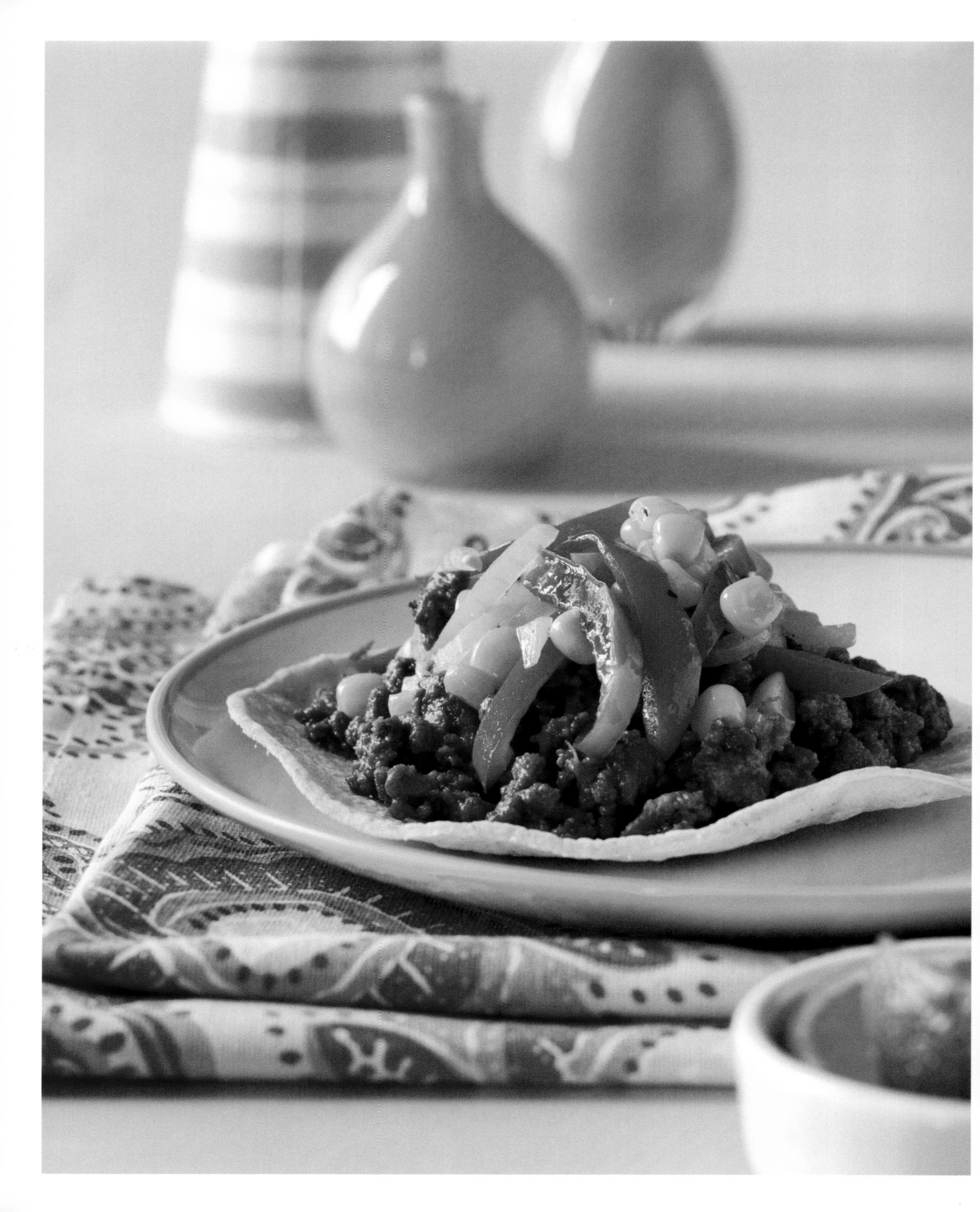

FAJITA TOSTADA

MEAT DISHES

PREP TIME: **15 MINUTES** COOK TIME: **30 MINUTES** YIELD: **4 SERVINGS**

INGREDIENTS

2 medium onions, thinly sliced

2 bell peppers (ribs and seeds removed), thinly sliced

1 ½ cups fresh or frozen corn kernels

2 tablespoons olive oil

1 teaspoon sea salt

1 teaspoon ground pepper

2 cups ground lean chicken, turkey or beef

½ cup low-sodium chicken broth

Fajita spice mix (recipe follows)

4 tortillas, corn or whole-wheat (6-inch)

DIRECTIONS

1 Preheat oven to 450 degrees. Combine onions, bell peppers, corn and 1 tablespoon olive oil in a large bowl; season with salt and pepper.

2 Place vegetables on a rimmed baking sheet lined with aluminum foil. Roast vegetables until tender and lightly browned, about 15–20 minutes.

3 Meanwhile heat remaining tablespoon olive oil in a nonstick skillet. Brown meat; add chicken stock and fajita spice mix. Combine and cook for 5–10 minutes, until most liquid has cooked out.

4 Combine vegetables and chicken in a large serving dish, discarding foil but reserving baking sheet.

5 Arrange tortillas on baking sheet. Dividing evenly, brush with remaining tablespoon oil and bake until edges are golden, 3–5 minutes.

6 Either top tortillas with meat and vegetable mix or serve separate and allow your guests to make their own.

FAJITA SPICE MIX

INGREDIENTS

1 tablespoon chili powder

1 ½ teaspoons cumin

1 teaspoon black pepper

1 teaspoon salt

1 teaspoon paprika

½ teaspoon dried oregano

¼ teaspoon garlic powder

¼ teaspoon onion powder

¼ teaspoon cayenne pepper

NUTRITION INFORMATION PER SERVING: Calories: 462, Calories from Fat: 213, Protein: 32 g, Carbs: 45 g, Dietary Fiber: 9 g, Sugars: 3 g, Fat: 24 g, Sodium: 1,503 mg

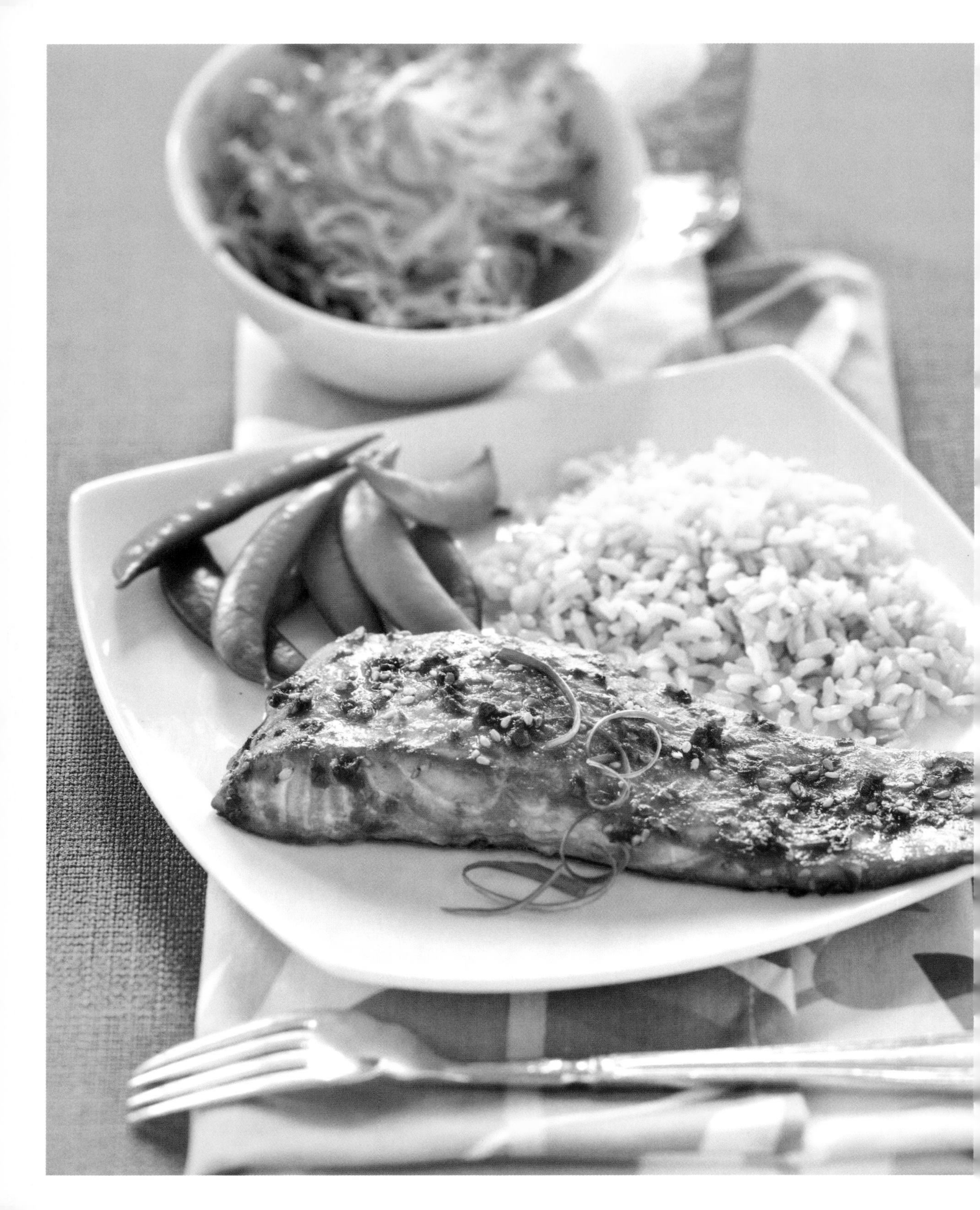

SPICE UP MY SALMON

FISH

PREP TIME: **10 MINUTES** COOK TIME: **13–15 MINUTES PLUS MARINATING TIME** YIELD: **4 SERVINGS**

INGREDIENTS

2 tablespoons low-sodium soy sauce

2 tablespoons wasabi paste or 1 tablespoon wasabi powder

1 ½ teaspoons toasted sesame seeds

1 ½ tablespoons ginger, minced

1 tablespoon minced garlic

1 tablespoon honey or molasses

1 teaspoon cayenne pepper

1 tablespoon olive oil

1 tablespoon rice vinegar

4 salmon fillets, each 4 ounces

DIRECTIONS

1 In a small bowl, combine all ingredients except salmon until well combined. Place in a zippered plastic bag; blend well. Add salmon, seal and toss to coat. Refrigerate for 1 hour.

2 Preheat oven to 400 degrees.

3 Place marinated salmon on a baking sheet lined with aluminum foil, discarding marinade.

4 Bake until fish flakes easily with a fork, about 13 minutes.

TIP: Add 1 ½ tablespoons red miso paste to the marinade for an extra kick! This salmon goes perfectly with your favorite brown rice.

NUTRITION INFORMATION PER SERVING: Calories: 315, Calories from Fat: 180, Protein: 23 g, Carbs: 11 g, Dietary Fiber: 0.2 g, Sugars: 6 g, Fat: 20 g, Sodium: 566 mg

GROWN-UP CHICKEN TENDERS

POULTRY

PREP TIME: **20 MINS** COOK TIME: **30 MINS** YIELD: **6 SERVINGS**

INGREDIENTS

- ½ cup flaxseed
- ½ cup oat bran
- 1 cup puffed rice
- 2 tablespoons onion powder
- 1 tablespoon garlic powder
- 2 tablespoons paprika
- 2 tablespoons dried thyme
- 4 tablespoons dried parsley
- 2 teaspoons salt
- 2 teaspoons pepper
- 2 cups oats
- 4 eggs
- ½ cup fresh lemon juice
- 4 boneless skinless chicken breast cut into strips

DIRECTIONS

1 Preheat oven to 350 degrees.

2 Prepare a baking sheet by lining it with parchment paper.

3 Combine flaxseed, oat bran, puffed rice and all spices in a food processor. Pulse until
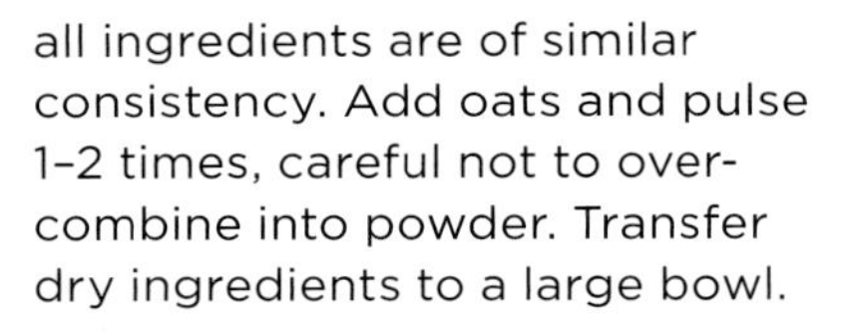
all ingredients are of similar consistency. Add oats and pulse 1–2 times, careful not to over-combine into powder. Transfer dry ingredients to a large bowl.

4 In a medium bowl, whisk egg and lemon juice until just combined.

5 One strip at a time, coat chicken first in egg mixture, then in dry ingredients. Place chicken on prepared baking sheet. Bake for 20–30 minutes until strips are golden brown.

6 If you want very crispy strips, broil for an extra 10 minutes.

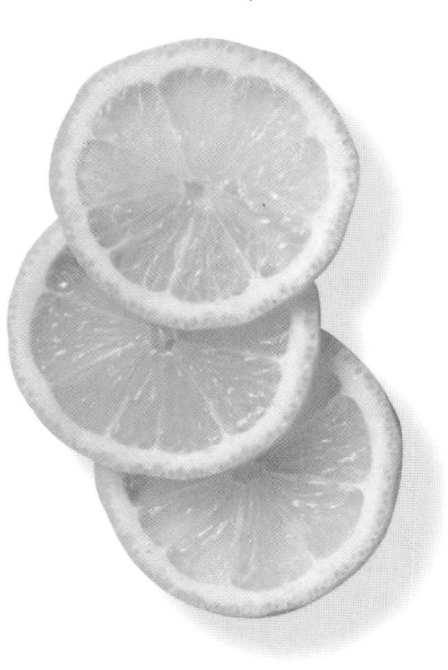

NUTRITIONAL VALUE PER SERVING: Calories: 380, Calories from Fat: 120, Protein: 31 g, Carbs: 39 g, Dietary Fiber: 10 g, Sugars: 3 g, Fat: 13 g, Sodium: 740 mg

JOE'S SLOPPY TURKEY

POULTRY

PREP TIME: **15 MINUTES** COOK TIME: **20 MINUTES** YIELD: **6 SERVINGS**

INGREDIENTS

1 tablespoon olive oil

2 cups grated carrots

1 large onion, finely diced

2 garlic cloves, minced

1 teaspoon sea salt

1 teaspoon pepper

3 tablespoons tomato paste

4 pounds lean ground turkey

5 plum tomatoes, diced

2 cups finely chopped button mushrooms (about 4 ounces)

1 tablespoon cider vinegar

1 tablespoon blackstrap molasses

1 tablespoon chili sauce or any mild hot sauce

1 tablespoon Worcestershire sauce

¼ cup water or low sodium chicken stock

6 whole-wheat rolls or 2 cups cooked brown rice

DIRECTIONS

1 In a large saucepan, heat oil over medium heat; add carrots, onion and garlic. Cook for 4–5 minutes until tender, season with salt and pepper.

2 Remove from heat, stir in tomato paste. Return to heat and add turkey. Cook turkey through for 5 minutes and break apart with wooden spoon.

3 Add tomatoes and mushrooms and cook with the lid on for 3–4 minutes, until they begin to soften. Add vinegar, molasses, Worcestershire sauce, chili sauce, water or stock and stir. Simmer for 8–10 minutes until liquid has reduced.

4 Serve on roll or over brown rice.

NUTRITIONAL VALUE PER SERVING: Calories: 623, Calories from Fat: 234, Protein: 65 g, Carbs: 36 g, Dietary Fiber: 6 g, Sugars: 8 g, Fat: 26 g, Sodium: 934 mg

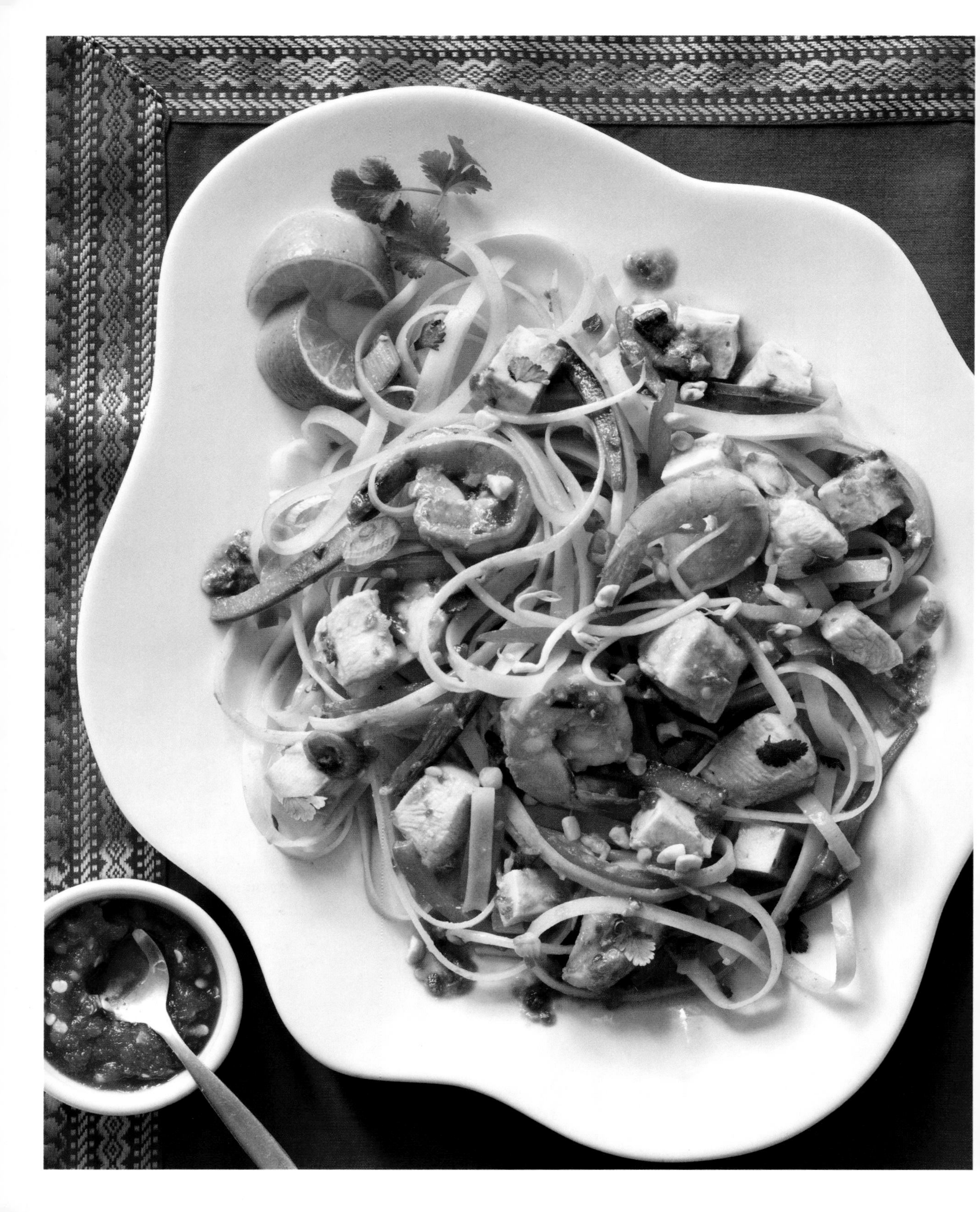

EASY PAD THAI

POULTRY

PREP TIME: **20 MINUTES** COOK TIME: **20 MINUTES** YIELD: **4 SERVINGS**

INGREDIENTS

2 cups flat rice noodles or vermicelli

⅓ cup chili sauce

¼ cup low-sodium soy sauce

¼ cup lime juice

½ tablespoon water

1 teaspoon chili paste or hot pepper sauce

2 tablespoons olive oil or coconut oil

4 shallots sliced

1 green bell pepper, sliced

1 red bell pepper, sliced

6 cloves garlic, minced

6 ounces chicken breast, cubed

6 ounces large shrimp, cubed

½ cup medium tofu, cubed

2 cups bean sprouts

6 green onions, sliced

½ cup chopped fresh coriander

1 egg, lightly beaten

½ cup chopped toasted peanuts (optional)

DIRECTIONS

1 In large bowl, soak noodles in warm water until flexible, about 15 minutes. Drain and set aside in a large bowl.

2 Meanwhile, prepare sauce: combine chili sauce, soy sauce, lime juice, water and chili paste in a small bowl and stir until well combined.

3 In wok, heat 1 tablespoon olive or coconut oil over medium-high heat; add shallots and green and red peppers and cook until softened, about 4 minutes. Add garlic.

4 Add remaining oil to wok; stir-fry chicken until white and shrimp until pink, about 2 minutes.

5 Coat in sauce and bring to a boil; reduce heat to medium.

6 Add tofu, bean sprouts, green onions, chopped coriander and noodles; stir-fry until noodles are tender, about 3 minutes.

7 Stir in egg; cook, stirring, until sauce is thickened, about 1 minute. Serve.

8 Garnish with peanuts if desired.

NUTRITIONAL VALUE PER SERVING: Calories: 476, Calories from Fat: 198, Protein: 32 g, Carbs: 46 g, Dietary Fiber: 7 g, Sugars: 10 g, Fat: 22 g, Sodium: 496 mg

MOUSSAKA

POULTRY

PREP TIME: **30 MINUTES** COOK TIME: **30 MINUTES** YIELD: **10 SERVINGS**

INGREDIENTS

2 medium eggplants, sliced into ¼-inch slices

1 teaspoon sea salt

1 pound ground turkey or chicken

1 white onion, diced

2 cloves garlic, minced

1 teaspoon ground cinnamon

½ teaspoon ground nutmeg

1 teaspoon pepper

4 cups whole peeled tomatoes, coarsely chopped

¼ cup tomato paste

¼ cup chopped fresh oregano

½ cup chopped fresh flat-leaf parsley

2 cups yogurt cheese (prepared ahead of time; see page 259)

¼ cup grated Parmesan cheese

2 egg whites

Olive oil cooking spray

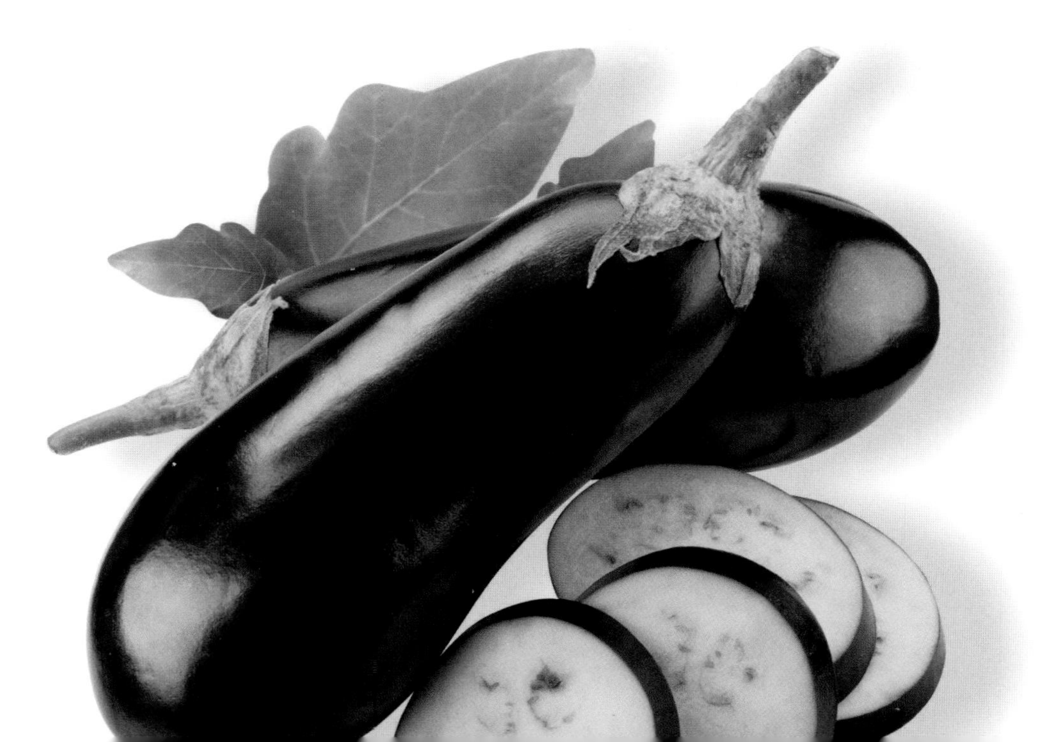

DIRECTIONS

1 Sprinkle salt on both sides of sliced eggplant. Place eggplant slices in a colander over a bowl; let stand 1 hour to drain.

2 Brown turkey or chicken in a saucepan over medium heat, about 5–7 minutes. Transfer to a medium bowl.

3 In the same saucepan cook onion and garlic. Stir in cinnamon, salt, nutmeg and pepper, cook until onion is tender, about 10 minutes.

4 Return turkey to saucepan. Add tomatoes, tomato paste and oregano. Bring to a boil; reduce heat to simmer over medium-low heat, until liquid has reduced and sauce has become thick, about 30 minutes.

5 Meanwhile, preheat broiler.

6 Once eggplant has drained, discard the liquid and rinse slices briefly under cold water, dry off immediately with paper towel and place on a baking sheet.

7 Coat eggplant in olive oil or spray and broil until browned, 2–5 minutes. Set aside.

8 Preheat oven to 400 degrees.

9 Add Parmesan and egg whites to prepared yogurt cheese. Whisk together briskly with a fork.

10 To assemble the moussaka, place a layer of eggplant on the bottom of a lightly oiled 9-by-13-inch lasagna baking dish. Cover with half the turkey sauce and ¼ of the yogurt cheese mixture. Repeat layers without yogurt cheese mixture. Cover with one final layer of eggplant and coat with remaining yogurt cheese mixture. Bake until top is bubbling and starts to brown, about 30 minutes.

11 Allow moussaka to cool and firm for about 10 minutes.

TIP: Don't like eggplant? Swap the eggplant with zucchini and have the same great flavor. Prepare your zucchini in the same manner as the eggplant.

NUTRITIONAL VALUE PER SERVING: Calories: 205, Calories from Fat: 54, Protein: 21 g, Carbs: 21 g, Dietary Fiber: 4 g, Sugars: 11 g, Fat: 6 g, Sodium: 445 mg

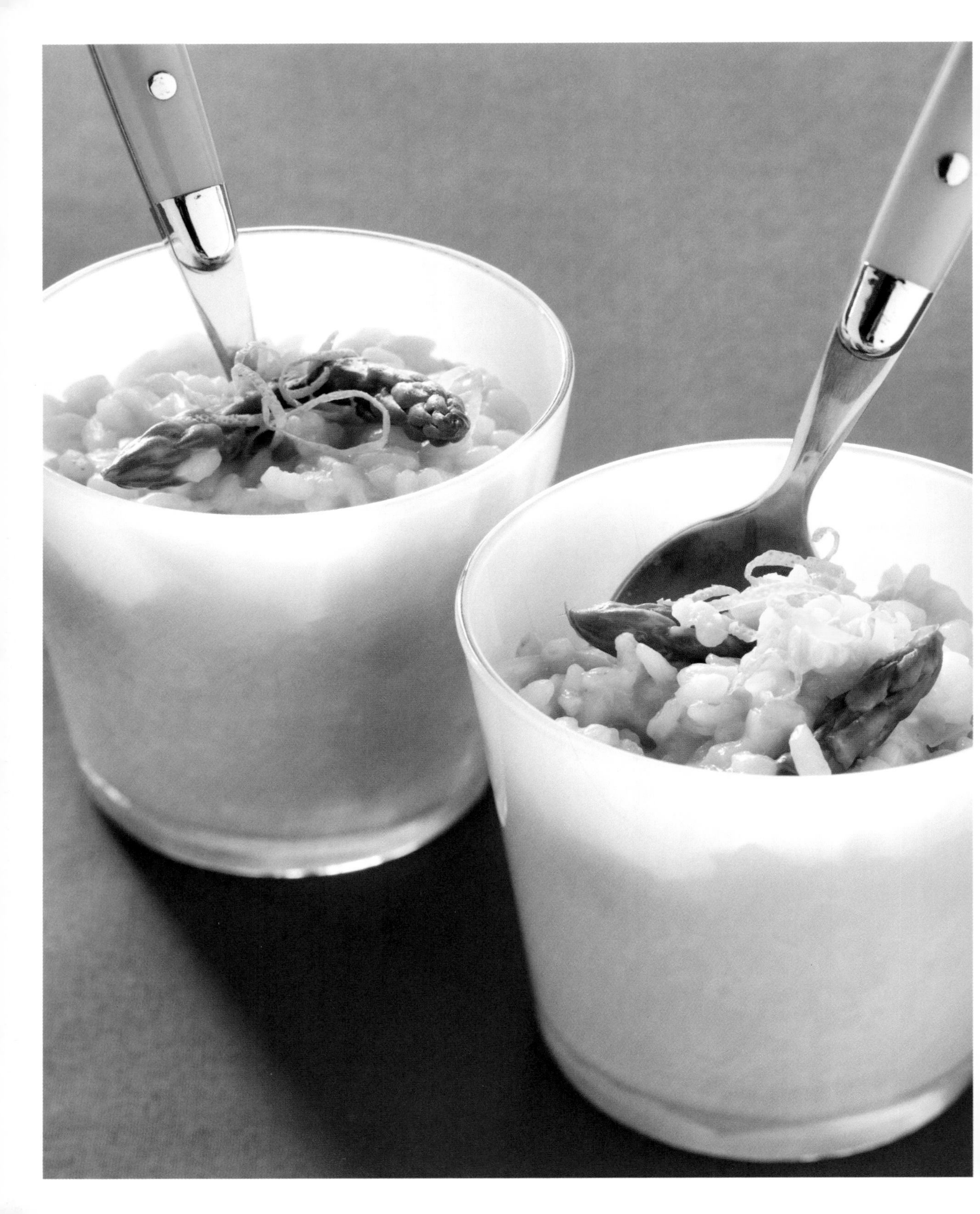

GARLICKY LEMON ASPARAGUS RISOTTO

MEATLESS DISHES

PREP TIME: **10 MINUTES** COOK TIME: **45 MINUTES** YIELD: **4 SERVINGS**

INGREDIENTS

1 pound asparagus

2 tablespoons olive oil

½ tablespoon butter

½ cup chopped shallots

1 cup arborio rice

3 cloves garlic, minced

1 sprig fresh rosemary or 1 teaspoon dried

2 ½ cups low-sodium chicken stock

1 tablespoon lemon zest

2 tablespoon lemon juice

¼ cup water

½ cup freshly grated Parmesan cheese (optional)

Salt and pepper

DIRECTIONS

1 Prepare the asparagus by breaking off tough ends. Cut into bite-size pieces, tips longer, base shorter.

2 Bring a saucepan with a quart of water to a boil.

3 Meanwhile, prepare a large bowl of ice water. Blanch asparagus pieces for 2 minutes, remove from saucepan with a slotted spoon and submerge in ice water until cool, about 5 minutes, reserving 1 cup of cooking water.

4 Drain asparagus.

5 In a large saucepan or skillet, heat olive oil and butter over medium heat. Add shallots and cook for 3 minutes until translucent. Add the rice, garlic and rosemary, and cook for 2 minutes more, stirring until evenly coated.

6 Meanwhile, in a saucepan bring stock to a simmer. Add lemon zest.

7 Add lemon juice and water to shallot pan and stir slowly, allowing the rice to absorb liquid. Once liquid is almost completely absorbed, add ½ cup of stock to the rice. Continue to stir until the liquid is almost completely absorbed.

8 Repeat this process using the remaining stock until the rice is tender but still firm to the bite. You may need more or less liquid: if more, use reserved asparagus water. Remove from heat. Gently stir in the Parmesan cheese and the asparagus. Add salt and pepper to taste. Serve immediately.

NUTRITION INFORMATION PER SERVING (WITH PARMESAN CHEESE): Calories: 260, Calories from Fat: 100, Protein: 12 g, Carbs: 29 g, Dietary Fiber: 3 g, Sugars: 3 g, Fat: 12 g, Sodium: 440 mg

PERFECT PASTA

MEATLESS DISHES

PREP TIME: **10 MINUTES** COOK TIME: **20–30 MINUTES** YIELD: **4 SERVINGS**

INGREDIENTS

2 cups green beans

2 bunches small asparagus

2 medium zucchini, halved and sliced into small slivers

1 package spelt, rice or whole-wheat fettuccine

¼ cup olive oil

7 whole garlic cloves

Salt and pepper

DIRECTIONS

1 Boil two pots of salted water, one small for vegetables and one large for pasta.

2 Prepare a large bowl with ice water and have a strainer or colander ready.

3 Place green beans in small pot and blanch for 3–5 minutes until just tender. Using a slotted spoon, remove beans, place in strainer and submerge in ice water until beans are chilled, about 4 minutes. Repeat with asparagus and then zucchini, using the same boiling water.

4 Place pasta in large pot and cook for 8–10 minutes.

5 Meanwhile, heat 3 tablespoons oil in a large skillet over medium high heat. Add 5 cloves of garlic, vegetables, salt and pepper. Coat vegetables in oil and allow to heat through, stirring occasionally, about 5 minutes.

6 Remove vegetables from pan and place in a large flat serving dish.

7 Heat remainder of the oil in the same pan over low heat, toss drained pasta and remaining garlic until coated. Add to serving dish, toss with vegetables and top with salt and pepper to taste.

If desired you can add protein to this recipe—for example, chicken, shrimp or scallops.

CHICKEN: 4 ounces chicken breast, diced. Heat a nonstick skillet over medium-high heat. Lightly coat chicken in olive oil and add salt and pepper. Cook for 3–5 minutes on either side until firm.

SHRIMP OR SCALLOPS: 4 large shrimp or scallops. Heat a nonstick skillet over medium-high heat. Lightly coat fish in olive oil and salt and pepper. Cook for 2–3 minutes on either side until opaque.

Serve on top of your perfect pasta for a complete Eat-Clean meal.

NUTRITIONAL VALUE PER SERVING (WITHOUT CHICKEN OR FISH): Calories: 429, Calories from Fat: 139, Protein: 20 g, Carbs: 58 g, Dietary Fiber: 17 g, Sugars: 1 g, Fat: 15 g, Sodium: 142 mg

SIMPLE SPINACH PESTO AND SIMPLE SALSA

SIMPLE SPINACH PESTO

PREP TIME: **10 MINUTES** COOK TIME: **2–3 MINUTES** YIELD: **12 SERVINGS (2 TABLESPOONS EACH)**

INGREDIENTS

1 pound flat-leaf spinach, trimmed and washed

½ cup packed flat-leaf parsley leaves

1 packed cup basil

1 teaspoon grated lemon zest

2 tablespoons lemon juice

1 teaspoon sea salt

1 teaspoon ground pepper

⅓ cup grated Parmesan cheese, plus more for serving (optional)

¼ cup pine nuts

2 garlic cloves

¼ cup olive oil

DIRECTIONS

Combine all ingredients except olive oil in a food processor until paste forms. With motor running, add oil until smooth and creamy, about 1 minute. Add Parmesan if desired, season with salt and pepper.

Toss pesto with your favorite whole wheat or spelt pasta, or enjoy over chicken or as a spread.

NUTRITIONAL VALUE PER SERVING (WITHOUT CHEESE): Calories: 82, Calories from Fat: 68, Protein: 3 g, Carbs: 2 g, Dietary Fiber: 1 g, Sugars: 1 g, Fat: 7 g, Sodium: 242 mg

SIMPLE SALSA

PREP TIME: **10 MINUTES** YIELD: **8 SERVINGS**

INGREDIENTS

1 can (19 ounces) black beans, drained and rinsed

1 cup corn kernels

1 cup grape tomatoes, diced

¼ cup white onion, finely chopped

¼ cup fresh cilantro, finely chopped

1 tablespoon lime juice

1 tablespoon lemon juice

½ teaspoon cumin

½ teaspoon sea salt

½ teaspoon pepper

DIRECTIONS

1 Combine all ingredients in a medium bowl.

2 Serve with Mexican Chipotle-Marinated Pork Tenderloin (see page 264) or over chicken with baked whole-grain tortilla or pita chips and a salad.

NUTRITIONAL VALUE PER SERVING: Calories: 90, Calories from Fat: 5, Protein: 5 g, Carbs: 17 g, Dietary Fiber: 5 g, Sugars: 1 g, Fat: 0.5 g, Sodium: 124 mg

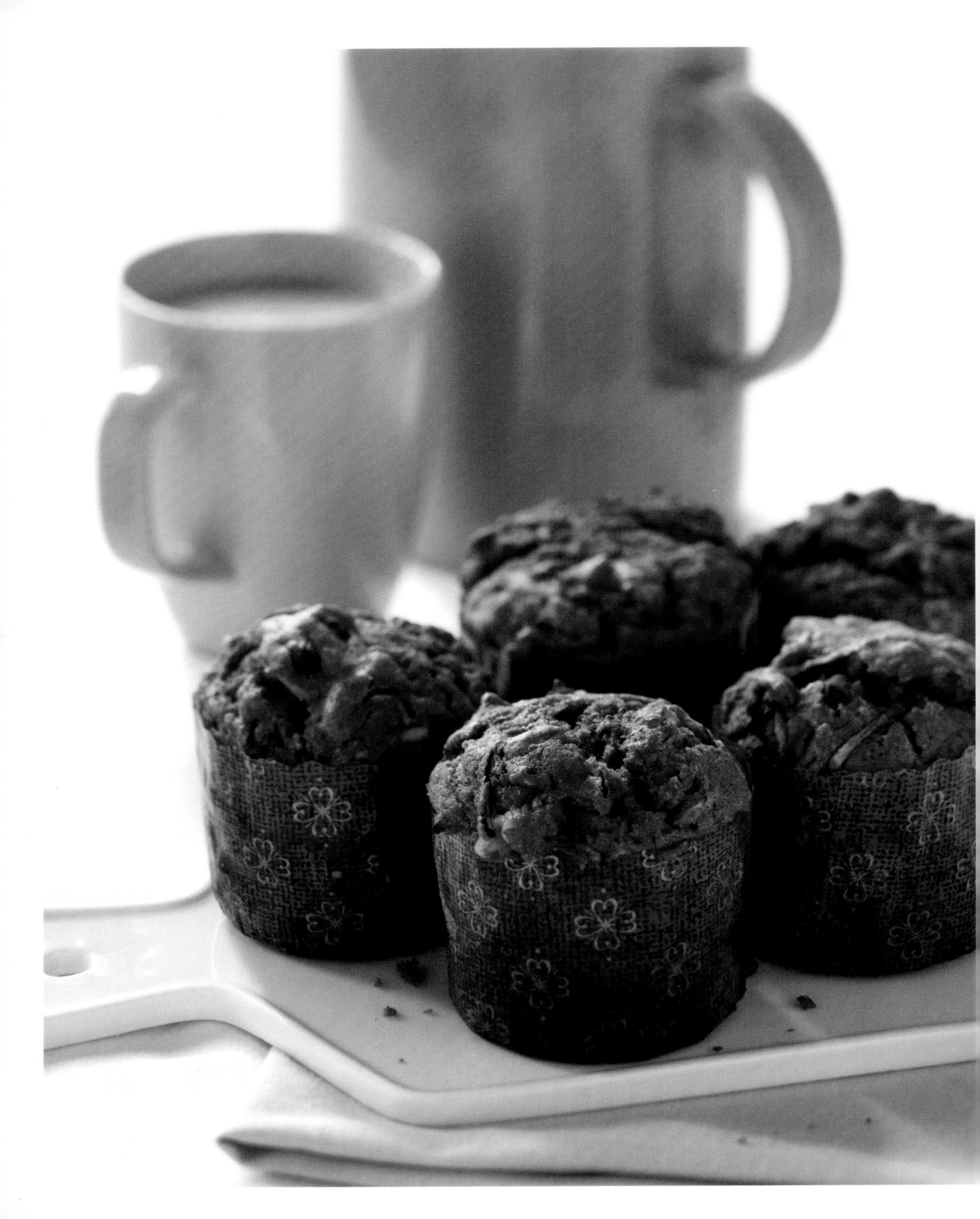

ZUCCHINI MUFFINS

SNACKS

PREP TIME: **20–25 MINUTES** COOK TIME: **25 MINUTES** YIELD: **24 MUFFINS**

INGREDIENTS

2 1⁄4 cups spelt or whole-wheat flour

1⁄2 teaspoon baking soda

1⁄2 teaspoon baking powder

1⁄2 teaspoon salt

1 1⁄2 teaspoons ground cinnamon

1⁄2 teaspoon nutmeg

2 large egg whites

1 egg yolk

1 teaspoon vanilla extract

1 tablespoon molasses

1 tablespoon honey

2⁄3 cup vegetable oil

2 cups finely shredded unpeeled zucchini

1⁄2 chopped nuts or dark chocolate chips (optional)

DIRECTIONS

1 Preheat oven to 375 degrees. Line a muffin tin with paper liners, set aside.

2 In a large bowl combine flour, baking soda, baking powder, salt, cinnamon and nutmeg.

3 In a mixing bowl with an electric mixer, beat egg whites on high to stiff peaks. Lightly fold egg whites into the flour mixture.

4 In a separate bowl combine egg yolk, vanilla extract, molasses, honey, vegetable oil and zucchini. Fold into flour mixture until just combined. Stir in nuts or chocolate chips if desired.

5 Fold egg white into zucchini mixture until just combined.

6 Fill muffin cups 3⁄4 full. Bake for 20–25 minutes until toothpick comes out clean.

7 Cool for 5–10 minutes before removing from paper liners.

TIP: Before you put in the egg yolk mixture the batter should be quite thick; if you find it is runny, add 1⁄4 cup of flour. You can swap grated carrot for zucchini—add 1⁄2 cup low fat plain yogurt and you have a delicious batch of carrot muffins.

NUTRITION INFORMATION PER SERVING (WITHOUT NUTS OR CHOCOLATE CHIPS):
Calories: 73, Calories from Fat: 23, Protein: 3 g, Carbs: 11 g, Dietary Fiber: 2 g, Sugars: 2 g, Fat: 3 g, Sodium: 83 mg

OAT AND GRANOLA BAR

SNACKS

PREP TIME: **15–20 MINUTES** COOK TIME: **25 MINUTES** YIELD: **14 SERVINGS**

INGREDIENTS

2 cups rolled oats

1 cup sliced almonds

½ cup wheat germ

½ cup honey

2 large egg whites plus 1 yolk

¼ cup olive oil

¼ cup sucanat or rapadura

2 teaspoons vanilla extract

½ teaspoon sea salt

1 ½ cups chopped dried fruit of your choice

½ cup natural nut butter (peanut or almond)

DIRECTIONS

1 Preheat oven to 350 degrees. Line baking sheet with parchment paper. Combine all ingredients except salt, dried fruit and nut butter on a baking sheet and toast, tossing occasionally, until golden brown, about 15 minutes. Set aside to cool. Lower heat to 300 degrees.

2 Meanwhile, line a 9-by-11-inch glass baking dish with parchment paper. Set aside.

3 Whisk the salt, dried fruit and peanut butter in a large bowl, add toasted mixture and combined until evenly coated.

4 Pour mixture in baking dish and press down evenly. Bake for 25 minutes. Cool for 10 minutes before cutting and serving.

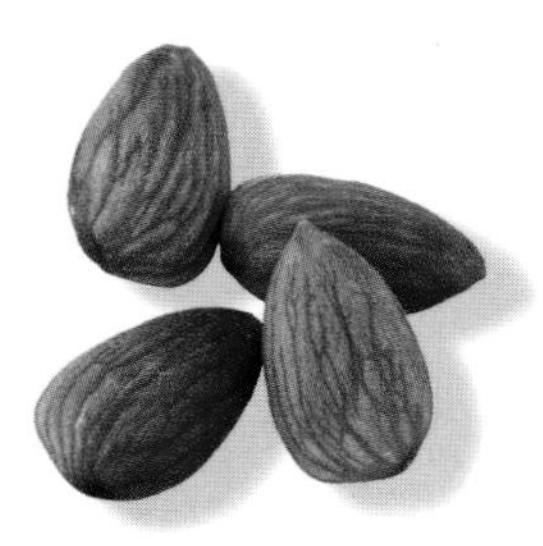

NUTRITIONAL VALUE PER SERVING: Calories: 277, Calories from Fat: 117, Protein: 7 g, Carbs: 41 g, Dietary Fiber: 5 g, Sugars: 10 g, Fat: 13 g, Sodium: 80 mg

OAT AND ROSEMARY ENGLISH CRACKERS

SNACKS

PREP TIME: **15–20 MINUTES** COOK TIME: **15 MINUTES** YIELD: **12 SERVINGS**

These crackers are like biscuits or cookies and make a great snack.

INGREDIENTS

1 cup oats

½ cup oat bran

½ cup spelt flour

1 teaspoon salt or garlic salt

1 teaspoon pepper

1 teaspoon rosemary

1 teaspoon baking powder

½ cup olive oil, plus more for coating

¼ cup warm water

Topping of choice, such as sea salt, chopped rosemary, Parmesan cheese

DIRECTIONS

1 Preheat oven to 350 degrees. Lightly grease two baking sheets.

2 Combine all dry ingredients in a food processor until oats are finely chopped. Pulse in olive oil until dough forms. If dough is too dry, pulse in water until dough forms.

3 Roll dough into 24 balls of 1-inch diameter and place on baking sheet. Using a fork, press the dough down in an X shape.

4 Lightly coat dough with olive oil and sprinkle with topping of your choice.

5 Bake for 10–15 minutes, until golden brown. Transfer to wire rack and cool.

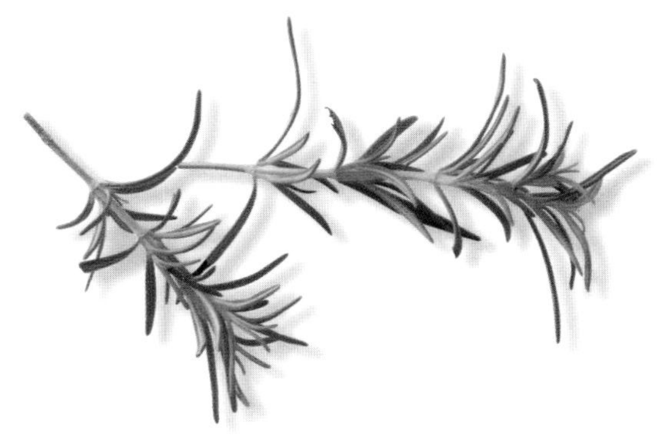

NUTRITIONAL VALUE PER TWO-CRACKER SERVING: Calories: 130, Calories from Fat: 90, Protein: 2 g, Carbs: 14 g, Dietary Fiber: 2 g, Sugars: 0 g, Fat: 10 g, Sodium: 207 mg

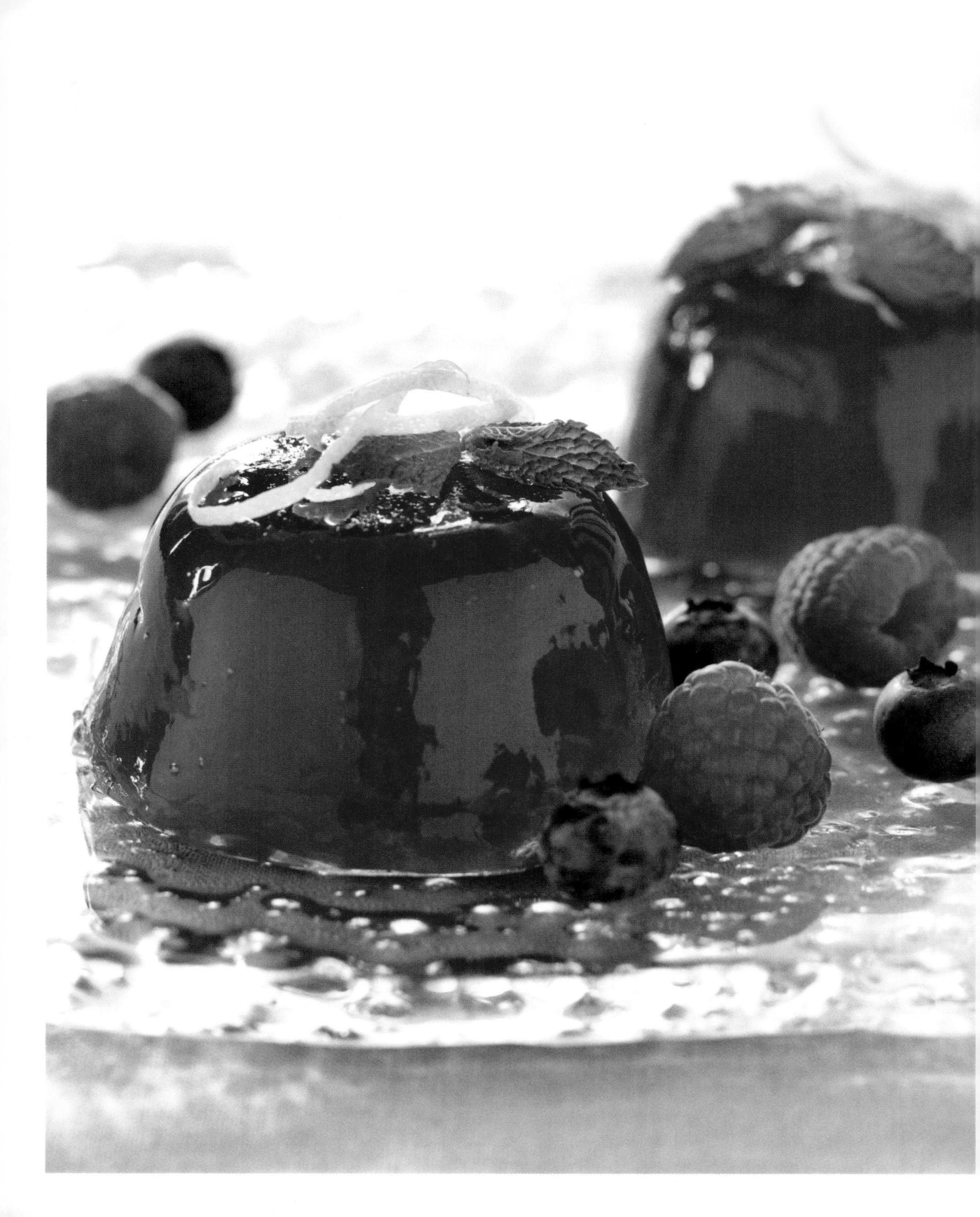

OH NO JELL-O

DESSERTS

PREP TIME: **10 MINUTES** COOK TIME: **20 MINUTES** YIELD: **8 SERVINGS**

INGREDIENTS

4 cups fresh berries of your choice

8 cups water

2 ⅓ cups fresh apple juice

1 tablespoon lemon juice

2 packets unflavored gelatin

3 tablespoons honey or sucanat

DIRECTIONS

1 Bring berries and water to a boil in a large pot. Lower heat and let mixture simmer until berries are very soft, about 15 minutes. Strain liquid through cheesecloth-lined colander into a large bowl. Press on berries to release all juice.

2 In a large saucepan, add ⅓ cup fresh juice and 2 packets of gelatin. Stir on low heat until gelatin is completely dissolved. Increase heat to medium and bring to a boil, add honey or sucanat and lemon juice and boil for 1 minute, stirring constantly.

3 Remove from heat and add 2 more cups of fresh juice, stirring constantly.

4 Transfer to large glass bowl or Tupperware, cover and refrigerate until set, about 30–60 minutes.

5 Serve with fresh berries.

NUTRITION INFORMATION PER SERVING: Calories: 99, Calories from Fat: 3, Protein: 2 g, Carbs: 24 g, Dietary Fiber: 3 g, Sugars: 12 g, Fat: 0.5 g, Sodium: 3 mg

GINGERBREAD RICE PUDDING

DESSERTS

PREP TIME: **5 MINUTES** COOK TIME: **40–50 MINUTES** YIELD: **8 SERVINGS**

INGREDIENTS

1 cup long-grain brown rice

6 cups vanilla soy milk

½ cup sucanat

1 tablespoon honey

3 egg whites plus 1 yolk

1 teaspoon pure vanilla extract

2 tablespoons grated fresh ginger

¼ teaspoon sea salt

1 teaspoon ground ginger

¼ teaspoon ground cinnamon

⅛ teaspoon nutmeg

½ cup golden raisins or crystallized ginger (optional)

DIRECTIONS

1 In a large saucepan, combine rice and 5 cups milk; bring to a boil. Reduce heat to medium; cover, simmer, stirring occasionally, until rice is tender, 15–17 minutes.

2 Stir in ground ginger.

3 Allow rice to sit for 30 minutes with the lid on to soften the rice grains.

4 Meanwhile, in a medium bowl, whisk together sugar, honey, eggs, ginger, salt, vanilla, cinnamon, nutmeg and remaining 1 cup milk.

5 Slowly pour egg mixture into rice mixture; cook over medium-low heat, stirring constantly, until pudding coats the back of a spoon, 3–5 minutes.

6 Remove from heat and pour into a 6-quart casserole dish or large bowl; let cool to room temperature. Cover and refrigerate at least 1 hour (or up to 3 days).

7 Serve pudding garnished with raisins, a sprinkle of cinnamon or crystallized ginger.

TIP: Keep an open mind—could be a breakfast dish as well. To boost nutritional value just add your favorite dried fruit.

NUTRITIONAL VALUE PER 1-CUP SERVING: Calories: 189, Calories from Fat: 32, Protein: 7 g, Carbs: 31 g, Dietary Fiber: 1 g, Sugars: 7 g, Fat: 4 g, Sodium: 156 mg

SWEET QUINOA

DESSERTS

PREP TIME: **10 MINUTES** COOK TIME: **40–50 MINUTES** YIELD: **4 SERVINGS**

INGREDIENTS

1 cup red quinoa, well rinsed and drained (do not skip this step since quinoa has a bitter coating that must be removed before cooking; otherwise it is unpalatable)

2 cups vanilla soy milk

¼ teaspoon sea salt

1 teaspoon ground cinnamon

¼ cup pure maple syrup

1 cup dried fruit of your choice

1 teaspoon pure vanilla

⅓ cup dry-roasted unsalted sliced almonds

DIRECTIONS

1 Place the quinoa, soy milk, sea salt and cinnamon in a medium saucepan, cover and bring to a boil over medium heat.

2 Reduce heat to low and simmer for 15 minutes.

3 Add maple syrup and simmer uncovered for 10 minutes. Remove from heat, add dried fruit and vanilla. Cover and let sit for 15 minutes to thicken. Fluff with a fork, mix in sliced almonds and serve.

TIP: This also makes for a tasty breakfast dish when you're in the mood for something sweet.

NUTRITIONAL VALUE PER SERVING: Calories: 455, Calories from Fat: 99, Protein: 12 g, Carbs: 83 g, Dietary Fiber: 8 g, Sugars: 20 g, Fat: 11 g, Sodium: 177 mg

Your Grocery List

FRUITS

- ☐ Lemon
- ☐ Lime
- ☐ Peaches or apples
- ☐ Berries

VEGETABLES

- ☐ Large onions
- ☐ Medium onions
- ☐ Small onions
- ☐ Scallions
- ☐ Shallots
- ☐ Carrots
- ☐ Celery
- ☐ Cucumber
- ☐ Cabbage
- ☐ Leeks
- ☐ Asparagus
- ☐ Zucchini
- ☐ Eggplants
- ☐ Spinach
- ☐ Kale
- ☐ Bean sprouts
- ☐ Red and green peppers
- ☐ Button mushrooms
- ☐ Plum tomatoes
- ☐ Grape tomatoes
- ☐ Fresh or frozen corn kernels
- ☐ Frozen peas

FRESH HERBS

- ☐ Garlic
- ☐ Basil
- ☐ Sprig rosemary
- ☐ Holy basil leaves
- ☐ Flat-leaf parsley
- ☐ Oregano
- ☐ Cilantro
- ☐ Coriander
- ☐ Chives
- ☐ Mint
- ☐ Ginger root
- ☐ Chilies
- ☐ Thai chilies

DRIED

- ☐ Nuts
- ☐ Cashews
- ☐ Almonds
- ☐ Sliced almonds
- ☐ Toasted peanuts
- ☐ Pine nuts
- ☐ Soy nuts
- ☐ Pumpkin and/or sunflower seeds
- ☐ Sesame seeds
- ☐ Nut butter (peanut or almond)

FRUITS

- ☐ Dried raisins
- ☐ Dried cranberries
- ☐ Chopped dried fruit
- ☐ Crystallized ginger

GRAINS

- ☐ Rolled oats
- ☐ Flaxseed
- ☐ Wheat germ
- ☐ Oat bran
- ☐ Quinoa
- ☐ Brown rice
- ☐ Long-grain brown rice
- ☐ Arborio rice
- ☐ Puffed rice

DAIRY

- ☐ Skim or soy milk
- ☐ Eggs
- ☐ Butter, margarine
- ☐ Yogurt cheese
- ☐ Regular firm tofu
- ☐ Medium tofu
- ☐ Parmesan cheese

CANNED

- ☐ Canned whole tomatoes in juice
- ☐ Red beans
- ☐ Black beans
- ☐ Chipotle chile in adobo
- ☐ Chickpeas

MEAT AND FISH

- ☐ Ground lean chicken breast
- ☐ Lean ground turkey
- ☐ Boneless skinless chicken breast halves
- ☐ Boneless, skinless chicken breasts
- ☐ 1 pound pork tenderloin
- ☐ Salmon fillets
- ☐ 12 ounces large shrimp

OTHER

- ☐ Wonton wrappers
- ☐ Rice-paper wrappers
- ☐ Whole-wheat or corn tortillas (6 inches each)
- ☐ Thick-sliced whole-wheat bread
- ☐ Whole-wheat rolls
- ☐ Rice noodles or soba noodles

SPICES

- ☐ Sea salt
- ☐ Pepper
- ☐ Red pepper flakes
- ☐ Cinnamon
- ☐ Cinnamon sticks
- ☐ Nutmeg
- ☐ Basil
- ☐ Thyme
- ☐ Rosemary
- ☐ Ground cloves
- ☐ Oregano
- ☐ Parsley
- ☐ Garlic powder
- ☐ Onion powder
- ☐ Garlic salt
- ☐ Celery seeds
- ☐ Coriander
- ☐ Allspice
- ☐ Paprika
- ☐ Cayenne pepper
- ☐ Cumin
- ☐ Chili powder
- ☐ Fennel seed
- ☐ Anise seed
- ☐ Wasabi paste or powder

LIQUIDS

- ☐ Low-sodium chicken stock
- ☐ Olive oil
- ☐ Coconut oil
- ☐ Peanut oil
- ☐ Toasted sesame oil

SWEETENERS

- ☐ Honey
- ☐ Molasses
- ☐ Maple syrup

PASTES

- ☐ Tomato paste
- ☐ Chili paste

VINEGARS

- ☐ Cider vinegar
- ☐ Rice-wine vinegar (not seasoned)
- ☐ Pear vinegar
- ☐ Balsamic vinegar
- ☐ Rice vinegar
- ☐ Sherry vinegar

SAUCES

- ☐ Worcestershire sauce
- ☐ Low-sodium soy sauce
- ☐ Oyster sauce
- ☐ Hot sauce
- ☐ Fish sauce
- ☐ Tabasco sauce

BAKING

- ☐ Spelt or whole-wheat flour
- ☐ Baking soda
- ☐ Baking powder
- ☐ Sucanat (or rapadura)
- ☐ Vanilla extract
- ☐ Chocolate chips
- ☐ Unflavored gelatin

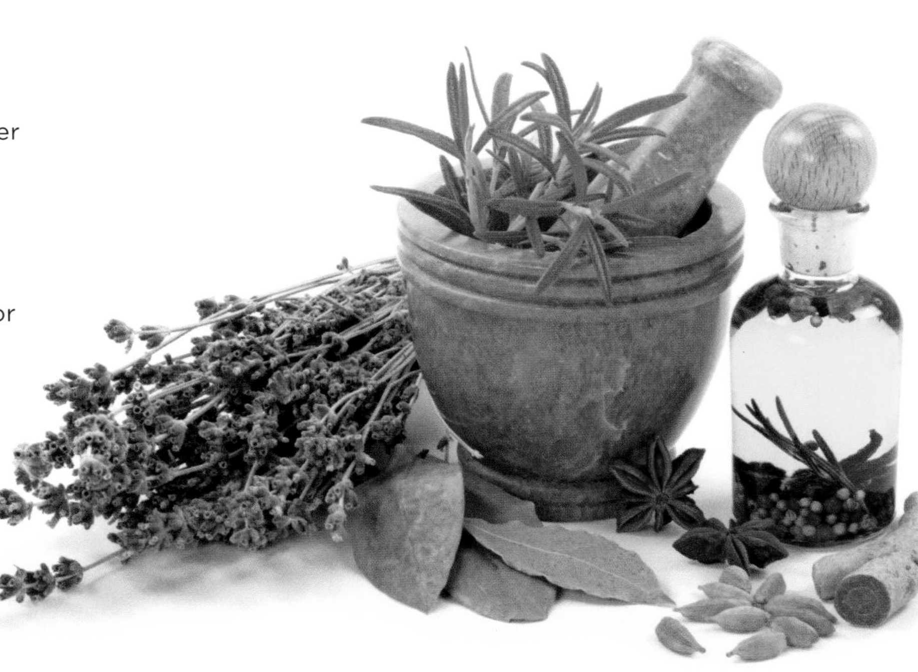

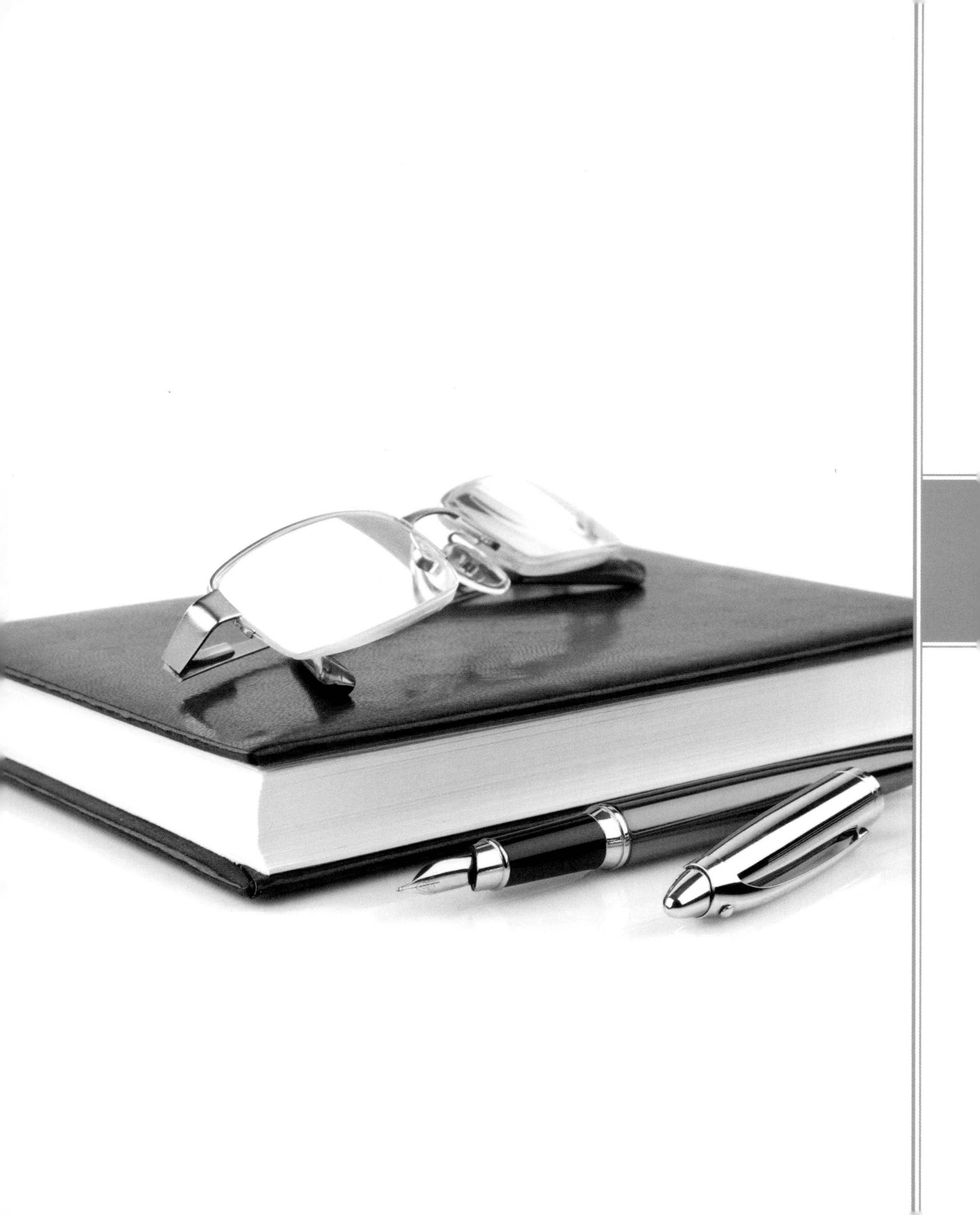

Best Body Now Journal 10

ONE OF THE BEST WAYS TO GUARANTEE SUCCESS IS TO KEEP track of your progress. And that's just what the Best Body Now journal will help you do. Writing down each commitment you make—and speed bump you encounter—on your journey will make you that much more dedicated to creating Your Best Body Now.

Your Best Body Now Diet Tracker

Studies have repeatedly shown that keeping track of your food intake on a daily basis is one of the most powerful weight-loss tools you can use. In fact, research published in the *American Journal of Preventive Medicine* shows that those who recorded how much they ate, as well as their exercise levels, increased their weight loss by as much as 50 percent. This is a strong argument for you to do the same while using the Best Body Now program to transform your health and your life. Make it a habit to record food consumption and your goals will soon be reached.

The Best Body Now diet recommends consuming several small meals a day, sufficient in protein, fresh fruits, vegetables and whole grains (see Chapter 4 for more). Use the following guide to help you monitor what you're eating and how often. You'll see that unhealthy habits, such as skipping meals and not drinking enough water, have nowhere to hide when you're tracking your progress. The notes section helps you outline successes, challenges and goals for the coming week. Photocopy a fresh page each week, log your results and you're on your way to your Best Body Now.

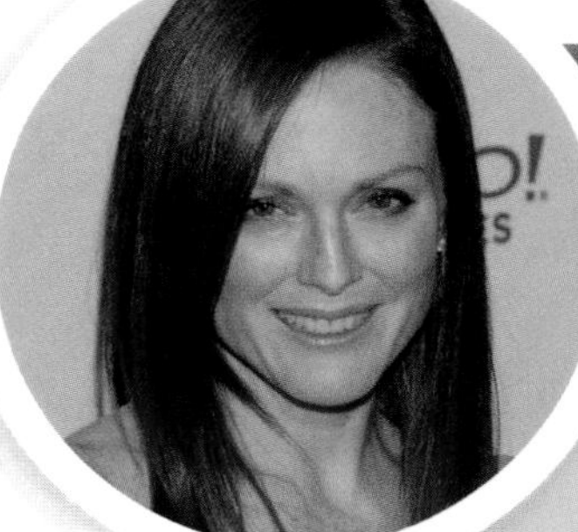

The "H" Factor: A-List Proof That Life Gets Better at 40

At forty-nine, Julianne Moore rocks the Best Body Now attitude with an ageless spirit. Rather than get caught up in the Hollywood face-lift circuit, she recently told Britain's *Observer Magazine* she's not interested in cosmetic work: "You're not going to look the same as you did at twenty-five. What are you going to do about it?" She's got three Oscar nominations (and thirty-eight other acting wins, plus forty-five additional nominations, according to IMDb) under her belt, two of them while she was in her forties. In 2003, she became one of just ten actors nominated for an Academy Award in both lead and supporting roles in the same year.

BREAKFAST	MIDMORNING	LUNCH	MIDAFTERNOON	DINNER	LAST MEAL
MONDAY					
WATER*:					
TUESDAY					
WATER:					
WEDNESDAY					
WATER:					
THURSDAY					
WATER:					
FRIDAY					
WATER:					
SATURDAY					
WATER:					
SUNDAY					
WATER:					

NOTES

BEST BODY NOW **CHALLENGES**

BEST BODY NOW **SUCCESSES**

NEXT WEEK'S **GOALS**

*GOAL: 8 GLASSES

Your Best Body Now Fitness Tracker

Use this to track workouts, exercises, weights, reps and sets (refer to Chapter 5 for recommended exercises). You can also monitor successes, challenges and goals for staying motivated. Photocopy a new sheet for each workout, log your results and you're on your way to your Best Body Now.

DAY:

BODY PARTS WORKED:

EXERCISE	SET 1		SET 2		SET 3		SET 4		SET 5	
Sets 4 and 5 are optional	Reps	Weight	Reps	Weight	Reps	Weight	Reps	Weight	Reps	Weight
Example: Triceps: kickbacks	12 reps	4 lbs	12 reps	4 lbs	12 reps	6 lbs				

NOTES

BEST BODY NOW SUCCESSES

CARDIO

BEST BODY NOW CHALLENGES

NEXT WORKOUT'S GOALS

Your Best Body Now Inspiration Tracker

Use this guide, customized by Dr. Gannon, to help drive your Best Body Now inspiration every day. It's a great way to outline your successes, challenges and progress, as well as your personal joy.

Today

Three things I'm grateful for:

What is the best thing that happened today?

What was my biggest challenge?
What can I do differently to sidestep or overcome it tomorrow?

I'm proud of myself for:

Daily Commitments

How successful was I today in meeting my Best Body Now commitments? Did I:

Take time for myself?

Surround myself with positive people?

Take emotional risks?

Eat Clean?

Work out?

Drink water?

Long-Term Goals

Am I being the person I want to be?

Am I living the life I want?

Am I acting the way I want to feel?

Am I enjoying the journey?

Where do I need extra encouragement?

What is my plan to get support?

What supportive, friendly words can I tell myself?

What do I like about the Best Body Now new me?

My Best Body Now notes:

Converting to Metric

Volume Measurement Conversions

U.S.	Metric
1/4 teaspoon	1.25 ml
1/2 teaspoon	2.5 ml
3/4 teaspoon	3.75 ml
1 teaspoon	5 ml
1 tablespoon	15 ml
1/4 cup	62.5 ml
1/2 cup	125 ml
3/4 cup	187.5 ml
1 cup	250 ml

Weight Conversion Measurements

U.S.	Metric
1 ounce	28.4 g
8 ounces	227.5 g
16 ounces (1 pound)	455 g

Cooking Temperature Conversions

To convert temperatures in Fahrenheit to Celsius, use this formula:

C = (F-32) times 0.5555

So, for example, if you are baking at 350° F and want to know that temperature in Celsius, use this calculation: **C = (350-32) times 0.5555 = 176.65°**

References

Abbas, S.; Nieters, A.; Linseisen, J.; Slanger, T.; Kropp, S.; Mutschelknauss, E.J.; Flesch-Janys, D.; and Chang-Claude, J.; "Vitamin D Receptor Gene Polymorphisms and Haplotypes and Postmenopausal Breast Cancer Risk," *Breast Cancer Research*; 2008; 10: R31.

Abbott, R.D.; Ando, F.; Masaki; K.H., Tung, K.H.; Rodriguez, B.L.; Petrovitch, H.; Yano, K.; and Curb, J.D.; "Dietary Magnesium Intake and the Future Risk of Coronary Heart Disease," *American Journal of Cardiology*; September 2003; 92(6): 665–9.

Al-Ghamdi, S.M.; Cameron, E.C.; and Sutton, R.A.; "Magnesium Deficiency: Pathophysiological and Clinical Overview," *American Journal of Kidney Diseases*; November 1994; 24(5): 737–52.

Altman, R.D.; and Marcussen, K.C.; "Effects of a Ginger Extract on Knee Pain in Patients with Osteoarthritis," *Arthritis and Rheumatism*; November 2001; 4(11): 2531–8.

Amagase, H.; Sun, B.; and Borek, C.; "Lycium Barbarum (Goji) Juice Improves In Vivo Antioxidant Biomarkers in Serum of Healthy Adults," *Nutritional Research*; January 2009; 29(1): 19–25.

American Academy of Neurology, "Cardiovascular Risk Factors in Midlife Strongly Linked to Risk of Dementia," www.aan.com.

American Academy of Neurology, "Controlling Cholesterol, Blood Pressure Adds Up to Prevent Stroke," www.aan.com.

American Academy of Neurology, "High Cholesterol in your Forties Increases Risk of Alzheimer's Disease," www.aan.com.

American Cancer Society, "Eat Right to Prevent Colorectal Cancer," www.cancer.org.

American Cancer Society, "Keeping Your Exercise Program on Track," www.cancer.org.

American Cancer Society, "Regular Exercise Late in Life Helps Reduce Breast Cancer Risk," www.cancer.org.

American Heart Association, "Fish and Omega-3 Fatty Acids," www.americanheart.org.

Anderson, J.W.; "Diet First, Then Medication for Hypercholesterolemia," *Journal of the American Medical Association*; July 2003; 290(4): 531–3.

Anderson, J.W.; "Whole Grains and Coronary Heart Disease: The Whole Kernel of Truth," *American Journal of Clinical Nutrition*; 80(6): 1459–60.

N.I.H., National Eye Institute, "Antioxidant Vitamins and Zinc Reduce Risk of Vision Loss from Age-Related Macular Degeneration," www.nei.nih.gov.

Arjmandi, B., M.D.; Khan, D., M.D.; Juma, S., M.S; and Svanborg, A., M.D., Ph.D.; "The Ovarian Hormone Deficiency-Induced Hypercholesterolemic Is Reversed by Soy Protein and the Synthetic Isoflavone, Ipriflavone," *Nutrition Research*; May 1997; 17(5): 885–94.

Arthritis Foundation, *Arthritis Today*, www.arthritistoday.org.

Assuncao, M.; Ferreira, H.; dos Santos, A.; et al; "Effects of Dietary Coconut Oil on the Biochemical and Anthropometric Profiles of Women Presenting Abdominal Obesity," *Lipids*; July 2009; 44(7): 593–601.

Assuncao, M.; Santos-Marques, M.J.; Carvalho, F.; Lukoyanov, N.V.; and Andrade, J.P.; "Chronic Green Tea Consumption Prevents Age-Related Changes in Rats," *Neurobiology of Aging*; May 1, 2009.

Aubrey, A.; "A Better Breakfast Can Boost a Child's Brainpower," npr.com; August 31, 2006.

Baer, A.; "40 Must-Have Foods for the 40-Year-Old Body," *Best Life Magazine*, May 2008.

Baird, D.D., et al; "High Cumulative Incidence of Uterine Leiomyoma in Black and White Women: Ultrasound Evidence," *American Journal of Obstetrics and Gynecology*; 2003; 188(1): 100–7.

Bar-Sela, G.; Epelbaum, R.; and Schaffer M.; "Curcumin as an Anti-Cancer Agent: Review of the Gap Between Basic and Clinical Applications," *Current Medicinal Chemistry*; November 24, 2009.

Bar-Sela, G.; Tsalic, M.; Fried, G.; and Goldberg, H.; "Wheat Grass Juice May Improve Hematological Toxicity Related to Chemotherapy in Breast Cancer Patients: A Pilot Study," *Nutrition and Cancer*; 2007; 58(1): 43–48.

Basaria, S.; Wisniewski, A.; Dupree, K.; Bruno, T.; Song, M.Y.; Yao, F.; Ojumu, A.; John, M.; and Dobs, A.S.; "Effects of High-Dose Isoflavones on Cognition, Quality of Life, Androgens and Lipoprotein in Post-Menopausal Women," *Journal of Endocrinological Investigation*; February 2009; 32(20): 150–5.

Bastianetto, S.; and Quirion, R.; "Natural Extracts as Possible Protective Agents of Brain Aging," *Neurobiologic Aging*; Sep–Oct 2002; 23(5): 891–7.

Bauer, J.; "Forgetful? Eat Memory-Boosting Foods," www.msnbc.com; May 16, 2007.

Bio-Medicine, "NHLBI Study Finds Hostility, Impatience Increase Hypertension Risk," www.bio-medicine.org.

Blum, D.; "The Plunge of Pleasure," *Psychology Today*, September 1, 1997.

Borst, P.; "Mega-dose Vitamin C as Therapy for Human Cancer?" *PNAS*; December 2008; 105(48): E96.

Breast Cancer Network of Strength, "Breast Cancer Statistics," www.networkofstrength.com.

Brody, S.; Preut, R; Schommer, K.; and Schümeyer, T.H.; "A Randomized Controlled Trial of High Dose Ascorbic Acid for Reduction of Blood Pressure, Cortisol, and Subjective Responses to Psychological Stress," *Psychopharmacology*; January 2002; 159(3): 319–24.

Champeau, R.; "UCLA/VA Study Finds Chemical Found in Curry May Help Immune System Clear Amyloid Plaques Found in Alzheimer's Disease," www.ucla.edu; October 3, 2006.

Chan, F.L.; Chen, S.; Lee, K.W.; Leung, L.K.; and Wang, Y.; "The Red Wine Polyphenol Resveratrol Displays Bilevel Inhibition on Aromatase in Breast Cancer Cells," *Toxilogical Sciences*; 2006.

Chen D.Z.; Qi, M.; Auborn, K.J.; and Carter, T.H.; "Indole-3-Carbinol and Diindolylmethane Induce Apoptosis of Human Cervical Cancer Cells and in Murine HPV16-transgenic Preneoplastic Cervical Epithelium," *Journal of Nutrition*; December 2001; 131(12): 3294–302.

Choi, H.Y.; Chong, S.A.; and Nam, M.J.; "Resveratrol Induces Apoptosis in Human SK-HEP-1 Hepatic Cancer Cells," *Cancer Genomics Proteomics*; Sep–Oct 2009; 6(5): 263–8.

Clarke, R.; "B Vitamins and the Prevention of Dementia," *Proceedings of the Nutrition Society*; February 2008; 67(1): 75–81.

Clarke, R.; "Vitamin B_{12}, Folic Acid and the Prevention of Dementia," *New England Journal of Medicine*; June 29, 2006; 354(2): 2816–9.

Clarke, R.; Birks, J.; Nexo, E.; Ueland, P.M.; Schneede, J.; Scott, J.; Molloy, A.; and Evans, J.G.; "Low Vitamin B-12 Status and Risk of Cognitive Decline in Older Adults," *American Journal of Clinical Nutrition*; November 2007; 86(5): 1384–91.

CNN, "Age, Exercise May Boost Memory," www.cnn.com, November 25, 2003.

Colcombe, S.J.; Erickson, K.I.; Scalf, P.E; et al.; "Aerobic Exercise Training Increases Brain Volume in Older Adults," *Journal of Gerontology Series A: Biological Sciences and Medical Sciences*; 61: 1166–1170.

Collins, K., R.D.; "Fight Cancer with Dark Green Vegetables," msnbc.com, April 8, 2005.

Columbia University Medical Center, "Researchers at Columbia University Medical Center Link Blood Sugar Levels to Normal Cognitive Aging," www.cumc.columbia.edu, December 2008.

Davidson, T.; and Swithers, S.; "A Pavlonian Approach to the Problem of Obesity," *International Journal of Obesity*; July 2004.

Davidson, T.; and Swithers, S.; "A Role for Sweet Taste: Calorie Predictive Relations in Energy Regulation by Rats," *Behavioral Neuroscience*; 2008; 122(1): 161–173.

Devlin, K.; "Cutting Back on Calories Can Help Improve Memory," telegraph.co.uk, January 2009.

Dhanasekaran, M.; and Ren, J.; "The Emerging Role of Coenzyme Q_{10} in Aging, Neurodegeneration, Cardiovascular Disease, Cancer and Diabetes Mellitus," *Current Neurovascular Research*; 2005; 2(5): 447–59.

Du, W.X.; Olsen, C.W.; Avena-Bustillos, R.J.; McHugh T.H.; Levin C.E.; and Friedman, M.; "Effects of Allspice, Cinnamon, and Clove Bud Essential Oils in Edible Apple Films on Physical Properties and Antimicrobial Activities," *Journal of Food Science*; September 2009; 74(7): M372–8.

Eby, G.A.; and Eby, K.L; "Rapid Recovery from Major Depression Using Magnesium Treatment," *Medical Hypotheses*; 2006; 67(2): 362–7.

Evans, R.C.; Fear, S.; Ashby, D.; Hackett, A.; Williams, E.; van der Vliet, M.; Dunstan, F.D.J.; and Rhodes, J.M.; "Diet and Colorectal Cancer: An Investigation of the Lectin/Galactose Hypothesis," *Gastroenterology*; June 2002; 122(7) 1784–92.

Epel, E.S.; McEwen, B.; Seeman, T.; Matthews, K.; Castellazzo, G.; Brownell, K.D.; Bell, J.; and Ickovics, J.R.; "Stress and the Body Shape: Stress-Induced Cortisol Secretion is Consistently Greater Among Women with Central Fat," *Psychosomatic Medicine*; 2000; (62): 623–32.

Gallessich, G.; "Scientists Show Certain Vegetables—Like Broccoli—Can Combat Cancer," University of California, Santa Barbara; www.ia.ucsb.edu.

Ghanbari, Z., M.D.; Manshavi, F.D., M.D.; and Jafarabadi, M., M.D.; "The Effect of Three Months' Regular Aerobic Exercise on Premenstrual Syndrome," *Journal of Family and Reproductive Health*; December 2008; 2(4): 167–71.

Gillman, M.W., M.D.; Rifas-Shiman, S., M.P.H.; Kleinman, K., ScD; Rich-Edwards, J.; and Lipschultz, S.E., M.D.; "Maternal Calcium Intake and Offspring Blood Pressure," *Circulation Research*; 2004.

"Gingko May Prevent Ovarian Cancer Cell Growth," Brigham and Women's Hospital; Newsroom; November 2005; www.brighamandwomens.org.

Goncagul, G.; and Ayaz, E.; "Antimicrobial Effect of Garlic (Allium sativum)" *Recent Patents on Anti-infective Drug Discovery*; November 23, 2009.

Green, D.M., Ph.D.; "Calcium Aceteate Treatment Causes Hypercalcemia and Vascular Calcification in Hemodialysis Patients," *American Journal of Nephrology*; Oct. 9, 2003.

Hall, C.; "Cabbage Extract Can Kill Cancer Cells," *Telegraph*; October 11, 2006; www.telegraph.co.uk.

Harvard Health Publication, Harvard Medical School, "Eating Nuts Promotes Cardiovascular Health," www.health.harvard.edu.

Harvard Health Publication, Harvard Medical School, "Yoga for Anxiety and Depression," www.health.harvard.edu.

Harvie, M.; Chapman, M.; Cuzick, J.; Flyvbjerg, A.; Hopwood, P.; Jebb, S.; Parfitt, G.; and Howell, A.; "The Effect of Intermittent Versus Chronic Energy Restriction on Breast Cancer Risk Biomarkers in Premenopausal Women: A Randomised Pilot Trial," *Breast Cancer Research*; 2008; 10 (Suppl 2): P53.

Hegsted, D.M.; "Calcium and Osteoporosis," *Journal of Nutrition;* 1986; 116(11): 2316.

Hegsted, D.M.; "Fractures, Calcium and the Modern Diet," *American Journal of Clinical Nutrition*; 74(5); 571–3, November 2001.

Hill, K.; "Exercise, Diet May Protect Against Colorectal Cancer," University of Wisconsin-Madison News; www.wisc.edu; May 15, 2006.

Howell, A.; and Harvie, M.; "Should Lifestyle Modifications Be Promoted to Prevent Breast Cancer?" *Breast Cancer Research* 2008; 10(Suppl 4); S11.

Hu, F.B., M.D.; Stampfer, M.J., M.D.; Manson, J.E., M.D.; Rimm, E., Sc.D.; Colditz, G.A., M.D.; Rosner, B.A., Ph.D.; Hennekens, C.H., M.D.; and Willett, W.C., M.D.; "Dietary Fat Intake and the Risk of Coronary Heart Disease in Women," *New England Journal of Medicine*, 1998; 338(13): 917.

Hu, F.B., M.D.; Stampfer, M.J., M.D.; Manson, J.E., M.D.; Rimm, E., Sc.D.; Colditz, G.A., M.D.; Rosner, B.A., Ph.D.; and Willett, W.C., M.D. "Dietary Fat Intake and the Risk of Coronary Heart Disease in Women," *BMJ*; November 1998; 17(7169): 1341–5.

Hughes, T.F.; Andel, R.; Small, B.J.; Borenstein, A.R.; Mortimer, J.A.; Wolk, A.; Johansson, B.; Fratiglioni, L.; Pedersen, N.L.; and Gatz, M.; "Midlife Fruit and Vegetable Consumption and Risk of Dementia in Later Life in Swedish Twins," *American Journal of Geriatric Psychiatry*; November 10, 2009.

Ingels, D., N.D.; "Sage May Be Effective for Mild to Moderate Alzheimer's," Heathnotes Newswire; July 10, 2003.

Jakicic, J.M., Ph.D.; Bess, M.H., Ph.D.; Gallagher, K.I.; Napolitano, M., Ph.D.; and Lang, W., Ph.D.; "Effect of Exercise Dose and Intensity on Weight Loss in Overweight, Sedentary Women: A Randomized Trial," *Journal of the American Medical Association*; September 10, 2003.

Javnbakht, M.; Hejazi, Kenari R.; and Ghasemi, M.; "Effects of Yoga on Depression and Anxiety of Women," *Complementary Therapies in Clinical Practice*; May 2009; 15(2): 102–4.

Jenkins, D.J.; Kendall, C.W.; Marchie, A.; Faulkner, D.A.; Wong, J.M.; de Souza, R.; Emam, A.; Parker, T.L.; Vidgen, E.; Lapsley, K.G.; Trautwein, E.A.; Josse, R.G.; Leiter, L.A.; and Connelly, P.W; "Effects of a Dietary Portfolio of Cholesterol-Lowering Foods vs Lovastain on Serum Lipids and C-reactive Protein," *Journal of the American Medical Association*; July 2003; 290(4): 502–10.

Jiang, Q.; Christen, S.; Shegenaga, M.K.; and Arnes, B.N.; "Gamma-Tocopherol, the Major Form of Vitamin E in the U.S. Diet, Deserves More Attention," *American Journal of Clinical Nutrition*; December 2001; 74(6): 714–22.

Jones, L.W.; Viglianti, B.L.; Tashjian, J.A.; Kothadia, S.M.; Keir, S.T.; Freedland, S.J.; Potter, M.Q.; Jung, M.E.; Schroeder, T.; Herndon, J.E. II; and Dewhirst, M.W.; "Effect of Aerobic Exercise on Tumor Physiology in an Animal Model of Human Breast Cancer," *Journal of Applied Physiology*; December 3, 2009.

Jordan, K.G., M.D.; "Ginkgo Biloba. A Treasure from the Past," *Life Extension Magazine*; May 2000; www.lef.org.

Kaplan, M.; Hayek, T.; Raz, A.; Coleman, R.; et al.; "Pomegranate Juice Supplementation to Atherosclerotic Mice Reduces Macrophage Lipid Peroxidation, Cellular Cholesterol Accumulation and Development of Atherosclerosis," *Journal of Nutrition*; August 2001; 131(8): 2082–89.

Kelly, J.; "Got Magnesium? Those with Heart Disease Should," webmd.com; November 9, 2000.

Kim, S.; Lee, I.; Lee, Y.; and Kim, E.; "Neuroprotective Effect of Ginkgo Biloba L. Extract in a Rat Model of Parkinson's Disease," *Phytotherapy Research*; October 2004; 18 (8); 663–6.

Kirchheimer, S.; "Coffee: The New Health Food?" www.webmd.com.

Kohama, T.; Heral, K.; and Inoue, M.; "Effect of French Maritime Pine Bark Extract on Endometriosis as Compared with Leuprorelin Acetate," *Journal of Reproductive Medicine*; August 2007; 52(8): 703–8.

Kris-Etherton, P.M.; Hu, F.B; Ros, E.; and Sabaté, J; "The Role of Tree Nuts and Peanuts in the Prevention of Coronary Heart Disease: Multiple Potential Mechanisms," *Journal of Nutrition*; September 2008; 138(9): 1746S–1751S.

Kooperman, S.; and Ackerman, L.; "Yoga for the 50+," American Senior Fitness Association, www.seniorfitness.net.

Lai, C.N.; Dabney, B.; and Shaw, C.; "Inhibition of In Vitro Metabolic Activation of Carcinogens by Wheat Sprout Extracts," *Nutrition and Cancer*; 1 (1): 27–30.

Lai, C.N.; "Chlorophyll: The Active Factor in Wheat Sprout Extract Inhibiting the Metabolic Activation of Carcinogens In Vitro," *Nutrition and Cancer*; 1979; 1(3): 19–21.

Lappe, J.; Travers-Gustafson, D.; Davies, M.K.; Recker, R.R.; and Heaney, R.P.; "Vitamin D and Calcium Supplementation Reduces Cancer Risk: Results of a Randomized Trial," *American Journal of Clinical Nutrition*; June 2007; 85(6): 1586–91.

Larson, E.B., M.D.; Wang, L., M.S.; Bowen, J.D., M.D.; et al. "Exercise Is Associated with Reduced Risk for Incident Dementia Among Persons 65 Years of Age and Older," *Annals of Internal Medicine*; January 2006; 144(2): 73–81.

Larsson, S.C., Ph.D.; Virtanen, M.J., M.Sc.; Mars, M., Ph.D.; Männistö, S., Ph.D.; Pirjo, P., D.Sc.; Albanes, D., M.D.; Virtamo, J., M.D.; "Magnesium, Calcium, Potassium, and Sodium Intakes and Risk of Stroke in Male Smokers," *Archives of Internal Medicine*; March 10, 2008; 168, No.5.

Larsson, S.C.; Bergkvist, L.; and Wolk, A.; "Magnesium Intake in Relation to Risk of Colorectal Cancer in Women," *Journal of the American Medical Association*; 2005; 293: 86–9.

Leitzmann, M.F.; Moore, S.C.; Peters, T.M.; Lacey Jr., J.V.; Schatzkin, A.; Schairer, C.; Brinton, L.A.; and Albanes, D.; "Prospective Study of Physical Activity and Risk of Postmenopausal Breast Cancer," *Breast Cancer Research*; 2008; 10; R92.

Lichtenstein, A.H.; Appel L.J.; Brands, M.; Carnethon, M.; Daniels, S.; "Diet and Lifestyle Recommendations Revision 2006: A Scientific Statement from the American Heart Association Nutrition Committee," *Circulation*; July 2006; 114(1): 82–96.

Lin, J.N.; Lin, V.C.; Rau, K.M; et al.; "Resveratrol Modulates Tumor Cell Proliferation and Protein Translation via SIRT1-Dependent AMPK Activation," *Journal of Agricultural and Food Chemistry*; November 2009.

Lita, L., Ph.D.; "Anti-Cancer Effects of Coconut Oil," www.coconutoil.com.

Lita, L., Ph.D.; "Thyroid-Stimulating, Antiaging Effects of Coconut Oil," www.coconutoil.com.

Liu, S.; Stampfer, M.J.; Hu, F.B.; Giovannucci, E.; Rimm, E.; Manson, J.E.; Hennekens, C.H.; and Willett, W.C.; "Whole-Grain Consumption and Risk of Coronary Heart Disease: Results from the Nurses' Health Study," *American Journal of Clinical Nutrition*; September 1999; 70(3): 307–8.

Lu, T.; Pan, Y.; Kao, S.Y.; Li, C.; Kohane, I.; Chan, J.; and Yankner, B.A.; "Gene Regulation and DNA Damage in the Aging Human Brain," *Nature*; June 24, 2004; 429 (6994): 883–91.

"Low-Carb (High-Protein) Diets," *U.S. News and World Report*; health.usnews.com.

Maglione-Garves, C.A.; Kravitz, L., Ph.D.; and Schneider, S., Ph.D. "Cortisol Connection: Tips on Managing Stress and Weight," www.unm.edu.

Massey, P.B., M.D., Ph.D.; "Lemon Balm Seen to Improve Memory Powers," *Daily Herald,* Natural Health Research Institute; January 15, 2007.

Massey, P.B., M.D., Ph.D.; "The Alternative Approach: The Amazing Power of Exercise," *Daily Herald,* Natural Health Research Institute; July 27, 2009.

Mathers, T.W.; and Becksrand, R.L.; "Oral Magnesium in Adults with Coronary Heart Disease of Heart Disease Risk," *Journal of the American Academy of Nurse Practitioners*; December 2009; 21 (12): 651–7.

Mayo Clinic, "Depression and Anxiety: Exercise Eases Symptoms," www.mayoclinic.com.

Mayo Clinic, "Stretching: Focus on Flexibility," www.mayoclinic.com.

Mayo Clinic, "Put on a Happy Face for a Longer Life," mayoclinic.com.

Mayo Clinic, "Aerobic Exercise: Top 10 Reasons to Get Physical," mayoclinic.com.

Mayo, W.; George, O.; et al.; "Individual Differences in Cognitive Aging: Implication of Pregnenolone Sulfate," *Progress in Neurobiology*; September 2003; 71(1): 43–8.

Mayo, W.; Lemaire, V.; Malaterre, J.; et al.; "Pregnenolone Sulfate Enhances Neurogenesis and PSA-NCAM in Young and Aged Hippocampus," *Neurobiologic Aging*; January 2005; 26(1): 103–14.

Marchant, D.; Greig, M.; and Scott, C.; "Attentional Focusing Strategies Influence Muscle Activity During Isokinetic Biceps Curls," *Athletic Insight*; 2008; 10(2).

Minton, B.; "Drink Tea and Reduce Risk of Breast Cancer by 37 Percent," naturalnews.com; February 16, 2009.

Mishra, G; Silva, I.; McNaughton, S.; McCormack, V.; Hardy, R.; Stephen, A.; and Kuh, D.; "Dietary Patterns Across the Life Course, Mammographic Density and Implications for Breast Cancer: Results from a British Prospective Cohort," *Breast Cancer Research*; 2008; 10(Suppl 2): 02.

Mitchell, M.; "Exercise Appears to Improve Brain Function Among Younger People," University of Illinois; December 18, 2006; www.news.illinois.edu.

Moiseeva, E.P.; and Heukers, R.; "Indole-3-Carbinol-Induced Modulation of NF-kB Signalling Is Breast Cancer Cell-Specific and Does Not Correlate with Cell Death," *Breast Cancer Research and Treatment*; June 2007; 109(3); 451–462.

Morris, M.C.; Evans, D.A.; Tangney, C.C.; Bienias, J.L.; and Wilson, R.S.; "Associations of Vegetable and Fruit Consumption with Age-Related Cognitive Change," *Neurology*; October 2006; 67(8): 1370–6.

"Mushrooms, Green Tea May Reduce Breast Cancer Risk," *The Nurse Practitioner*; December 2009; 34(12): 52.

Myers, D.; "The Secrets of Happiness," *Psychology Today*, July 1, 1992, psychologytoday.com.

National Institutes of Health, National Institute of Neurological Disorders and Stroke, "Brain Basics: Understanding Sleep," www.inds.nih.gov, May 21, 2007.

National Institutes of Health, Office of Dietary Supplements, "Dietary Supplement Fact Sheets," http://ods.od.nih.gov, March 2010.

National Uterine Fibroids Foundation, "Cancer," http://www.nuff.org/health_cancer.htm.

Nelson, J., M.S., R.D.; and Zeratsky, K., R.D.; "Vitamin D: Benefits in Pregnancy and Beyond," www.mayoclinic.com; January 17, 2009.

Nozue, T.; Kobayashi, A.; Uemasu, F.; Takagi, Y.; Sako, A.; and Endoh, H.; "Magnesium Status, Serum HDL Cholesterol, and Apolipoprotein A-1 levels," *Journal of Pediatric Gastroenterology and Nutrition*; 1995; 20: 316–8.

Obikoya, G., M.D.; "Vitamin B–9 (Folic Acid) Benefits," Vitamins & Nutrition Center, www.vitamins-nutrition.org.

Ogunleye, A.A.; and Holmes, M.D.; "Physical Activity and Breast Cancer Survival," *Breast Cancer Research*; 2009; 11: 106.

Ogunleye, A.A.; Xue, F.; and Michels, K.B.; "Green Tea Consumption and Breast Cancer Risk or Recurrence: a Meta-analysis," *Breast Cancer Research and Treatment*; May 2009.

Oregon State University, Linus Pauling Institute, Micronutrient Information, www.lpi.oregonstate.edu.

Oregon State University, "OSU Study Finds Elderly Women Can Halt Bone Loss," May 1, 2000, www.oregonstate.edu.

Ortiz-Ortiz, M.A.; Morán, J.M.; Ruiz-Mesa, L.M.; Niso-Santano, M.; Bravo-San Pedro, J.M.; Gómez-Sánchez, R.; González-Polo, R.A.; and Fuentes, J.M.; "Curcumin Exposure Induces Expression of the Parkinson's Disease-Associated Leucine-Rich Repeat Kinase 2 ($LRRK_2$) in Rat Mesencephalic Cells," *Neuroscience Letters*; January 4, 2009; 468(2): 120–24.

Osterweil, Neil; "Fighting Forties Flab," WebMD.

Our Bodies Ourselves, "Ten Myths about Women's Health Over 40," www.ourbodiesourselves.org.

Panickar, K.S.; Polansky, M.M.; and Anderson, R.A.; "Cinnamon Polyphenols Attenuate Cell Swelling and Mitochondrial Dysfunction Following Oxygen-Glucose Deprivation in Glial Cells," *Experimental Neurology*; April 2009; 216(2): 420–7.

Palmer, L.F., "Milking Your Bones," *Dynamic Chiropractic*, Jan. 1, 2002; 20(1).

Parker-Pope, T.; "Unlocking the Benefits of Garlic," *New York Times*; December 5, 2009.

Parry, B.M.; Lawrence, J.M.; Storey, L.; Brown, J.E.; Clarke, D.B.; Horton, S.M.; Stilwell, J.M.; and Rainsbury, R.M.; "Food Choice and Phytoestrogen Consumption in Women Previously Treated for Postmenopausal Breast Cancer," *Breast Cancer Research*; 2008; 10(Suppl 4): S11.

Patil, C.S.; Singh, V.P.; Satyanarayan, P.S.; Jain, N.K.; Singh, A.; and Kulkarni, S.K.; "Protective Effect of Flavonoids Against Aging- and Lipopolysaccaride-Induced Cognitive Impairment in Mice," *Pharmacology*; October 2003; 69(2): 59–67.

Paturel, A., M.S., M.P.H.; "Spices and Herbs May Help You Avoid Disease," www.cnn.com, December 28, 2006.

Paturel, A., M.S., M.P.H.; "Your Heart, Your Belly and Alzheimer's: People with So-Called Metabolic Syndrome May Be at a Higher Risk of Developing Alzheimer's Disease and Dementia," American Academy of Neurology, www.aan.com.

Peterson, D.W.; George, R.C.; Scaramozzino, F.; LaPointe, N.E.; Anderson, R.A.; Graves, D.J.; and Lew, J.; "Cinnamon Extract Inhibits Tau Aggregation Associated with Alzheimer's Disease In Vitro," *Journal of Alzheimer's Disease*, July 2009; 17(3): 585–97.

Physical Activity and Public Health Guidelines, American College of Sports Medicine, www.acsm.org.

Pick, M., OB/GYN, NP; "Anxiety in Women—Causes, Symptoms and Natural Relief," www.womentowomen.org.

Pledgie-Tracy, A.; Sobolewski, M.D.; and Davidson, N.E.; "Sulforaphane Induces Cell Type-Specific Apoptosis in Human Breast Cancer Cell Lines," *Molecular Cancer Therapeutics*; March 2007; 6(3): 1013–21.

Prasad, A.S.; "Zinc: Role in Immunity, Oxidative Stress and Chronic Inflammation," *Current Opinion in Clinical Nutrition and Metabolic Care*; November 2009; 12(6); 646–52.

Preuss, H.G., M.D., "Oregano Oil May Protect Against Drug-Resistant Bacteria, Georgetown Researcher Finds," Georgetown University Medical Center, October 6, 2001.

Puetz, T.; Flowers, S.; and O'Connor, P.J.; "A Randomized Controlled Trial of the Effect of Aerobic Exercise Training on Feelings of Energy and Fatigue in Sedentary Young Adults with Persistent Fatigue," *Psychotherapy and Psychosomatics*; 2008; 77: 167–74.

Roberts, E.; "Pregnenolone—from Selye to Alzheimer and a Model of Pregnenolone Sulfate Binding Site on the GABAA Receptor," *Biochemical Pharmacology*; January 1995; 49(1): 1–16.

Rose, P.; Huang, Q.; Ong, C.N.; and Whiteman, M.; "Broccoli and Watercress Suppress Matrix Metalloproteinase-9 Activity and Invasiveness of Human MDA-MB-231 Breast Cancer Cells," *Toxicology and Applied Pharmacology*; December 2005; 209(2): 105–13.

Ryder, K.M., M.D.; Shorr, R.I.; Bush, A.J., Ph.D.; Kritchevsky, S.B., Ph.D.; Harris, T., M.D., M.P.H.; Stone, K., Ph.D.; Cauley, J., Dr.P.H.; and Tylavsky, F.A., Dr.P.H.; "Magnesium Intake from Food and Supplements is Associated with Bone Mineral Density in Healthy Older White Subjects," *Journal of the American Geriatrics Society*; 2005; 53(11).

Sabaté, J.; "Nut Consumption, Vegetarian Diets, Ischemic Heart Disease Risk, and All-Cause Mortality: Evidence from Epidemiologic Studies," *American Journal of Clinical Nutrition*; September 1999; 70(3): 500S–503S.

Sasazuki S.; Inoue, M.; Miura, T.; Iwasaki, M.; and Tsugane, S.; "Plasma Tea Polyphenols and Gastric Cancer Risk: A Case-Control Study Nested in a Large Population-Based Prospective Study in Japan," *Cancer Epidemiology Biomarkers and Prevention*; February 2008; 17(2): 343–51.

Schmitz, K.H.; Lin, H.; Sammel, M.D.; et al.; "Association of Physical Activity with Reproductive Hormones: The Penn Ovarian Aging Study," *Cancer Epidemiology, Biomarkers and Prevention*; 2007; 16(10): 2042–7.

Shechter, M.; Merz, C.N.; Paul-Labrador, M.; Meisel, S.R.; Rude, R.K.; Molloy, M.D.; Dwyer, J.H.; Shah, P.K.; and Kaul, S.; "Oral Magnesium Supplementation Inhibits Platelet-Dependent Thrombosis in Patients with Coronary Artery Disease," *American Journal of Cardiology*; 1999; 84: 152–6.

ScienceDaily, "Brain Malfunction Explains Dehydration in Elderly," December 18, 2007, www.sciencedaily.com.

ScienceDaily, "Diet Linked to Cognitive Decline and Dementia," November 12, 2007, www.sciencedaily.com.

ScienceDaily, "Exercise Reduces Menopausal Symptoms and Improves Quality of Life," March 22, 2006, www.sciencedaily.com.

ScienceDaily, "Exercise, Rest Reduce Cancer Risk," November 30, 2008, www.sciencedaily.com.

ScienceDaily, "Green, Black Tea Can Reduce Stroke," March 4, 2009, www.sciencedaily.com.

ScienceDaily, "Hot Cocoa Tops Red Wine and Tea in Antioxidants; May Be Healthier Choice," November 6, 2003, www.sciencedaily.com.

ScienceDaily, "Slow Exercise (Not Fast) Is Better for Menopausal Women," July 8, 2008, www.sciencedaily.com.

ScienceDaily, "Walk Away Menopausal Anxiety, Stress and Depression," January 4, 2008; www.sciencedaily.com.

Shiraki M.; Shiraki Y.; Aoki, C.; and Miura, M.; "Vitamin K_2 (Menatetrenone) Effectively Prevents Fractures and Sustains Lumbar Bone Mineral Density in Osteoporosis," *Journal of Bone Mineral Research*; 2000; 15(3): 515–23.

Shrubsole, M.J.; Lu, W.; Chen, Z.; Shu, X.O.; Zheng, Y.; Dai, Q.; Cai, Q.; Gu, K.; Ruan, Z.X.; Gao, Y.T.; and Zheng, W.; "Drinking Green Tea Modestly Reduces Breast Cancer Risk," *Journal of Nutrition*; February 2009; 139(2): 310–6.

Spiegel, K.; Tasali, E.; Penev, P.; and Van Cauter, E.; "Brief Communication: Sleep Curtailment in Healthy Young Men Is Associated with Decreased Leptin Levels, Elevated Ghrelin Levels, and Increased Hunger and Appetite," *Annals of Internal Medicine*; December 7, 2004; 141 (11): 846–50.

Stone, G.D.; Wang, L.S.; Zikri, N.; Chen, T.; Hecht, S.S.; Huang, C.; Sardo, C.; and Lechner, J.F.; "Cancer Prevention with Freeze-Dried Berries and Berry Components," *Seminars in Cancer Biology*; October 2007; 17(5): 403–10.

Shukla, M.; Gupta, K.; Rasheed, Z.; Khan K.A.; and Haqqi, T.M.; "Consumption of Hydrolyzable Tannins-Rich Pomegranate Extract Suppresses Inflammation and Joint Damage in Rheumatoid Arthritis," *Nutrition*; Jul–Aug 2008; 24(7–8): 733–43.

Sierpina, V.; Wolschlaeger, B.; and Blumenthal, M.; "Gingko Biloba," *American Academy of Family Physicians*; September 2003.

Yoshitake, T.; Iizuka, R.; Yoshitake, S.; Weikop, P.; Müller, W.E.; Ögren, S.O.; and Kehr, J.; "Hypericum perforatum L. (St. John's Wort) Preferentially Increases Extracellular Dopamine Levels in the Rat Prefrontal Cortex," *British Journal of Pharmacology*; June 2004; 142(3): 414–8.

Tamborlane, W.V., M.D.; Weiswasser, Janet W.; Fung, T.; Held, N.; and Liskov, T.P.; *Yale's Guide to Children's Nutrition*; www.med.yale.edu; 1997.

The Magnesium Online Library, Mgwater.com, "Magnesium Linked to Aging Mystery and Calcifications."

The National Coalition for Women with Heart Disease, "Myths and Truths on Women and Heart Disease," www.womenheart.org.

"The Problem with Trans Fat," *Washington Post,* February 25, 2003, washingtonpost.com.

University of Maryland Medical Center, Medical Reference, "Coenzyme 10," www.umm.edu.

University of Maryland Medical Center, Medical Reference, "Cysteine," www.umm.edu.

University of Maryland Medical Center, Medical Reference, "Green Tea," www.umm.edu.

University of Maryland Medical Center, Medical Reference, "Licorice," www.umm.edu.

University of Maryland Medical Center, Medical Reference, "Magnesium," www.umm.edu.

University of Maryland Medical Center, Medical Reference, "Stress," www.umm.edu.

University of Maryland Medical Center, Medical Reference, "Vitamin K," www.umm.edu.

U.S. Department of Health and Human Services, "The Fibroid Registry," www.ahrq.gov.

U.S. Department of Health and Human Services, "Women: Stay Healthy at Any Age," www.ahrq.gov.

Vance, J.; Wulf, G.; Tullner, T.; McNevin, N.; and Mercer, J.; "EMG Activity as a Function of the Performer's Focus of Attention," *Journal of Motor Behavior*; 2004; 36; 450–9.

"Vitamin C: Stress Buster," *Psychology Today*, April 25, 2003, www.psychologytoday.com.

Vitamin D Council, "Understanding Vitamin D Cholecalciferol," vitamindcouncil.org.

Volz, T.; and Schenk, J.; "L-arginine Increases Dopamine Transporter Activity in Rat Striatum via a Nitric Oxide Synthase-Dependent Mechanism," *Synapse*; 2004; 54(3): 173–82.

WebMD, "Exercise May Help Prevent Breast Cancer," February 16, 2007.

WebMD, "High Cholesterol Risk Factors" September 26, 2009.

Weil, A., M.D., "In the News: Berries Fight Cancer," www.drweil.com.

Weninger, S.C.; and Yankner, B.A.; "Inflammation and Alzheimer's Disease: The Good, the Bad, and the Ugly," *Natural Medicine*; May 2001; 7(5): 527–8.

Wiklund, L.; Pousette, J.; and George, M.; "Magnesium Intake, Drinking Water, and Risk of Colorectal Cancer," *Journal of the American Medical Association*; January 2005; 293 (1): 86–9.

Winkels, R.M.; Brouwer, I.A.; Clarke, R.; Katan, M.B.; and Verhoef, P.; "Bread Cofortified with Folic Acid and Vitamin B-12 Improves the Folate and Vitamin B-12 Status of Healthy Older People: A Randomized Controlled Trial," *American Journal of Clinical Nutrition*; August 2008; 88(2): 348–55.

Women's Health, "Eat to Beat Stress: Nine Foods That Will Keep You Calm," December 2007.

Women's Heart Foundation, "Women and Heart Disease Facts," www.womensheart.org.

Wong, G.Y.; Bradlow, L.; Sepkovic, D.; Mehl, S.; Mailman, J.; and Osborne, M.P.; "Dose-Ranging Study of Indole-3-Carbinol for Breast Cancer Prevention," *Journal of Cellular Biochemistry Supplement*; 1997; 2–29; 111–6.

Yan, X.J.; Qi, M.; Yancopoulos, S.; Madaio, M.; Satoh, M.; Reeves, W.H.; Teichberg, S.; Kohn, N.; Auborn, K.; and Chiorazzi, N.; "Indole-3-carbinol Improves Survival in Lupus-Prone Mice By Inducing Tandem B- and T-Cell Differentiation Blockades," *Clinical Immunology*; June 2009; 131(3); 481–94.

Yankner, B.A.; "A Century of Cognitive Decline," *Nature*; March 9, 2000; 404(774): 125.

Helpful Websites

eatcleandiet.com, the online destination for the Eat-Clean Diet® series, including tips, tools and inspiration from a community of people who share your journey.

drmichellegannon.com, website for inspiration expert Dr. Michelle Gannon.

drtrevorborn.com, website for beauty expert Dr. Trevor Born.

loraccosmetics.com, website for beauty expert Carol Shaw.

Oxygen fitness magazine, www.oxygenmag.com.

Toscareno.com, the online destination for my books, news, blog and more.

uzzireissmd.com, website for hormone expert Dr. Uzzi Reiss.

Index

C

D

E

F

G

H

L

M

N

O

P

Q

R

S

T